# Health Science and College Life

# Contributing Authors

**BRIDGETTE ALLEN**
Photographic Consultant

**WILLIAM T. BREESMAN, M.D. — Chronic Disease**
Cardiologist
Lewistown, Pennsylvania

**ALEXANDER FRANCO, M.D. — Planning your Family — Pregnancy, Childbirth, and Abortion**
Staff Physician
Ritenour Health Center
Obstetrician
The Pennsylvania State University

**JOHN A. HARGLEROAD II, M.D. — Communicable Diseases**
Director of University Health Services
The Pennsylvania State University

**MARY W. HICKS, PH.D. — Human Sexuality: A Developmental Overview**
Associate Professor, Department of Child and Family
Southern Illinois University

**GUY S. PARCEL, PH.D. — Communicable Diseases**
Assistant Professor of Pediatrics
University of Texas Medical School
Galveston

**ALICE SHOEMAKER, R.D. — Nutrition, Consumer Health**
Nutrition Consultant
Bureau of Nutrition Services
Arizona Department of Health Services

**HARRY C. STAMEY, M.D. — Mental Health**
Medical Director
Geisinger Medical Center
Danville, Pennsylvania

**WM. J. STONE, ED.D. — Physical Fitness**
Associate Professor of H.P.E.R.
Director of Human Performance Laboratory
Arizona State University

**RICHARD H. WAGNER, PH.D. — Environmental Hazards and Man's Health**
Consulting Ecologist
San Francisco

**ANITA YANOCHIK, R.D. — Nutrition, Consumer Health**
Chief, Bureau of Nutrition Services
Arizona Department of Health Services

# Health Science and College Life

**Brice W. Corder**
Arizona State University

**Ronda Kerr Showalter**
Lewisburg, Pennsylvania

Second Edition

Wm. C. Brown Company Publishers
Dubuque, Iowa

**HEALTH**

Consulting Editor
*Robert Kaplan*
*The Ohio State University*

**PHYSICAL EDUCATION**

Consulting Editor
*Aileene Lockhart*
*Texas Woman's University*

**PARKS AND RECREATION**

Consulting Editor
*David Gray*
*California State University, Long Beach*

Copyright © 1972, 1975 by Wm. C. Brown Company Publishers

Library of Congress Catalog Card Number: 74—18561

ISBN 0—697—07367—X

Printed in the United States of America

# Contents

# Foreword

Many people believe that the importance of health education is declining as our society becomes increasingly mechanized and medical science continues to advance its frontiers. This is simply not the case. The importance of health education continues to grow. The health problems of society are, of course, changing but the importance of our personal health to our efficiency in whatever we do, to our personal happiness, and even to our survival, is not changing. The development of proper habits, attitudes, and knowledge concerning health is still an essential part of any person's education.

Survey courses in health, which are a part of the standard curriculum in most colleges and universities, present a basic problem of textbook selection. Textbooks often fall into one of two extreme categories. In many cases the text is so closely related to the course that it has little or no value to the student except as a part of the course; it is nothing more than a prepared notebook. At the other extreme we find textbooks which are so general in scope that the student is frustrated in attempts to use the text in relation to the course.

This book attempts to find a desirable middleground between the two undesirable extremes. The topics covered were selected as those of greatest value and interest to students after extensive student surveys and consultations with physicians and faculty in health-related fields. Each topic is covered in depth in a scholarly and timely fashion which should make the book a useful reference, independent of the course for which it was designed.

Dr. Robert J. Scannell

# Preface

This second edition of HEALTH SCIENCE AND COLLEGE LIFE is aimed at the college student in an era of complex living. Our belief that the student, rather than the subject matter, is the focal point of education led us to consult students as to the essential content for their text. The topics were selected after surveying men and women students enrolled in required health classes. Final decisions were made after consulting the members of the local medical society and the staff of The Pennsylvania State University's Health Center for their opinions as to the health needs and interests of young adults. These findings have subsequently been reinforced by results of similar surveys throughout the country. Content was then selected based not only on interests, but on needs and abilities to comprehend the various areas.

It is our belief that the college student of today wants more than a health lecture about his anatomy. He wants and needs factual information pertaining to current health problems. A personal health course at the college level should teach the student how to recognize and prevent illness, how to improve his well-being, and how to prolong and improve the quality of his life.

This book is designed not only to present important health facts, but also to stimulate the students thinking. As adults, college students face new and increasingly more complex problems and situations. It is an objective of this book to motivate an individual toward sound decision making that will lead to intelligent self-direction in his health behavior. Positive health behavior is accomplished through development of a positive attitude and actualized through application of sound information. One is health activated once health becomes a major principle in his life. The utilization of the kind of information found in this text should be viewed as a tool in achieving that principle. But, rather than health being an end in itself, it is a means of realizing one's potential as a human being.

The contributing authors have added expertise and insights. They were selected for their qualifications and for their dedication to working with young people. A glance at the contents of any health text will reveal that the scope of health science involves many important subject areas. Thus, professionals working daily in those areas can provide the most perceptive and an assured quality of information.

# Health Science and College Life

# 1

# The Meaning of Health

## General Concept

Good health is a sound mind and body encompassing the physical, social, mental, and emotional well-being of each individual.

## Outcomes

1. The student should be able to define the nature and meaning of health.
2. The student should be able to explain the need for health education.
3. The student should be able to apply effective health practices to his everyday life style.

### Health—A Quality of Life

In a busy world in which we must concern ourselves with the realities of racism and poverty, inflation and the high cost of living, technology and the energy crisis, science and space exploration, streaking and campus frivolity, and a society which is slowly becoming dehumanized, we are also confronted with health problems that extend the complexities of living a full and useful life. The country is attempting to solve the urgent problems of overpopulation, the emotional dilemmas of many individ-

1

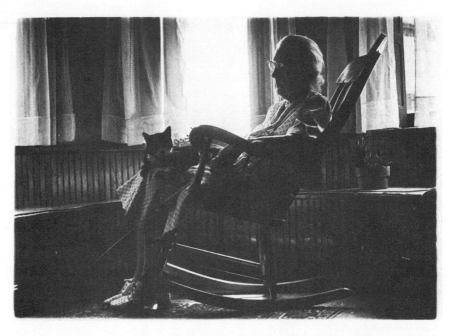

How long and how well one may live may depend upon the daily health practices established in one's youth.

uals—the problems of aging, destructive behavior, accidents, crime, obesity, smoking, drug abuse, and alcoholism.

For many college students, health is taken for granted. The academic world frequently appears to emphasize grades, examinations, degrees, and vocational placement. Our society requires its youth to make decisions about employment, graduate school, marriage, and a family. It is easily forgotten that without physical and mental well-being, one may be unable to achieve the goals he sets for himself. An old Egyptian saying described health as being "a crown upon a well man's head as only seen by a sick man."

The idea of health itself is a human value judgment. It is an enabling value rather than a definitive purpose. To achieve it is to be in the condition that allows fulfillment of one's potential.

The real dilemma is the contest between the value assigned to health and the value asssigned to competing activities that may be antagonistic to health. Both political and economic stability are prerequisite to the health of the population. General education and specific health-related education, for parents and teachers, are essential to the fostering of those determinants of health that are personally controlled by the individual.

Periodically, as when a person walks across campus and sees a handicapped person, for example, he may appreciate his own measure of good health. But such incidents are soon forgotten and the moments of appreciation are dismissed.

The health problems facing college students are always in the process of change. Fifty years ago, students thought of their health only in terms of a biological being. As an organism, this being needed nurturing and care. Many students still associate "health" with disease or with anatomical structures and physiological systems. The health-educated individual, however, is aware that health encompasses more than simply a scientific knowledge of disease and the body.

To a parent, in many instances, health is two-dimensional. A parent may neglect his own health, but be continuously aware of the health of his children. A parent may take every precaution to see that his children's health is not hampered. He may guide and direct their behavior and practices in his everyday living, providing he has adequate health knowledge. A dichotomy exists, however, when a parent fails to measure his own degree of wellness, or allows his habits to abuse his own well-being.

A health educator, be he or she a teacher, a physician, or a nurse, views health in still a different light—one focused upon education and preventive measures. It is his aim to motivate and improve health habits, knowledge, and attitudes. Misconceptions still dominate our thinking, and, in turn, affect our beliefs and behavior. For instance, there are those who think that cancer is a single disease entity, that venereal disease may be transmitted by toilet seats, or that a chiropractor is a licensed medical doctor. It is the responsibility of those in positions related to the area of health education to guide, inform, and direct the individual into intelligent self-direction. Once an individual acquires the correct information, he may change his attitudes and perhaps his practices, if necessary. The Commission on Philosophy for School Health Education states:

To educate in health means to make a good life in spite of handicaps, and more significantly to help each person seek that state of affairs which moves him toward an optimal stage of development . . . to aid the individual to avoid the misbalance, the disease, and the accidents of life.[2]

2. Commission on Philosophy for School Health Education, *"A Point of View for School Health Education."* Washington, D.C.: NEA, 1962.

## Definitions

Workable definitions are of importance for the study of health. Here are some:

## Health

The World Health Organization of the United Nations describes health as a "state of complete physical, mental, and social well-being, and not merely the absence of disease or infirmity." This definition is the one most widely accepted, although it assumes that the individual is in *good* health when it uses the term "well-being." An individual is still experiencing health even when not well. Health may imply a condition of body and mind with all parts functioning adequately.

The Committee on Terminology of School Health Education describes health as:

A state of feeling well in body, mind, and spirit together with a sense of reserve power. It is based upon normal functioning of the tissues and organs of the body, a practical understanding of the principles of healthful living, and a harmonious adjustment to the physical and psychological environment, together with an attitude which regards health not as an end itself, but a means to a richer life as measured in constructive service to mankind.[3]

In most definitions of health, the intent or degree of wellness is implied. One might describe *wellness* as being a certain quality of life which moves the individual to best serve himself and his community, and to be a contributing member to society. Men such as Berthet interpret health "as a plentitude of life, the balanced output, the total harmony of the human being, adapted as perfectly as possible to the demands of our modern world and its permanent evolution."[4]

The characteristics of good health imply buoyancy, pleasure, vigor and zest, the ability to relax, few emotional "hang-ups," acceptable size, weight, and appearance, and the absence of disabling remediable defects.

---

3. Committee on Terminology of School Health Education, *Journal of the American Association for Health, Physical Education and Recreation* 22 (September, 1951):7.

4. Etienne Berthet, "The Disproportion of Man," *Man in His Biological Environment,* International Conference on Health and Health Education, June 30–July 7, 1962, Philadelphia, Volume 2, p. 128.

Anderson describes the quality of health in terms of levels:

*A Level*—Very high level but not perfect health; freedom from disabling remediable defects with pronounced vigor and buoyancy. This category demands adjustment to everyday situations.

*B* Level—Freedom from disabling defects but lacking the degree of buoyancy and vigor of "A."

*C* Level—Individuals may pass as being well, but lack vitality, functioning at a minimum rather than a maximum. They are not sick, but drag in appearance and behavior.

*D* Level—Characteristic of chronic infection or other apparent or concealed factors and a low level of health.

*E* Level—Obviously an ill individual.[5]

A person may fluctuate from time to time in the various levels, but every individual should strive for the "A" level.

## Health Instruction

Health instruction is the dissemination of health facts and concepts in a structured environment, utilizing mental powers to ascertain health-related information. Health instruction refers to a design that provides a sequential arrangement of learning experiences.

Sitting in a classroom reading or hearing a lecture given on alcohol would be an example of health instruction. One may excel in health knowledge, however, but fail to *apply* that knowledge. One may take an examination on alcohol and not miss a single question, but if the person is a heavy drinker and becomes an alcoholic, was his individual health *educated* as well as *instructed*?

The objective of health instruction is to close the gap between what is *known* in the health field and what is *practiced* by the public. It must be remembered, however, that information which is acceptable today may be obsolete tomorrow. Hence, the principal purpose of health instruction is that of equipping students to cope with the inescapable facts of change by fostering the ability to solve problems which change produces, and to develop the basic skills for doing so. Such basic skills would include:

1. Thinking critically
2. Solving problems intelligently

5. C. L. Anderson, *School Health Practice*, (St. Louis: C. V. Mosby Co., 1964), p. 48.

3. Developing self-reliance
4. Demonstrating self-direction
5. Assuming responsibility for continued learning
6. Examining issues and values
7. Understanding how knowledge is best discovered and used

These skills are not acquired in a vacuum. Rapid medical advances and new knowledge require *continuing* efforts to bridge the gap between knowledge, practices and attitudes.[6] Health instruction is the planned or opportunistic imparting of formal and informal knowledge. It comes from the extrinsic learning environment where the individual is taught and receives and learns information.

## Health Education

Health education is the summation of experiences that influence an individual's attitudes, behavior, and knowledge as related to himself and the community in which he lives.

A student cannot be instructed to apply values. He must form individual values, values which will often be reflected in his actions. Given health instruction, a person becomes health-educated when he utilizes this information and applies it to his living pattern. For example, if a student learns about the effects of alcohol in class, attends a fraternity party and sees alcohol being consumed as well as the effects that alcohol has, he adds to his experiences. If he decides to drink moderately at a social event thereafter, he becomes health-educated when he shows his values pertaining to drinking by means of conduct and control. John Dewey believed that "an individual learns best by doing." In other words, exposure and experience, when coupled with knowledge, increase the breadth of our educational process. Colleges and universities ideally should provide opportunities for mature development by which a student can gain a deeper insight into his environment.

Values in health should be appraised in terms of changing times. Each generation will test the values they have inherited and will usually try a new value structure of their own. The same concept applies to health values, as society places different degrees of approval or disapproval on certain health practices. To drink moderately is socially acceptable but detrimental to health; yet smoking tobacco is now socially

---

6. Commission on Philosophy for School Health Education, *"A Point of View for School Health Education."*

undesirable because of the mass media's pointing out of the cancer potential. Ten years ago smoking was a social must. Therefore neither society nor peers are always capable of creating correct health values. Every individual must decipher information from experiences and knowledge to formulate his own values. People of all ages fail to practice their values and often suffer medical consequences. Health education may contribute by serving as a basis or foundation from which to help clarify health values. Knowing and applying may serve youth in recognizing the full potential of being and the profoundness of man, rather than in accepting a superficial existence.

The ultimate goal of health education, then, is to liberate man's potential energies and creativity so as to formulate a scheme of values that will make for better living. If a person fails to apply what he knows, he is not truly educated.

## School Health Program

A school health program embodies the prepared course of action established by the institution. Health programs include health services, health instruction, and education for healthful campus living.

A genuine deep zest for living is an important component of health.

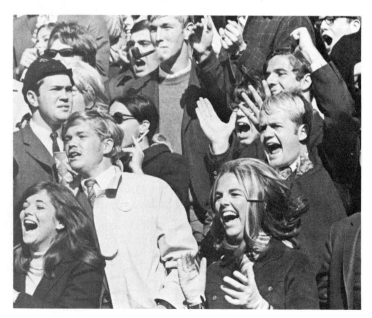

From the medical services provided at the university infirmary to the food preparation and menus in the dormitories, each aspect of the program functions as a part contributing to the whole to make for a healthy campus environment and a healthy student population.

## Public Health Program

A public health program encompasses all of society's attempts to handle health problems in such a way as to follow E. A. Winslow's concept of prevention of disease, extension of life, and the promotion of general well-being.[7]

## Historical Significance

School health education was developed on the fundamental principle that an educational institution should prepare a person to meet the demands of life and to promote his own well-being. Health as an applied science has gradually developed as our educational system has evolved.

The Egyptian civilization was the first to stress healthful living in the enforced building of earth closets, construction of public drainage systems and emphasis on simple personal hygiene. The Hebrews contributed the first formal health codes in their Mosaic Laws. The Jewish custom of refraining from consumption of pork evolved from the observation that people became ill from eating pork; thus, the introduction of a zoonosis.

The Greeks stressed the importance of physical fitness in achieving a sound mind and body. However, the Greek populace experienced only a limited level of health. The Romans did not experience a high level of health, although they did construct aqueducts and sewage systems. Even today in the city of Rome, garbage and sanitation are major public health nuisances.

Health status in colonial America posed serious threats to arriving immigrants; the average life span of a colonist was only twenty-nine years of age. The country was besieged by smallpox and diphtheria. It was not until Jenner discovered the smallpox vaccine that the principles of immunization were to contribute to scientific progress.

7. E. A. Winslow, "The Untilled Fields of Public Health," *Science* 51:23, 1920.

The modern era of health in this country has been fourfold in sequence. In the miasmic period (1850–80), people believed that disease was caused by noxious odors; witchcraft prevailed. In the bacteriological phase (1880–1920), Pasteur and Koch found through their research that a specific organism caused a specific disease. The groundwork was completed and Pasteur developed the rabies vaccine while VonBehring invented a diphtheria vaccine. Death rates in the United States began to decline rapidly.

The positive health period (1920–60), developed as a result of national concern about the large numbers of men failing to pass army physical examinations, and the nation ushered in a campaign to promote higher degrees of healthiness. New types of health personnel were introduced, such as sanitarians, health educators, social workers, audiometrists, and epidemiologists, to name but a few. The period reached a climax when President Kennedy motivated the youth of tomorrow to improve their physical health. To do so, a national campaign to try a fifty-mile hike as a determining criterion for good physical conditioning was instituted.

The social engineering phase (1960—) continues to describe and depict the public's health approach today. There are new priorities: heart transplants, a cure for cancer, mental illness, dental caries, the pill and the morning after pill, drugs, alcoholism, and sex education. Man, because of his communal coexistence in an advanced scientific and polarized world, will always be confronted with health problems. The question of what these problems of tomorrow will be, remains to challenge us today. But more important is our understanding and striving to solve those health problems that face us now.

## Health Problems Today

With modern medicine, newer drugs, more research, and an increase in longevity it would appear that Americans have reached adequate to maximum degrees of healthful living. This is not a safe assumption to make, however, since even though many Americans are living longer, they are not necessarily living better. Health education and preventive medicine must struggle to improve the quality of longevity. These additional years should be made full and productive. Scientific discovery only benefits individuals when they utilize their knowledge.

Recently the federal government under the auspices of the Food and Drug Administration and the Department of Health, Education, and Welfare studied opinions and practices in health matters. Over 2800 individuals were randomly selected in the country to complete a thorough, detailed, fifty page questionnaire. The results revealed many surprising misconceptions:

1. Vitamin pills give pep and energy.
2. A daily bowel movement is essential to good health.
3. Over-the-counter diet pills work effectively.
4. Arthritis and cancer are caused by vitamin and mineral deficiencies.
5. All vitamins are harmless. (Actually, excessive intake of vitamin D produces toxicity in man).
6. Organic or natural foods are more beneficial than those which are not.
7. One in eight of the respondents admitted to self-medication for health problems existing beyond two weeks.

The study revealed little correlation between health beliefs and practices. Few respondents had organized sets of health values. Robert Kaplan, professor of health education at The Ohio State University, points out ideas about health are most often handed down by word-of-mouth, through folklore, and experiences of family and acquaintances. He also states a predominant belief which affirms that "whatever ailment you have, there is a medicine for it, so why suffer?"[8] This belief, coupled with the idea of individuals wanting immediate relief, frequently poses problems. The government study indicated a pressing need for application and knowledge of health values.

In the past years health has been discussed as a three-dimensional quality taking individualized forms; yet today our health programs do not reflect these concepts. Many individuals find it easier to philosophize passively about health values rather than to practice them. It is clear that health is not an absolute and its interpretation remains static, regardless of analysis, knowledge, and evaluation. Health is becoming interpreted to be a personal quality which may enable one to utilize his full potential within his society. Everyone is subject to change and, as a result, we grow, mature, age, become educated, and have numerous experiences which

8. William Furlong, "You and Your Dangerous Health Practices," *Today's Health,* Oct. 1972, p. 60.

broaden our social relationships. All of these forces are vital ingredients affecting our life-style and well-being. Environment alone is a changing, often threatening force which will affect our health status.

Even in the ideal form, time, and different situations will impose varying emphases on one's life-style. In describing health status, Read asserts:

> There is not time enough in the day for the full development of one's physical, mental, and social potential. The dedicated athlete, the true intellectual, or the involved community leader may excel in his specialty, but only at the cost of doing something less than his best in other areas of living. And like a work of art, the true quality of one's health becomes impossible to measure objectively.[9]

Man will have to realize that static solutions do not function effectively in a dynamic environment which continuously confronts our health status. In the future, as in the present, man will have to continually re-evaluate his health beliefs and practices. Obviously more strategy and effort will be necessary to lose weight, stop smoking, or refrain from driving after drinking, for example, in order to counteract the present reliance on taking medication or getting a pill for health problems. All of these factors including the development of a sound health philosophy are mandatory if individuals are to succeed in attaining a healthful balance in everyday living, one which is valued then exemplified in active practice.

In the following chapters, selected problems pertinent to college students will be explored. Basic information will be presented, but it is up to the individual student to determine its relevance to his own needs and to form positive attitudes and practices. Only then can one become health-educated.

## Questions for Study and Discussion

1. How do most college students look upon their individual health?
2. Why is the biological emphasis alone in health instruction inadequate?

9. Donald Read, *New Directions in Health Education* (New York: MacMillan Co., 1971) p. 117.

3. What are some of the ingredients of your own personal philosophy of health?
4. How do health instruction and health education interrelate?
5. What do you forsee to be the major health problems of your children?
6. Why is a minimal operating level of wellness unsatisfactory for today's mode of living?
7. Is there currently a keen national interest in the field of health?
8. How does one formulate values and then reflect them in behavior?

## References

Anderson, C. L. *School Health Practices.* St. Louis: C. V. Mosby Co., 1964.

Berthet, Etienne. "The Disproportion of Man," *Man in His Biological Environment,* vol. 2. Philadelphia: International Conference on Health Education, 1962.

Commission on Philosophy for School Health Education. "A Point of View for School Health Education." Washington, D.C.: NEA, 1962.

Committee on Terminology of School Health Education. "Report on Terminology of School Health Education," *Journal of the American Association for Health, Physical Education and Recreation* 22 (September 1951):7.

Furlong, William, "You and Your Dangerous Health Practices," *Today's Health,* February, 1972:60.

Joint Committee on Health Problems in Education of the National Education Association and the American Medical Association. "Health Appraisal of School Children." Washington, D.C., 1964.

Read, Donald, *New Directions in Health Education.* New York: Macmillan Co., 1971.

Subcommittee on Health Curriculum. "Philosophical Platform." College of Health, Physical Education and Recreation, The Pennsylvania State University, 1969.

Wheatley, George and Hallock, Grace. *Health Observation of School Children.* New York: McGraw-Hill, Inc., 1965.

Winslow, C. E. A.: "The Untilled Fields of Public Health." *Science* 51 (1920):23.

World Health Organization. "Health Education, A Selected Bibliography." United Nations Educational, Scientific and Cultural Organization, 1956.

# 2

# Mental Health

## General Concept

A healthy mind is one that does its job well.

## Outcomes

A student should be able to:
1. Understand the purpose and functioning of the mind
2. Recognize the characteristics of a properly functioning mind
3. Recognize symptoms of malfunction
4. Have sufficient mental health himself to
    a. Adjust to daily life in a realistic way
    b. Have a reasonable degree of zest for living
5. Know and make use of available resources should he feel that he or his acquaintances need advice or other help

The usual student coming to college for the first time has already achieved a high degree of mental health, as evidenced by his ability to live with reasonable satisfaction in his home environment. When he leaves this environment, he leaves behind his comfortable surroundings, his old friends, his parents, his pets, all that is familiar to him, and he is faced with that most frightening of human experiences—change. It is to be hoped that he will be able to adjust adequately. He will bring with him certain mental tools, certain personality traits which will help him tolerate change. Attitudes and activities that have proven effective before will be used by him again as he makes an effort to blend his old environment into the new.

In the final analysis, the new student's ability to overcome his fears and to settle down to effective college life will depend on that elusive quality we call mental health.

## What Is Mental Health?

There are all sorts of definitions of mental health. Eaton and Peterson describe a mentally healthy adult as "a person who is free of psychiatric disease, has a general feeling of well-being, functions at or near his full biological capacity, is competent in dealing with his environment, and

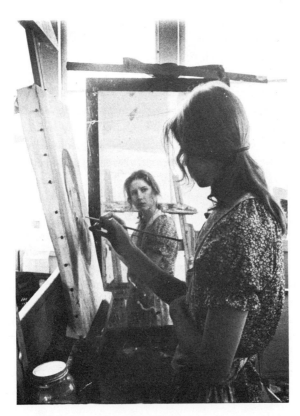

Self-identity and a positive self-image are necessary for sound mental health.

has good ego strength."[1] Others, such as Kolb, have approximated this definition, and there are almost as many definitions as there are definers.

Put more simply, a healthy mind is one that does its job well. Such efforts at simplification often raise more questions than they answer, however, and this definition is no exception. To understand it, we must understand the function of the mind. This subject has been debated by philosophers from the beginning of time, with poets, artists, theologists, and teachers all having their favorite theories. Even among psychologists and psychiatrists, who like to feel that they are scientists, opinions clash —frequently with high emotion. There are social theories, learning theories, systems theories, and more. It is beyond the scope of this chapter to fully discuss these ideas, but the reader should have some familiarity with them and he is referred to various texts for a complete study.

For our purposes, let us think for a few moments as biologists. From this viewpoint we see the human body as a vastly complicated interconnection of systems, each influencing and being interdependent upon the others. The lungs oxygenate the blood; the heart pumps it around the body; the liver and kidneys remove waste products. Each of these systems is closely connected with the others and is regulated by *feedback mechanisms* which tell it how it is doing, causing it to speed up or slow down much as the thermostat in our home controls the furnace.

Picture for a moment a series of five or six open containers resting on a table. If these could be interconnected through a system of piping, water poured into one of the cans would fill all the others to the same level. Should there be an outlet at the bottom of one of the cans, water will pass through that outlet at a rate proportional to the pressure of the water level in the cans. Additions or subtractions to the water level in any one can will affect all the others almost instantly. Thus it is with the mental system of thoughts, emotions, sensations, and memories: Anything which affects one component will affect the others and will, through this interaction, affect the behavior which emerges from the central part of the system.

A control center is needed to govern all this, some sort of computer capable of gathering data through the sense organs, storing that data in memory banks, and then using it as necessary to plan activity. This is the purpose of the mind.

1. Merrill T. Eaton, Jr. and Margaret H. Peterson, *Psychiatry* (New York: Medical Examination Publishing Co., 1967), p. 90.

## How Does It Work?

Our computer is so fantastic in its capabilities that a full comprehension of its function is difficult. Perhaps a simple example will help. If a child accidentally places his hand on a hot stove, he will jerk it away immediately. This occurs through reflex nerve action carrying pain to the spinal cord which then activates motor centers to move the hand. The purpose of the reflex system is to prevent injury, and it is activated automatically.

Such reflex activity is common to all forms of life, but in humans the situation is much more complicated. The pain sensation will continue on to the brain where it will be felt consciously as pain. Our little boy may, in addition to his immediate pain, remember that his mother has told him not to be in the kitchen alone. This will stir up fear or guilt, emotions based on memories of what happened when he was caught misbehaving previously. He may be ashamed of himself for doing such a foolish thing, or angry that someone left the stove turned on. At any rate, he is likely to be uncomfortable. Hoping to avoid such discomfort in the future, he will develop the ability to anticipate danger, being more watchful as to where he puts his hands and more conscious of safety measures such as turning off the stove or cautioning others to do so. He will gradually *learn* which of the various possibilities open to him should be followed, working it out through trial and error.

Our computer is remarkably well equipped for this learning pro-

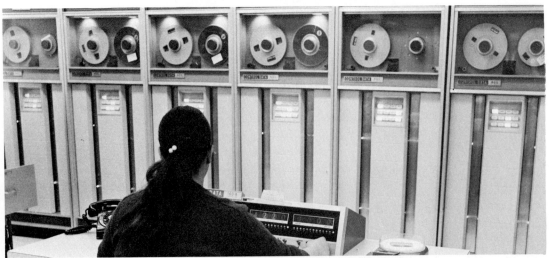

UPI

The human mind in many ways is like a computer.

cess. Any action we take will cause a reaction in ourselves and in our environment which is sensed, run through the computer, and compared to previous actions. Thoughts and emotions are again stimulated and the feedback goes round and round, simultaneously modifying activity and storing memories of all the action and its results. In any given situation, sooner or later an effective way is found to relieve discomfort. When the same or a similar situation is met with in the future, the mind will remember and will try the same solution. If it works again and again, our computer decides that this is an effective method. To avoid having to consciously think about it each time, the mind takes a shortcut and relegates this particular bit of behavior to an automatic status which we call a *habit*. It can be summoned into action as needed, depending on the stimuli which are sensed. A good example of this is the simple task of walking. The young infant learning to walk must concentrate on every movement, because each one creates new sensations and new dangers. With time, however, he learns which movements work satisfactorily and these soon become automatic, so that he no longer has to think about all the details. The same is true of talking, eating, and many other automatic functions.

We human beings like to believe that we handle new situations through conscious thought, bringing our experience and intellect to bear on these problems and solving them in a very intelligent way. We are certainly capable of this and when we are functioning at our most mature level we do it to some extent. A great deal of human mental activity however, goes on beyond our awareness. We would have complete chaos if we were aware of all the processes going on in our minds at any one time. To avoid this, much of our thinking is sidetracked into that area we call the *unconscious,* as we focus or *concentrate* on only that mental activity which requires our immediate attention. This unconscious material continues to exert an influence on our behavior which is as great or greater than that of conscious thought. Supporting evidence comes through study of parapraxias (slips of the tongue), dreams, symbolic activity, and the return of forgotten material to consciousness through the use of drugs such as sodium pentothal. This theory of unconscious determinants of behavior has been rejected by some people but remains the cornerstone of modern dynamic psychiatry.

## Personality Development

So far we have described learning in terms of physical activities. Many of these take place in the very young child, perhaps before the age of two.

Mastery of motor activity is most important during this period of life. As a child gets older, however, his mental activity expands, with thoughts and emotions assuming much more importance. The same principles of learning apply in this area of development. The child may find that certain activities bring him love and security, thus decreasing his mental pain. He may find that if he is a pleasant, conforming child, his mother will respond accordingly with attention and praise. He may then make such a pleasant, smiling attitude a basic habitual part of his activities. On the other hand, it may seem useful to him to be aloof and distant from people, thus avoiding direct confrontation and this, too, may become a basic part of his mental tool kit. He will experiment with this or that action in every area of human activity and, through trial and error, will find a set of tools which are useful to him. As they become habitual, a certain type of person begins to emerge. The sum total of the mental habits that the individual characteristically uses in all kinds of life situations is what we call his *personality*.

Personality development is a lifelong process and any attempt to judge an individual's mental health must take into consideration his age. We do not expect a ten-year-old to exhibit the maturity of a sixteen-year-old, and, in fact, we are concerned if he precociously does so. Erikson has described what he calls the psychological tasks of various ages.[2] He feels that each age has specific problems which must be solved if the individual is to function adequately at that level and to move on to further development. In the next few paragraphs we will be speaking of mental health from the standpoint of the adult, and later on we will make special reference to college students and their specific problems.

## What Does a Healthy Mind Do?

To evaluate this we must separate the functions of the mind into their component parts and inspect each one individually. In a professional psychiatric examination, this is done in great detail, but we don't think of this when dealing with our friends on an everyday basis. If their behavior is what we have come to expect of them and of any reasonable adult, we simply accept them as being "within normal limits." The following material is included to give the student a bit deeper concept of the functioning of a healthy mind.

2. Erik H. Erikson, *Childhood and Society,* 2nd ed. (New York: William Norton and Co., Inc., 1963), pp. 247–274.

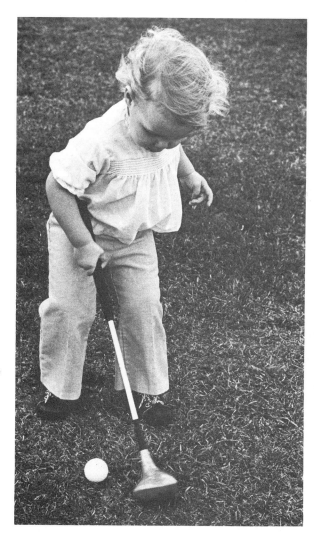

Mastery of motor activity
is very important before the
age of two.

## Assessment of Reality

In order to survive in our environment, we must constantly be getting
accurate information as to what this environment is all about. We receive
this data through our sense organs such as eyes, ears, etc., but this is only
a beginning. As this information is received, it must be interpreted. We
must be able to understand what other people are saying, what their
words and actions really mean. If we misinterpret this, we will have less
accurate information upon which to base decisions. The student who

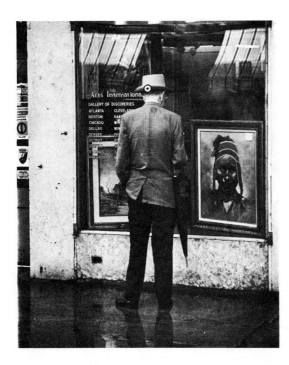

When minor mental frustrations begin to mount, one should try to relax. Taking a walk or talking with a friend are healthy mental outlets.

constantly feels that every criticism from his professors is based only on their personal dislike of him is bound to have lots of trouble. It can be hoped that he will be able to see them more realistically and, as he forms opinions as to their individual assets and liabilities, he will open the way to better control his relationship with them.

This assessment extends beyond just people. We make decisions about *things*, those inanimate parts of our life such as money, time, work, and so forth. Someone once said that the person who is habitually late is showing his hostility, the one who always comes early does so because of his anxiety, and the extremely punctual person is merely obsessive-compulsive. Under this guideline, we could never be right, but it is true that an individual who is always late or always early is not using his time realistically. Getting him to realize this, however, is often very difficult.

An even more difficult area in which to be realistic is in our opinion of ourselves. Very early in life we begin to wonder who we are, and we form an image of ourselves based on our best judgment at that time. Our capabilities, our inferiorities, our fears, hopes, etc., all play a role. It is painful to face defects in ourselves and it is rather natural for human beings either to deny these or to disguise them in some way. No matter how hard we try, we usually end up fooling ourselves to some extent. Nonetheless, the total of all these opinions we carry around with us is our *self-image.* We constantly compare this with our *ideal image,* that picture of what we think we should be, to find out how we measure up. If our self-image comes close to our ideal image, we have some regard for ourselves, which we call *self-esteem.* If we miss by a large margin, we are likely to be depressed or anxious or guilty. Struggling with these painful feelings requires time and effort better spent on studying, relaxation, and other more appropriate activities of life.

## Relationship to Others

What we decide about ourselves and others will determine how we relate to them. Will we be comfortably close to important people, or perhaps too close and too dependent? Will we have to remain aloof? A healthy person is free to do as the situation demands; to be close to people with warmth and love; to be aloof, even stern when necessary; occasionally to be properly suspicious, even angry. We should be able to move *toward* people as in friendship, courtship or marriage, but we should be able to tolerate loneliness *away* from people. Occasionally, we must act *against* people. A healthy mind is free to move in any of these directions, as warranted.

## Control of Impulses

As mentioned before, any stimulus stirs up thoughts and in turn come memories and emotions. The emotions are just links in the chain, but they seem to be the push behind our actions, the things that make us get up and move. Hunger is a basic instinct, but it is the anxiety that accompanies it which forces us to go hunting. This urge to action is called an *impulse.*

If we are to live together in any kind of fruitful society, impulses have to be controlled. Anger, sadness, love, hate, fear, despondency, annoyance—all are shades of human feeling and they make us want to *do* something, such as hit, or kiss, or run away. These actions are appropriate at times but certainly not all the time, and some sort of control of them must be established.

A newborn infant is a bundle of primitive impulses frustrated by his physical inabilities. As he grows, he develops mobility; as he moves around, he runs up against mother who says "no" to him, his first experience with that painful word. From age one to three, it must seem to the youngster that he isn't permitted to do much of anything. All sorts of impulses are stirred up and the potential for trouble is quite high. Motivated finally by his anxiety relative to displeasing mother, he "learns" how to handle his impulses through some compromise.

Some people never do learn this adequately, while others learn it too well, becoming rigidly over-controlled. If adequate controls are built in, the child can tolerate his frustrations, putting up with small doses of discomfort in favor of the long-term advantage.

He does this through varied techniques. He may, for example, *sublimate* his angry impulses into play, venting his hostility on the football field. Later he may handle it through his profession, becoming a professional ballplayer, lawyer, policeman, or a surgeon. This is over-simplified, of course, and the reader is again referred elsewhere for a more complete account of psychological *defense mechanism*.

## Thought Processes

Nothing in human activity is more readily taken for granted than the mysterious ability we call thinking. It just seems to be there and go on automatically, with one thought leading to another in a logical, coherent sequence. Let something go wrong, however, and we will immediately become painfully aware of it. The student preparing for an exam finds that he can't keep his thoughts away from a certain young lady, and he complains that he can't concentrate. Perhaps after he marries her and the romance fades, he may, as an aftermath to a quarrel, forget his wedding anniversary, and that spells trouble. Listen dispassionately sometime to a dorm discussion of politics or religion and you will quickly see ordinarily rational minds caught up in emotional positions from which they will not budge. All of us at times have felt anxious or depressed but have been unable to figure out why. Something in the computer is interfering, preoccupying the mind and making productive thought difficult. Such distractions are fleeting in the healthy mind, which is able to tolerate frustration and to eliminate extraneous thoughts. There is an organization to the thinking process which leads to a precise clarity of great beauty in and of itself. Properly harnessed and in tune with the emotions, it leads to productivity and creativity of the highest order. This is mental health.

## Attitudes about Life

As the child grows, all of these different processes begin to merge into a complete picture which we call his personality. As described earlier, he develops certain characteristic ways of handling his problems. With adequate performance in these areas he has what we call a healthy or mature personality. He will be able to take responsibility for himself and his actions. He will think and feel and act with a sense of harmony, with minimum interference of conflictual material. He will function at a level close to the limits of his biologic potential and, perhaps more importantly, he will experience much of the time a genuine deep zest for living. This is mental health.

## Mental Health in the College Student

Many things happen in the life of a college student which make him wonder sometimes about his sanity. This is understandable in view of the stresses under which he is placed, and it might be useful to talk about some of the problems which the normal student will face.

Since no child training is perfect, no student will come to college equipped with a computer which has all the answers. One fact that students (or anyone, for that matter) have trouble accepting is that they are just what the name implies—students. Not just in an academic sense but in the broad concept of living. The undergraduate years start in late adolescence and merge into early adulthood. According to Erikson, the psychological task of adolescence is to establish a sense of identity, to decide upon and become comfortable with the type of person you are going to be. This is part of the learning or maturing process, and it should be recognized by students, parents, and administrators that students are not yet fully mature and should not be expected to be.

We do expect, however, that students are fairly well along in this maturing process. College admissions personnel attempt to assess emotional health of candidates as well as their academic abilities, hoping to admit students who are most likely to benefit from the educational opportunity. These administrators realize that heavy responsibilities will fall on the new student and they do not wish to admit anyone who might be overwhelmed by such stresses.

### The Beatles' Music Has More Than a Beat

Beatle music has come under serious criticism from the establishment. Television personality Art Linkletter, testifying on October 24, 1969, before a hearing of the House of Representatives in Washington, D.C., declared the Beatles as leading advocates of an acid drug society . . . but the Beatles have concerned themselves with more than the drug culture. . . .

Aside from their musicianship, the Beatles' popularity stems from the fact that they deal, in most of their songs, with true (real life) social, emotional, and psychological issues facing the youthful listener. Often their lyrics summarize the unspoken word in individual or group therapy. . . . Examples of this can be found by examining the lyrics of the following eight songs:

1. "A Little Help From My Friends":
   The lyrics of this melody deal with the universal human need for acceptance and understanding. . . .

2. "Try To See It My Way":
   This lyric concerns itself with communication empathy, the concept that tranquility may be established if communication becomes possible.

3. "I'm Only Sleeping":
   Here the Beatles present a testimonial for day-dreaming. . . .

## Change

Perhaps the greatest of these stresses is the marked change which starts when the student leaves home and goes to college. Change is always frightening to people. Whether we live in a large city or a small town, we tend to do the same as other animals have been shown to do—we develop a small, circumscribed environment which we call our community. We become comfortable in a certain way of life, deriving that comfort from

4. "Real Nowhere Man":

The lack of self-identity is the psychological issue discussed in these lyrics. . . .

5. "Yesterday":

. . . The song lyrics suggest that regression to childhood would remove one from the agony of adolescence.

6. "Act Naturally":

Fantasy—this lyric suggests that success is possible without effort. . . .

7. "She's Leaving Home":

This all-time Beatle hit suggests that parents in the final analysis aren't really interested in the welfare of the child, but only about the image of their capability as parents. . . .

8. "While My Guitar Gently Weeps":

This hauntingly beautiful melody concerns itself with the phenomenon of futility. The lyric is perhaps the heaviest of all Beatle dialogue since it reflects on the growing concern of the youthful generation that things (the organization of society) are out of control. . . .

J. V. Toohey, "Beatle Lyrics Can Help Adolescents Identify and Understand Their Emotional Health Problems," in *Student Guide to Personal Health* by Betty J. Bachmann, Thomas L. Dezelsky, and Jack V. Toohey (Dubuque, Ia.: Kendall/Hunt Publishing Company, 1971), pp. 102–103. Reprinted by permission of the authors.

family, friends, familiar surroundings, etc. Most young people have some small area that is uniquely their own, perhaps their bedroom or a clubroom. Self-identity is linked to this area with decorations, posters on the wall, collections of books and records. The student begins to know who he is and where he stands with peers, adults and authority figures. More practically, he knows the barber, the auto mechanic, the doctor, and begins to feel comfortable with the idea that he is secure and that he can get help when he needs it.

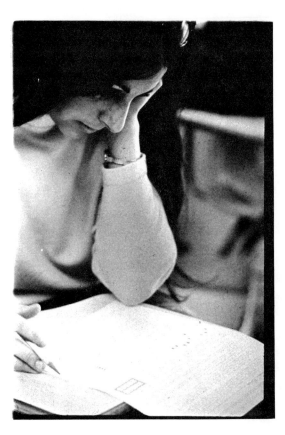

The mature, emotionally stable college student is able to cope with academic pressures and maintains a sense of harmony while still being challenged.

Suddenly all this changes. At college he is thrust into a large dormitory, perhaps rooming with someone he has never met. He must sleep in a strange room, find his way around in an unfamiliar town, trying frantically to find hidden classrooms without being late. He eats in a strange dining room which serves food that he is not accustomed to. Result? Anxiety.

Gradually the unfamiliarity fades away. New friendships are negotiated and new identifications forged. Association with professors replace those comfortable links with previous authority figures. Even new targets for minor aggressions present themselves. Some comfortable things are brought from home; pictures of family and girl friends are prominently displayed and a quick glance at these is reassuring. Phone calls home are frequent at first and then diminish. Favorite wall decora-

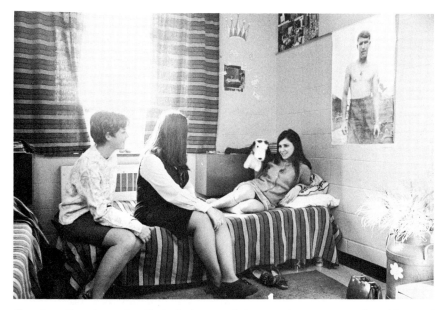

Once in college the student finds the impact of change giving way to new friendships and new identifications.

tions can be transferred, and in many other practical ways the gap is bridged, with the impact of change diminishing.

The changes go much deeper than these material trappings. Perhaps the most noticeable is the emphasis which college life places on individual responsibility. This changeover from a passive to an active role in controlling one's own life should begin early and progress steadily, but it undergoes a marked acceleration in college. Simple decisions of when to go to bed, when to get up, when to study, and when to play are suddenly left completely up to the student. College administrators are abandoning their role of *in loco parentis,* responding to demands of students and parents alike. It is questionable whether this has been a wise move, but it is a fact.

## Mental Health

In college a student must decide how diligently to apply himself to his educational pursuits. No one will push him to study and should he fall into academic difficulty, it is primarily his own problem to extricate himself. Help is available but is not handed to him as it might have been earlier. Choices of study courses are advised but not dictated. Planning of his entire day is suddenly thrust upon him. If our new student likes to stay up late and sleep in, this may bother his roommate who has a different pattern. Conflict stirs up friction, with resultant heat. Mother and dad are not around to referee, but problems have to be resolved if the atmosphere in the room is to be at all comfortable. With open dorms and coed dorms becoming more frequent, the difficulties are compounded.

## Identity

The development of new friendships is another area which can be troublesome. We are social creatures and all of us do place importance upon the opinion which other people have of us, though some people attempt to deny this. It is pleasant to be liked by others and it is unpleasant to have them think ill of us. The sense of personal identity which we discussed earlier is highly dependent upon what others think of us.

As new students struggle with this problem, initial politeness gives way to a strong atmosphere of competition. The animal kingdom is a vertical one, with the individual constantly struggling to maintain or improve his position relative to others. Like it or not, the same is true of the human animal. We are certainly entitled to an equal opportunity under the law to realize our potential, but most objective observers would agree that men are not equal in terms of what that biological potential is. Young people are at least vaguely aware of this and, as they progress in new relationships in college, they attempt to stake out their own positional claim. Who is the prettiest, who is the best athlete, who got the best grades on the college boards? Many students were academic leaders or athletic leaders in their high school classes but find themselves faced with other students of equal caliber, and the person used to being number one may indeed have to try harder yet still not succeed to that position. Most of us cannot be number one, but we are certainly at least vaguely aware of how we compare and we are properly concerned about it. Healthy competition is stimulating and therefore useful, but too much can be devastating.

## Moral Code

Pressures for acceptance by one's peers will often come into direct conflict with the individual's moral code. This code, a vaguely defined set of rules for living, has been building for years, but it is put to a real test in college. Perhaps for the first time all the props of previous support and enforcement are removed and the student is left entirely on his own. Drugs, sex, alcohol, dishonesty, rebelliousness, aggressivity, intimacy, all are open for exploration. Experimentation, while dangerous, is to be expected. Old values are tested, modified, perhaps rejected if found wanting. Out of this polishing process will come a working model which, it can be hoped, will be satisfactory for adult living.

Elsewhere in this book are chapters concerning the practical considerations of alcohol, drugs, and sex. The student is well advised to seek all the data available about these problems, but the final decision remains uniquely his own. His moral code, like all good systems of laws, should be sufficiently flexible to enable comfort and relaxation, but firm enough to promote social order in his life. An overly strong need for acceptance by one's peers can result in disruption of this system.

## Societal Code

Allied to this ethical sense are our attitudes about social problems, as we develop a code of ethics for society. Students today are remarkably more informed (and misinformed) about their world than ever before. They are interested in this world and anxious to take part in directing it, and this is as it should be. We must keep in mind, however, that all our thoughts are molded by past experience. What we believe relative to war, for example, is affected *to some degree* by our previous relationships with parents, friends, anger, fighting, and authority figures. This influence may be such as to increase our wisdom, but it can cause us to think in ways which are purely *rationalizations,* seemingly reasonable ideas which are actually designed by our computer to avoid pain.

It is important to know one's self well enough to avoid being overly in control of such hidden wants and impulses. Observe yourself the next time you get into a discussion of political matters with a friend. It will probably start with both of you making rather intelligent comments, but as the discussion turns into an argument, emotion begins to play a role and the heat mounts. Somewhere about here, the whole affair changes from a learning situation to a contest, and the goal becomes the winning of the contest or the destruction of the opponent, rather than the dispensation and acquisition of knowledge. Thus statements are brought out which have relatively little bearing on the problem but which make telling emotional thrusts, and the Vietnam conflict extends to a small war in your dormitory room. The angry impulse has won out over the conscious rational attitude. Judgments made under such conditions will not likely be very beneficial to society.

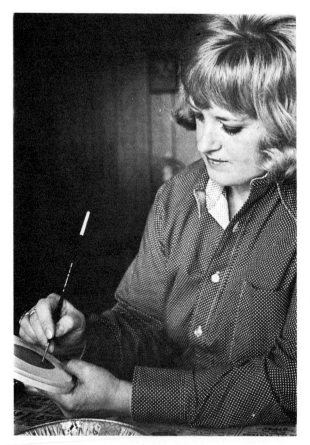

Creative outlets can channel our mental frustrations into constructive results.

## Frustration

College is a time of great frustration, much of it arising because the student is no longer a child entitled to the advantages of childhood, nor is he a socially productive adult with all the privileges and responsibilities of that state. Such frustration is extremely unpleasant, but we must learn that life is not always pleasant and that negative emotions such as anxiety and guilt are a necessary part of our makeup, serving as warning signals. We must learn to expect and accept ups and downs of emotion, with sometimes rather violent swings of mood. On the whole, however, maturity brings with it an ability to handle problems with reasonable equanimity. If this does not emerge, something may be wrong.

Out of all these problems which bombard the computer will come

---

### Schizophrenia and Culture

Schizophrenia is not one disease but many. It varies particularly with the cultural background of the individual. A study was conducted by Marvin Opler to compare cultural effects on the schizophrenic patients at Franklin D. Roosevelt Veterans Administration Hospital. The two control groups were comprised of 30 Irish and 30 Italian patients. After being given a battery of 13 psychological tests, each was the subject of extensive historical research. The findings revealed that the Irish and Italian schizophrenics had two distinct behavioral patterns. The Irish were fearful of females, low in self-esteem, tortured by feelings of guilt and inadequacy, and sunk in paranoid delusions. On the other hand, the Italian schizophrenics exhibited a hostility towards male figures, overtly homosexual behavior, extremely impulsive and excitable states, and moods of depression or uncontrolled elation sometimes resulting in assaultive and destructive behavior. Each of the patterns bore the imprint of the underlying cultural family experience and patterns of stress.

Marvin K. Opler, "Schizophrenia and Culture," *Scientific American*, August 1957, pp. 3, 5, 7.

some sort of action, determined primarily by the effectiveness of the computer. Along with the action will come a rather generally sustained emotion which we call a *mood*. Such a mood can be pleasant or unpleasant and will generally reflect the direction in which the mind is going. If most of the problems are being solved satisfactorily, the previously described zest for living will be present and the underlying mood will be a comfortable one. Should the general mood be one of sadness or despair, or in some other way uncomfortable, it may be indicative of trouble in the sphere of mental health.

## Trouble

As the student struggles to adapt to his new environment, problems arise if there are difficulties anywhere in the system we have been describing. Should the computer itself be defective through some type of brain damage, it will be handicapped in functioning adequately. It is unusual to see any major brain damage in college students, because such damage will usually cause mental retardation or other learning problems of sufficient severity to preclude a successful academic career. As our diagnostic techniques are refined, however, we discover more and more people with minor degrees of brain damage which have caused some degree of adaptational difficulty. Perhaps this damage was genetically transmitted, or the result of injury at birth. Illnesses such as encephalitis, or accidental injury to the skull and brain, as in automobile accidents, can cause brain damage with sometimes tragic results. Drugs certainly result in temporary toxic damage to the computer, with resultant malfunction and in some cases permanent damage. If the "hardware" is damaged, the machine will not function efficiently.

The majority of the problems that we find, however, have their source outside the area of physical malfunctioning. Trouble comes when the stresses placed upon the computer are too great for it to handle, either because those stresses are much too severe for anyone to cope with or because the computer itself is not equipped with the data to react satisfactorily. For example, a student will occasionally experience a run of misfortune in which there might be troubles at home, physical illness in himself or his family, financial problems beyond his control, etc. The resulting anxiety will make it difficult for him to study and his grades will go down. His anxieties will then increase and a vicious circle has begun. Everyone has his breaking point and unless some of these external pressures are relieved, the computer will blow a fuse—in the form of mental symptoms—possibly breaking down completely.

Relatively minor stresses can stir anxiety if the computer is not prepared to handle that particular problem. A student whose background in high school math is inadequate cannot handle advanced calculus without trouble. Likewise, one who has not solved problems in comfortably relating to people will be highly anxious in social situations. Thus we see that the tolerable level of stress varies with the individual's innate strength at that moment.

## Symptoms

Usually before the breaking point is reached, danger signals appear, warning that the system is overloaded. These signals take many forms and are usually recognized as *symptoms* of disturbance.

**Decreased Performance.** Perhaps the most common signal in students is the sudden worsening of academic performance. Previously good grades which suddenly drop certainly indicate that something is wrong. Inability to concentrate, excessive moodiness or irritability, a feeling of apathy, and an impulse to withdraw, all contribute to this decrease in performance.

**Worsening of Preexisting Personality Problems.** There is a natural tendency in people under stress to dip into their old collection of personality traits in an effort to handle it. A student who has always been more comfortable in a passive role will become more so, while the aggressive will become more aggressive. Sometimes such maneuvers work but more often than not they are exaggerated until they become maladaptive. Passivity in excess leads to procrastination, withdrawal, and dropouts. Too much aggressiveness can change to militancy, rebellion, and even violence. A careful look at the more extreme activist groups will frequently reveal serious emotional difficulties rather thinly disguised under the cloak of efforts at social improvement. Conversely, this does not by any means imply, as some would have it, that all people strongly working for the social good are in the grip of some sort of emotional illness. Fortunately this is usually not the case, but it does happen with sufficient frequency to bear consideration.

**Physical Complaints.** Multiple physical complaints may be the visible tip of the iceberg of mental trouble. Sleeplessness and loss of appetite are frequent problems, along with excessive fatigue unrelieved by rest. Headaches or intestinal distress are often seen, along with various types of "pressure" sensations, palpitations, and many more symptoms. Vague *somatic* complaints which don't fit any known physical pattern frequently indicate emotional disturbance. Most physicians are aware of such *psychophysiologic* problems and can be of great help in diagnosis and treatment of them.

**Poor Interpersonal Relationships.** Occasionally a student seems to suffer a state of alienation from others, with lack of enthusiasm, often coupled with frantic grasping for relief through drugs, alcohol, or promiscuity. The previously described pressure for acceptance plays a role here. A student may feel uncomfortable in any role and will consequently flit back and forth from one group to another, joining clubs and dropping out, constantly changing his social group. The building of strong ties with classmates, ordinarily a source of great gratification, suddenly seems impossible. Under it all, of course, is a pervasive sense of very unpleasant tension.

**Mood Changes.** Any persistent unrealistic mood may indicate trouble. Constant anxiety, fright, or uneasiness is not within normal expectancy. Fears of being disliked or ideas that people are talking about us cause great discomfort. Even positive ideas if carried too far are maladaptive. Euphoria, hypomania, or an overdeveloped sense of optimism can lead to a downfall.

Another frequent symptom is depression. This is a vague feeling of sadness coupled with ideas of hopelessness or despair. Usually it is not too severe but if it becomes persistent and if it is accompanied with pessimistic thoughts and fears, it can be serious. The outcome of extreme depression is suicide, and suicide is a major cause of death in young people. Since everyone has suicidal ideas on occasion, one should not be overly concerned about them. If they are persistent, however, they must be ken seriously and dealt with promptly.

**Failure of Adaptation.** As I have mentioned before, the natural state of the healthy mind is one of growth and maturity, giving a sense of fulfillment and gradual movement forward. Any sign of serious interruption of this progress toward adult productivity can be regarded as possible mental disturbance.

Adaptation has become almost a bad word in some circles, probably because it is confused with conformity. As young people struggle to develop a sense of identity, they rightly realize that they must break away from rigid conformity to the dictates of their past. They do this by a

# The Facts About Suicide

The Directors of the Los Angeles Suicide Prevention Center constantly stress the importance of educating as many people as possible to act on the warning signs posted by almost every potential suicide by urging them to seek professional help before it is too late. To this end, they suggest corrections for eight prevalent myths about suicide. The following true statements are worth remembering:

1. Some people who talk about suicide do commit suicide. Eight of ten suicides give definite warnings. Suicide threats must be taken seriously.

2. Suicide does not happen impulsively. Studies show that the suicidal person gives many clues to his intentions, often over a long period of time.

3. Suicidal people are not fully intent on dying. It is wrong to say "why bother because we can't stop them anyway?" Most suicidal people are undecided about living, and any suicide attempt is usually also a cry for help to save a life.

4. People are not suicidal for life. Hundreds of case histories show that a person brought through a suicidal crisis can go on to live a long and useful life.

5. Improvement does not necessarily mean the suicidal risk has passed. Many suicides take place in the three months following the beginning of "improvement." This is a time to be especially vigilant.

6. Suicide attacks all economic and occupational classes. Suicide is highly "democratic" and is spread proportionately throughout all levels of society.

7. Suicidal people are not necessarily mentally ill. The suicidal person is extremely unhappy, but this may result from a temporary emotional upset or a complete loss of hope.

8. Suicidal tendencies are not inherited. Suicide is an individual matter and can be prevented.

Excerpt from Joseph N. Bell, "Lifeline for Would-Be Suicides," *Today's Health,* June 1967, published by the American Medical Association. Reprinted by permission of the publisher and the author.

gradual series of changes, for example, short hair to long hair, clean-shaven to beards, often taken to extremes but gradually molded back to a compromise level satisfactory to the individual. Each new stage has aspects of rigid conformities of its own, as we see in high school students who give up their parents' ideas in favor of very strict compliance to the dictates of their peers. Gradually a sense of individuality emerges. All of this is carried out for the purposes of adaptation, that is, of learning how to live with reality in a reasonably comfortable way. We don't have to conform in every way but neither can we always do our own thing. Can you imagine a country such as ours with 220,000,000 people each doing his own thing?

**Psychosis.** All of the symptoms thus far described can be present in varying degrees of severity. Should they get severe enough that the student is completely separated from reality, living in a world of his own, we speak of him as *psychotic*. Such persons suffer from *hallucinations, delusional thinking,* and many other evidences of bizarre mental functioning. Fortunately, these are rare in college but they do occur and are usually promptly recognized and referred to appropriate sources of professional help. Problems do arise in distinguishing this type of patient from the individual we would ordinarily classify as eccentric, a person who is functioning reasonably well but whose personality is such that he does not seem to fit in to the main stream of college life. These people are frequently ostracized by their peers and this adds greatly to their problems. Caution is urged in considering everybody to be mentally ill should he not conform to our particular way of viewing life.

## Help—How to Get It

### Prevention

The best solution to any problem is to prevent it in the first place. There are many things we can do to prevent mental illness and many of these have already been mentioned. Association with friends, a proper balance of mental and physical activities, sports, hobbies, vacations, recreation of various sorts—many things are used by all of us to relax. As we evaluate ourselves more adequately, we learn the limits of our abilities and we learn not to exceed such limits, thus avoiding intolerable degrees of ten-

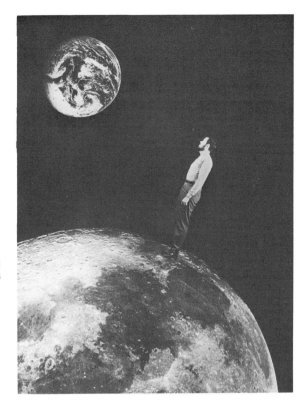

The psychotic is completely separated from reality and lives in a world of his own.

sion. We learn how many hours we can study without a break and we learn how closely we can relate to other people without becoming too uncomfortable. Such simple matters are very good preventive devices and most of us use them every day.

## Self-help

Should trouble arise in spite of these things, there are many self-help mechanisms which we can use. Most of these lie in the area of changing our computer input, that is, reducing the stresses under which we find ourselves. Perhaps the dropping of a troublesome course, or obtaining academic help through a tutor is a good example of this. Taking off for a long weekend or consideration of the changing of one's major course of study can do wonders in this regard. Technically this is called "manipulation of the environment."

Self-help involves some danger, however, simply because the thinking which has gotten us into trouble may not, at the moment, be sufficiently *objective* to get us out. At times like these it pays to make use of those close relationships we have built up with others. Talk to friends, parents, and other advisers. Two heads are often, though not always, better than one. It is surprising how often another person who is not emotionally involved in the problem can see things more clearly.

## Professional Help

There are times when more definitive measures are needed. Most colleges are aware of this and have set up sources of help. Academic advisers are experienced in the understanding of emotional problems, particu-

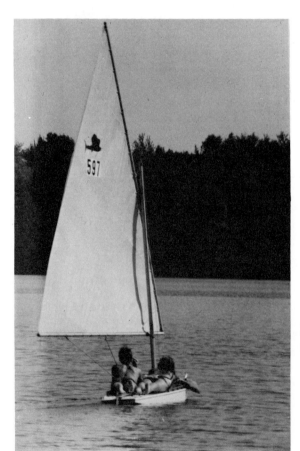

Allotting sufficient time for recreation is one means of preventing mental illness.

larly as related to academic performance. The student health service of a college is usually manned by nurses and physicians who are becoming more aware of and better trained in the problems of mental disturbance. Counseling services are available. These are staffed and directed by people with advanced degrees in psychology who are well-versed in the workings of the mind and are particularly interested in the student and his problems. Many colleges employ psychiatrists—medical doctors specializing in the diagnosis and treatment of mental disturbance.

Administrators have wisely realized that if such resources are to be useful, strict rules regarding confidentiality of information must be observed. This frees the student to discuss his personal problems, secure in the knowledge that this information will go no further. There can be no chance of jeopardizing his college career through involvement of administrative personnel. Should the student disclose plans for suicide or other life-threatening actions, the counselor has every right to get parents or administrators involved, but beyond such emergency situations, any competent professional will guarantee absolute confidentiality.

---

### Portrait of a Neurotic

John constantly talked about the great trips he was going to take to the South Seas. Whenever his friends asked him about his trips, they found that he had not yet gone because of various problems that had arisen, thus forcing John to postpone his trip. The problems always were outside of John's control, however his plans continued to grow in importance and complexity. He attended travelogues and read many books about the South Seas. Gradually, his friends noticed that among strangers his descriptions of his travel plans sounded less and less like plans and more and more like real past travels. Friends who pointed this out to John were soon dropped. As the years passed, John lost most of his old friends. However, he was very popular among his new friends because of his wide travels and worldly manner.

Frank Cox, *Psychology* (Dubuque, Ia.: Wm. C. Brown Company Publishers, 1970), p. 343.

---

**Psychotherapy.**   A reduction or a change in the environmental stresses pressing down upon the student are frequently all that is necessary. In a fairly sizeable number of problems, however, the trouble comes primarily from inside the computer. The thoughts and memories and emotions are perhaps unrealistic, inaccurate, or exaggerated. Medications can help in problems of this sort, but there are times when a more intensive, time-consuming effort must be made to alter the data in the computer. We speak of this type of effort as psychotherapy.

This therapy, often called "talk therapy," is an effort to help a person learn more about the inner workings of the mind. Exploration of his early mental development is undertaken to find out why he feels as he does. If areas are discovered in which his present mental activity is based upon mistaken or exaggerated beliefs or memories, he is helped to break loose from those misconceptions. Such treatment can be obtained from psychiatrists, psychologists, or allied mental health professionals, either privately or in governmentally funded clinics such as the community mental health centers which are being established throughout the country.

There are many types of psychotherapy, including individual (one-to-one therapy), group therapy, marital therapy, and family therapy. These vary in the approach that they use and the intensity with which they work.

**Psychoanalysis** is perhaps the most intensive of these therapies, usually involving an hour of treatment per day, perhaps five days per week. Its goal is to undertake a complete exploration of the personality in great depth and to make major changes in that personality. Such therapy is useful in a limited number of disturbances, but it is generally not needed and frequently impractical for the usual run of problems.

It will, of course, be bewildering to the student to attempt to decide what sort of treatment, if any, he might need. Anyone having such questions concerning his own mental state should feel free to contact any of the sources of help which have been described. In addition, ministers or family physicians can be of great help. There is plenty of help available and the student is urged to overcome his natural reticence and seek such aid if he feels he needs it.

**Caution.**   All sorts of mental health movements with varying degrees of competency are springing up in our society. Encounter movements as seen in various T-groups have become quite popular. These no doubt have their use, but their safety and efficacy are still in doubt. College campuses are fertile soil for the growth of such groups and the student should be very cautious about getting involved in any such undertaking. This writer's personal experience would indicate that there may be serious problems arising from such unsupervised therapeutic activity, no matter how well intended. Should this type of treatment prove effective and safe, it will be accepted into the treatment scene, but until such time as it is adequately tested, it would seem more prudent to follow the more usual channels to help.

## Closing the Communication Gap

Much is said today about a generation gap between young and old, with some magical dividing line at age thirty. It seems to me we are actually talking about a communication gap, a situation in which some people find themselves unable to talk to others adequately. Aligning the generations against one another is certainly thinking in generalities and does not clearly describe the problem. Communication gap exist when there are serious differences between people of any age, including people of exactly the same age. They exist in bad marriages, in bad teacher-student relationships, and in any other area where there are problems between people. Part of mental health is the ability to communicate adequately with others; thus a serious gap can exist only between those who are not healthy. Efforts to truly understand others and to evaluate our own ideas in the light of theirs will effectively close most gaps. As a rule of thumb, if one is having trouble with other people, it pays to think first of "What am I doing to cause this friction?" rather than "What is that so-and-so doing?"

## Summary

We have attempted in this chapter to outline some concepts regarding the functioning of the mind and the paths toward mental health or, conversely, toward mental illness. Many of these topics are controversial and the reader is urged to pursue the matter in more detail, keeping a healthily open mind to all theories. We hope the student is left with the conviction, however, that no matter what theory one may use, the truly royal road to mental health lies within himself. It is assumed that he came to college with a relatively high degree of maturity and that if he continues to grow, to polish his skills in this area, he will indeed have that interesting, enjoyable life which can only come with mental health.

## Questions for Study and Discussion

1. What environmental pressures create tension and stress for college students?
2. How can one control frustrations and depression?
3. How do mind and body affect one another?
4. Where on campus may one seek help if depressed or disturbed?
5. Why is there still the presence of social stigma surrounding mental illness?
6. What are some sound practices for maintaining good mental health?
7. Are "freaks" mentally disturbed since many do *not* adjust to reality?
8. Do you feel mental illness will decrease or increase in the next five years?
9. Why are some mental disturbances only neurotic and others psychotic?
10. What significance does education have on interpretation of mental health and mental illness?

## References

Eaton, Merrill T., Jr. and Peterson, Margaret H. *Psychiatry.* Medical Outline Series. New York: Medical Examination Publishing Co., 1967.

Kolb, Laurence C. *Noyes' Modern Clinical Psychiatry.* 7th ed. Philadelphia, Penn.: W. B. Saunders Co., 1965.

*American Handbook of Psychiatry,* vol. 1. Arieti, ed. New York: Basic Books, Inc., 1959.

Erikson, Erik H. *Childhood and Society.* 2nd ed. New York: William Norton and Co., Inc., 1963.

Ardrey, Robert. *The Social Contract.* New York: Atheneum Publishers, 1970.

# Communicable Diseases

**3**

## General Concept

Communicable diseases are those which are spread from one person to another by indirect or direct contact, and which may lead to serious health problems if not detected and treated in the early stages.

## Outcomes

The student should be able to:
1. Explain the principles of communicable diseases, pathogens, and treatment
2. Identify the mode of transmission and the effects of various micro-organisms
3. Avoid spreading or carrying of infectious disease and seek early treatment if necessary

## Causes of Disease

Communicable diseases are so-called because they are diseases which can be transmitted from man to man by various means, either directly or indirectly. Although diseases had been recognized as entities and the

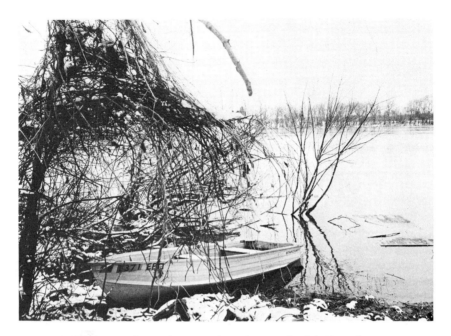

Polluted waters frequently serve as hosts for spreading infectious disease.

natural history of many diseases described before the latter part of the seventeenth century, it was not until then that Antonj van Leeuwenhoek saw a germ for the first time. Almost 200 years passed before Louis Pasteur showed that different kinds of fermentations were consequences of the activities of different kinds of organisms, and scientific thought made the transition to the possibility that different diseases could be caused by different micro-organisms. Lister (1827–1912), an English surgeon, was one of the first to use this concept of **antisepsis*** in surgery. It remained, however, for Robert Koch (1843–1910), a German physician, to develop the experimental methods necessary to the proof of the causal relation between bacteria and infectious diseases. Because of his great contribution to the knowledge and understanding of their relationship, a group of propositions have been known as Koch's postulate, although proof that he actually stated them as such is lacking. There are four of these:

1. The bacterium must be observed in every case of the disease
2. The bacterium must be isolated and grown in pure culture

* *Note:* Any term that appears in ***boldface*** print is defined in the glossary at the end of this chapter.

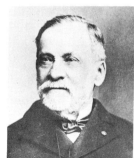

Louis Pasteur

UPI

3. The bacterium, in pure culture, must, when inoculated into a susceptible animal, give rise to the disease
4. The bacterium must be observed in and recovered from the experimental animal

In any disease which seems to be a contagious, communicable disease, these postulates are followed in the attempt to identify the causative organism. There are inherent and peculiar difficulties encountered at each step, so that often suspicion arises as to the very nature of a disease. **Infectious mononucleosis** is a case in point. So far no causative organism has been recovered, no experimental transmissions of the disease have conclusively been made, and yet we use the term "infectious." Recent work has shown a **serologic** relationship to a virus, but no virus has been recovered at any time which fulfills Koch's Postulates.

## Microorganism

Today many microorganisms have been recognized as the causative agent of disease, and these are identified by **morphologic** chemical and cultural means. They are viruses, rickettsia, bacteria, protozoa, and fungi.

Viruses are too small to be seen by an optical microscope, but much has been learned about them with the aid of the electron microscope and chemical analysis. They replicate only in living tissue—in fact, they become so much an integral part of a cell that no drug can affect the virus without also affecting the cell. To the present time the best method of controlling viral disease has been by immunization, not the use of antibiotics, which are useless against viruses. There is a wide range of viruses affecting man: from the common cold, influenza, measles, mumps, through poliomyelitis and smallpox.

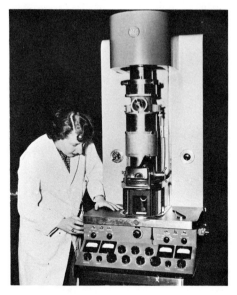

Much has been learned about viruses with the aid of the electron microscope.

UPI

Rickettsia are organisms somewhat larger than viruses and smaller than bacteria and with some of the characteristics of each. Rickettsia for the most part can multiply only in living tissue, but are affected by the broad spectrum antibiotics such as tetracycline and chloramphenicol. The diseases caused by these organisms, such as Rocky Mountain spotted fever and typhus, are transmitted by arthropods, the tick and louse respectively.

Bacteria are organisms which do not necessarily depend on living tissue in order to multiply. Because antibiotics are so effective, the greatest strides have been made in controlling infectious diseases caused by bacteria. Most of these known organisms are not pathogenic (disease-producing) to man and some are pathogenic only when growing in certain tissues of man. Some **streptococci** are normal inhabitants of the throat of man, but can, if growing in the vascular system cause a very serious illness. The diseases caused by bacteria are many: boils, pneumonia, syphilis, "strep" throat and meningitis.

Protozoa are one-celled animals capable of causing many diseases in man and animals. Some of the more well known diseases caused by these organisms are malaria, sleeping sickness, and amoebic dysentery. As in rickettsial diseases, insects may play a great part in the infection of man;

for example, the importance of the tsetse fly in sleeping sickness and the anopheles mosquito is well known. Generally, protozoas are not a serious problem in the United States, but *trichomonas hominis* is universally found. It frequently is the cause of severe itching and a serious vaginal discharge in the female, but causes little or no symptoms in the male. Although it can be transmitted by intercourse, it is not considered a venereal disease, since it is most often acquired from contaminated toilet seats, clothing, or bed clothes.

Fungi are simple vegetable forms, some species of which are capable of causing disease in man. Two main forms are usually responsible; yeasts and molds. Yeasts cause such diseases as **histoplasmosis, coccidioidomycosis,** and **monila infections.**

Monila infections, caused by fungus, can be the source of much discomfort. In the mouth of infants it is known as thrush; when it attacks the area between the fingers it is known as "bartenders' itch"; in skin folds at the inguinal area, "jockey itch"; when it appears as fissuring at the corner of the mouth, it is known as perleche; around the fingernail it is called paronychia; it also causes monilial vaginitis, which is probably the most common cause of vaginal discharge in women.

*Monila* is more commonly seen in diabetes, but the most important aspect is the marked frequency with which infections due to *Monila* are found after the use of penicillin and broad-spectrum antibiotic therapy for other diseases. It is easily recognized that this is one of the reasons antibiotics are not used as freely today as they were at one time, especially in such diseases as the common cold, where antibiotics have shown no effect on the primary viral infection.

Thus there are various types of microorganisms capable of causing disease, but to do so these microorganisms must be transmitted from their host to man. The host is most commonly man, but animals, plants and soil may act as the reservoir host wherein the microorganism is capable of living and, most often, multiplying. Transmission can be by direct contact, through vectors such as mosquitoes and flies, by inhalation of moisture droplets and dust, or by ingestion of contaminated food or drink.

Because of the unique growth characteristics of these disease-causing organisms, only certain transmission methods will apply to a certain organism. The **spirochete** causing syphilis soon dies if not on living human tissue, preferably mucus membrane, but the spore of tetanus may lie dormant for years in dry soil ready to cause infection if introduced beneath the skin on man. Transmission of a disease organism to man does not necessarily mean that a disease will follow. The barriers of the body must be penetrated and the resistance of body defenses overcome before a disease can become established.

Many known and unknown factors enter into the resistance of the body to disease. The skin, gastric juice, body secretions and their enzymes, cilia and other nonspecific barriers protect man from the entry of organisms. Various specific and nonspecific reactions occur within the body to combat invading organisms. Nonspecific reactions occur such as fever, which, by raising the body temperature, can create an unfavorable environment for an organism (giving rise to the term "friendly fever"); and increased blood flow at the site of invasion brings **leucocytes** which phagocytize (eat) organisms and interfere with viruses entering other cells.

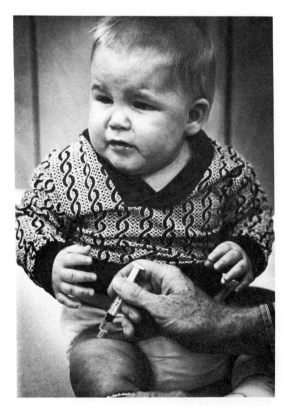

Active immunization can be produced by the inoculation of a killed or attenuated organism into the body.

Specific reaction to an invading organism is known as the **antigen-antibody** reaction. When pathogenic organisms are introduced into the body, they will act as an antigen and cause the production of a specific antibody, which will react in some way. This is known as active immunization. Passive immunization, as contrasted with the active form, is the transference of antibody from one individual to another. Antibody can be passed by the mother to her child across the placental barrier or through the nursing process, thus giving the child some protection during the early months of life. Tetanus antitoxin and immune globulin injections are other examples of passive immunity. Active immunity

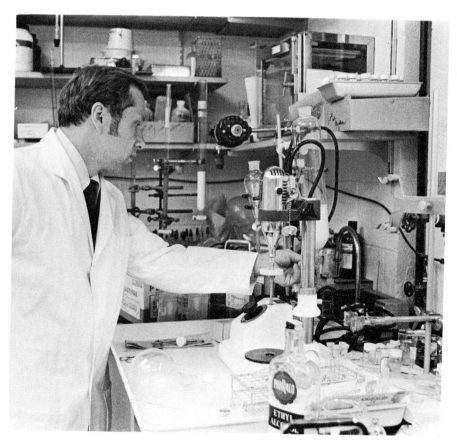

Modern advances in scientific procedures have resulted in a more exacting identification of disease producing agents.

gained by having the disease is usually permanent, whereas passive immunity is temporary. Active immunization can also be produced by the inoculation of a killed or attenuated organism into the body. Polio vaccines and tetanus toxoid vaccines are examples of this type of active immunization, which, although prolonged, may not be permanent. It must be remembered that immunity is a relative phenomenon and that an overwhelming invasion may overcome the immunologic defense.

## Epidemiology

Epidemiology is the phase of medical science and public health that deals with the dynamics of disease, incidence, cause, and control in human populations. In relation to communicable diseases, the possibilities of control can be demonstrated by illustrating the spread of disease as six links in a "chain of infection." These six steps must all take place and in a specific order if a new infectious disease is to take place. Any method that creates a break in the "chain of infection" will prevent the occurrence of the infectious disease process.

The first link in the chain is the causative agent or pathogenic organism. This agent will fall into one of the classifications of organisms described earlier. If a method can be found to destroy the agent, this link can be broken and prevented from starting a new infection. The process of sterilization is an example of attempts to control the spread of disease by destroying the causative agent.

The second link is the reservoir or source of the causative agent. If the reservoir can be identified and eliminated, the link can be destroyed and the spread of the disease controlled. For example, rabies, a disease commonly found in warm-blooded animals, can be controlled by destroying the animal identified as a carrier.

The third link is a mode of escape from the reservoir. The mode of escape for most pathogens is usually through the body's natural openings. Many viral infections, such as colds and influenza, could be controlled by having the infected individual cover his nose and mouth to eliminate a means for the agent to leave the body.

The fourth link is a mode of transmission. Although most infectious diseases are spread by direct contact, the spread of some disease requires an insect host (vector). This link can be eliminated by isolating the infected individual, thereby limiting his contact with other people. Malaria has been brought under control in many parts of the world by destroying the female anopheline mosquito, the insect host for the causative agent.

The fifth link is a mode of entry. In general, the modes of entry are the same as the modes of escape. To cause a new infection, the pathogen must gain entry into the new host at a site where it can survive.

The last link in the chain of infection is the susceptible host. This link has been eliminated for many diseases through immunization, making the individual nonsusceptible to the agent. Diseases such as diphtheria, pertussis, tetanus, polio, rubella, measles, smallpox, and mumps have been controlled through this process.

Infectious diseases may be classified in several ways. Sometimes they are classified by **etiology,** thus we have the viral diseases; sometimes by the bodily systems involved, for example, the respiratory diseases; and sometimes by the way they are transmitted, for example, venereal diseases. Let us examine the venereal diseases in a little more detail, because the highest incidence is in people of college age, and they can illustrate many of the aspects previously discussed.

The word "venereal" stems from Venus, the Goddess of Love, and accurately describes the mode of transmission. Included in the group are syphilis, gonorrhea, granuloma inguinale, and lymphogranuloma venereum.

## Syphilis

It is believed that syphilis was introduced into Europe by the returning men of Columbus' first voyage to America. Medical writings as well as bones showing evidence of the disease would seem to confirm this. The disease is caused by the spirochete *treponema pallidum* which is **anaerobic** and requires moisture and tissue for survival. The physiologic secretions (vaginal, salivary, and seminal fluid) collected in all stages of the disease, both early and late, have been shown in controlled experiments to be noninfectious. The blood, however, may contain the organisms in abundance in the early years of infection and at irregular intervals in later years. By this method the organisms may be transmitted to the fetus or be deposited in the vagina by menstrual blood.

Transmission of syphilis, therefore, is a lesion-to-lesion affair except by means of the blood. Syphilis, other than congenital syphilis, passes through several stages. During the incubation period of about 3 weeks (limit 10–60 days) there are no symptoms. Then, at the site of inoculation, a chancre will develop which is not painful. Usually this lesion is around the genitals, but may be inside the urethra or vagina, at the rectum, or inside the mouth. The lesion varies widely, but the typical lesion can be described as an eroded surface with serious discharge, painless, raw-ham-colored, single, firm, with rolled border and accompanied by rubbery regional lymph-glands. The lesion lasts from 1 to 5 weeks.

The secondary stage appears from 2 to 10 weeks later and is manifest by a generalized eruption which lasts 2 to 6 weeks. This rash can also vary widely, but is usually pustular in nature and widespread over the body. The spirochete is found in all the lesions, so this is the most contagious stage. Symptoms are so painless, and the lesions so often mistaken for something else, that it has been estimated that 40 to 60 percent of infected persons go undiagnosed.

Syphilis then passes into a latent stage lasting two to ten or more years in which there are no signs or symptoms. Finally it progresses into the late or symptomatic stage when various systems of the body may be affected (cardiovascular, central nervous system, etc.).

Diagnosis depends on clinical course plus finding the organism in the lesion in the first and second stage and/or by serologic testing. The immune response which occurs about one to two weeks after the primary lesion can be evidenced by several serologic tests, and is probably the most common way the diagnosis is made. Many states, as a method of controlling the disease, require that this test be done before a marriage license is issued.

Penicillin is the most effective method of treating syphilis, although other antibiotics can be used in those persons allergic to penicillin. Previously, treatment lasted for years, but now, in most cases, it lasts less than two weeks. With the advent of a quick, effective treatment it was hoped that the disease could be eliminated, but since 1955 there has been an increased incidence. Perhaps if it were transmitted in some other fashion, it would be eliminated by now, but unfortunately many infected persons are uncooperative in naming contacts.

If the diagnosis is primary syphilis, all possible source contacts up to three months prior to the onset of symptoms should be examined, and if secondary or early latent syphilis, for a 6- to 12-month period prior to diagnosis. As mentioned above, approximately 50 percent of infected persons are unaware of their disease; they are the real beneficiaries of

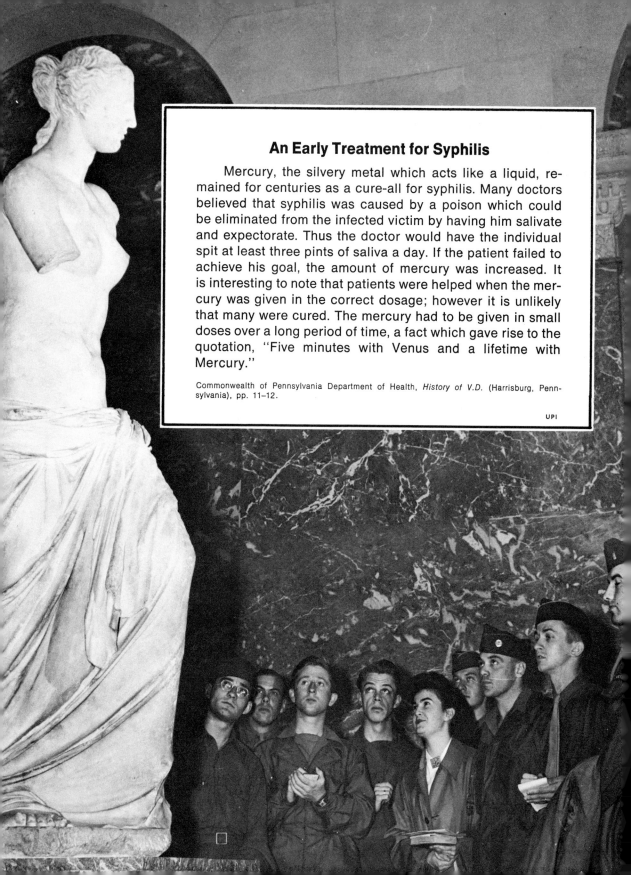

## An Early Treatment for Syphilis

Mercury, the silvery metal which acts like a liquid, remained for centuries as a cure-all for syphilis. Many doctors believed that syphilis was caused by a poison which could be eliminated from the infected victim by having him salivate and expectorate. Thus the doctor would have the individual spit at least three pints of saliva a day. If the patient failed to achieve his goal, the amount of mercury was increased. It is interesting to note that patients were helped when the mercury was given in the correct dosage; however it is unlikely that many were cured. The mercury had to be given in small doses over a long period of time, a fact which gave rise to the quotation, "Five minutes with Venus and a lifetime with Mercury."

Commonwealth of Pennsylvania Department of Health, *History of V.D.* (Harrisburg, Pennsylvania), pp. 11–12.

UPI

having the condition brought to light. Not only should the source be sought, but spread contacts should be identified and examined. There is a difference of opinion on the management of a spread contact: whether to treat on the basis of epidemiology or obtain a definite diagnosis. Serologic testing should be done for 3 months following sexual exposure before the diagnosis can be rejected.

Transmission of syphilis is usually by heterosexual contact. Spreading by homosexual practice will often involve a greater number of contacts per infected individuals because of greater promiscuity.

Among those who have the responsibility of controlling venereal disease, there is a difference of opinion regarding the questioning of contacts. One group feels that treatment should be rendered and no questions asked, that the possible embarrassment would deter the individual from seeking prompt attention. The other group believes that the job is only started when an individual is brought to treatment, that the disease can never be controlled until the reservoirs are removed. Certainly the wisest and most charitable person will seek prompt attention for himself and be considerate of others.

## Late Syphilis

Following spontaneous healing of secondary syphilis or inadequately treated cases, no symptoms will make themselves evident for a varying period of time—2 to 20 years. Tertiary syphilis may appear in the form of nodular or ulcerative lesions. The form the lesion takes is believed due to the host response. The ulcerative lesions are the result of greater sensitivity and the nodular form are due to lesser sensitivity. The lesions are not contagious, but may last for years unless specific treatment is instituted.

Late benign syphilis may attack the cardiovascular system, where it may leave permanent cardiovascular damage, or it may attack the liver or central nervous system. If the disease progresses to the brain, it may leave an atrophic condition or psychosis such as **paresis.** Columbus returned to Europe where he was declared insane as a result of paresis. He died fourteen years later.

## Gonorrhea

Although gonorrhea, meaning "flow of seed," was named by Galen in 130 A.D., and although its venereal nature was known before that, it was not until 1860 that it was known as a separate disease from syphilis. In 1879 A. Neisser discovered that the disease-producing organism was a diplococcus and named it gonococcus. Later it was named neisseria gonorrhea.

Infection with the organism varies somewhat, depending on whether the host is male or female. **Asymptomatic** gonorrhea exists both in the male and female, but much more commonly in the female. Pariser and Farmer have reported studies which show 36 percent of female sex partners of known gonorrhea patients to have asymptomatic infection. Twenty-six percent of the male sex partners of known gonorrhea patients had asymptomatic gonorrhea when urethral and prostatic secretions were cultured.

In the male, **urethritis,** with urgent and frequent urinations and a purulent discharge, are the first symptoms. The incubation period is approximately two to eight days, but may be longer. If untreated, the discharge will clear in several weeks except for a slight mucoid discharge noted in the morning. Spread of the infection can occur into the prostate seminal vesicle or **epididymis.** Stricture and retention of urine may ensue as a consequence of infection, and epididymitis can cause sterility.

Infection in the female can also cause a urethritis, but it frequently is of short duration and mild. Normally the Bartholin and Skenes glands secrete a fluid for lubricating the vulva and vaginal areas for intercourse. When gonorrhea invades this area, abscesses may form. The cervix may excrete a purulent discharge. These signs and symptoms may go unnoticed in a female, since secretions are normal during sexual arousal and menstruation. Therefore, the condition may be permitted to advance to the fallopian tubes, causing a condition, **salpingitis,** which is characterized by abdominal pain and fever, and can result in sterility.

Twenty percent to 40 percent of women will have involvement of the rectum with the symptoms of **proctitis.** The two most common extragenital areas of gonococcal involvement are the eyes and the joints. Prior to the obligatory use of silver nitrate into the eyes of all new-borns, there was a high incidence of blindness due to gonococci **ophthalmia.**

Arthritis, with hot, swollen joints, is the most frequent extra-genital involvement. It usually occurs within three weeks of infection and may represent a spread or an immune response.

Penicillin is the drug of choice in the treatment of gonorrhea, though the broad-spectrum antibiotics are frequently used. A strain of gonococcus resistant to many of the antibiotics has been found in service personnel returning from Vietnam. Prontosil, a sulfa drug, was introduced in 1932 and found to be very effective against the gonococcus. Drug laws of the day allowed over-the-counter purchase of the drugs and self-treatment was prevalent. Self-treatment was often in quantities sufficient to control the symptoms, but not to eradicate the infection. There was subsequent development of resistant strains of gonococci that were not controlled until the development of penicillin in 1939. It was this experience that helped promote the legislation controlling the use of many of our drugs today.

Control measures for gonorrhea are the same as for syphillis. The need for greater control is also evident in the fact that the cases reported in the United States in 1963 were 270,000 and in 1968, 431,000. Since the majority of cases go unreported, the true incidence is presently estimated at 1,500,000 cases per year. The age group with the highest incidence is 15 to 24 years of age.

## Lymphogranuloma Venereum

Lymphogranuloma venereum is a venereal disease caused by virus. Approximately 3 to 30 days after exposure, the disease is manifest by a small painless ulcer which may go unnoticed. Spread of the infection is through the lymphatics, and large matted glands in the inguinal area become noticeable and are called "Buboes." Abscess formation with draining sinuses may develop if untreated. Scarring with contractures are common in the area of the rectum.

Serologic testing is possible for the diagnosis and treatment is best accomplished with the sulfonamides or tetracycline.

Although the disease occurs everywhere, it is more commonly found in the tropics. Surveys taken during World War II showed one-third of the adult Negro population of the South was infected, but the number of cases reported in recent years is much less.

## Granuloma Inguinale

Granuloma inguinale is an **indolent granulomatous** and ulcerative disease usually localized to the genitalia and caused by a plemorphic coccobacillus called the "Donovan body." The initial lesion is a painless nodular infiltration which ulcerates. The lesion spreads by direct extension, is highly destructive to the skin and subcutaneous tissue, and secondary infection with other microorganisms is common.

The disease may be prevented by adequate washing with soap and water after exposure and the infection usually responds to any of several broad-spectrum antibiotics.

## Epidemiology of Venereal Disease

The "chain of infection" has its implications for the venereal diseases, specifically syphilis and gonorrhea. The agents are delicate organisms that exist in man primarily in the genital-urinary tract and mucus membranes. The agents can be destroyed by penicillin and other broad-spectrum antibiotics. Since the reservoir is man, this link in the chain cannot be destroyed. The mode of escape and mode of entry is through the genital-urinary tract. This link can be reduced to a limited extent through the use of a rubber sheath (condom) during sexual contact. Since mode of transmission is direct sexual contact with an infected individual, potential control of syphilis and gonorrhea could be made possible by limiting sexual contact to individuals who are not infected and by prohibiting infected individuals from sexual contact until they have been successfully treated. Since there is no effective immunization for the veneral diseases at this time, each individual is considered to be a susceptible host.

## Magnitude of the Problem

Through the application of epidemiological methods, many infectious diseases that once plagued man have been controlled and are no longer a threat to health and life. In spite of extensive medical knowledge of the cause, treatment, and control of venereal diseases, they persist as a major health problem in the United States. While the incidence of other infectious diseases has steadily decreased since 1964, reported cases of gonorrhea infections have increased from 290,603 in 1964 to 809,700 in 1973. The picture is even more disturbing when one considers the fact that the majority of gonorrhea infections are not reported to public health agencies. The U. S. Public Health Service estimates that the actual number of gonorrhea cases occurring in the nation is close to 2½ million. Most gonorrhea infections occur in the group under 25 years of age. Indications are that one in every 50 teenagers and one in every 25 in the twenty to twenty-four age group contracts gonorrhea. The U. S. Public Health Service revealed the number of reported new syphilis cases in 1973 to be 25,080. This number represents an increase of 8.1 percent over the previous year. If any of the other communicable diseases presented an equal threat to health, our society would become very much alarmed and demand control action.

Why then has venereal disease persisted, and in fact increased? The V.D. problem is more than a medical problem, it is also a social problem. Complacency and indifference are active factors in making control difficult. Venereal disease is often thought to be confined to lower classes, and many individuals consider the possibility of contracting V.D. too remote to consider before engaging in sexual activity. The fact is that V.D. cuts across all social strata and should always be considered a possibility in all nonmarital sexual activity.

Venereal disease is often referred to as a social disease. Many of our negative sexual attitudes make control difficult. Society, in general, does not approve of nonmarital sex and often views V.D. as a deterrent to sexual promiscuity. Out of fear and guilt, many people will fail to seek early treatment. This stigma is also responsible for the large number of V.D. cases that go unreported every year. Lack of knowledge and the high mobility of our population are other factors that contribute to making it difficult to control the venereal diseases.

## What Needs to Be Done

Since control of venereal disease begins with the individual, any sexually active person should be familiar with the symptoms of syphilis and gonorrhea and see a physician whenever any suspicious signs appear. Epidemiology begins with the physician, who will diagnose and prescribe treatment. The treatment of only obviously infected persons who see a physician is not sufficient for control or eradication, however. All of the sexual contacts of the individual must be examined and, if necessary, treated in a process known as "contact tracing." The infected patient is interviewed confidentially to find out to whom he has been exposed. These contacts are also interviewed and persuaded to be examined by their own doctors or in a clinic. The process continues as *their* contacts are located and interviewed. It should be emphasized that interviews are done by highly trained professionals and conducted in a confidential and dignified way.

Venereal disease spreads rapidly and can involve many people during the incubation period. The average number of contacts during this period is approximately five, but numbers as large as seventeen or more have been reported. This makes control even more difficult because each contact in turn develops his or her own line of contacts. Since the key to successful control is rapid, complete reporting of all sexual contact, the final responsibility for eradicating this disease resides within each individual.

## Infectious Mononucleosis

Infectious mononucleosis is a viral disease characterized by irregular fever, sore throat, swelling of lymph glands in the neck, and occasionally a rash. There may also be associated weakness and fatigue and in some cases pain or discomfort in the upper abdominal area due to enlargement of the spleen. Mononucleosis is sometimes referred to as "the kissing disease" or "students' disease" because it is spread by very close contact and most frequently affects young people between the ages of fifteen and thirty. The incubation period varies from two to six weeks and is communicable from before symptoms appear to the end of fever and clearing of any lesions.

There are no specific preventive measures for mononucleosis, but if at any time an individual suffers from any combination of the above symptoms, a physician should be consulted. The treatment consists primarily of complete rest, and sometimes antibiotics for any secondary infections. If recognized and treated early, mononucleosis will clear up in a short period of time. But if the symptoms are ignored and the disease allowed to progress, there may be liver damage which may lead to serious complications.

## Infectious Hepatitis

Another disease common among young people, especially those living in close quarters such as dormitories or barracks, is hepatitis, a viral disease localizing in the liver and producing liver damage. The onset is usually abrupt and characterized by the following symptoms: fever, weakness, nausea, abdominal discomfort, and jaundice. If jaundice develops, the skin and whites of the eyes become yellow, the urine is much darker, and the stools are light in color. The mode of transmission is considered to be person-to-person contact, presumably by the fecal-oral route. The agent may be found in feces and urine. Some outbreaks have been related to contaminated water and food. The agent is also present in circulating blood prior to onset of jaundice and for a few days later. This last factor may lead to the spread of the disease by inoculation of infected blood or blood products or by contaminated needles and syringes (a problem prevalent among illicit drug users).

Preventive measures consist of good sanitation and proper personal hygiene, with special emphasis on sanitary disposal of feces, proper sterilization of syringes and needles, or the use of disposable units for injections. The treatment is primarily bed rest and isolation. Early treatment is important because without proper care hepatitis may develop into a chronic and prolonged disease causing permanent liver damage. An additional control measure should include investigation of contacts. There is no vaccine for active immunization, but passive immunization should be given to those exposed to the disease.

## Glossary

**Anaerobic:** thriving without air

**Aneurism:** a sac which forms by the dilation of the walls of an artery or of a vein and fills with blood

**Antigen:** any substance which when introduced into the blood or tissues incites the formation of an antibody

**Antisepsis:** the prevention of poisoning by the destruction of microorganism and infective matter

**Aortic insufficiency:** lack of adequate function of the main trunk from which the entire arterial system proceeds

**Aortitis:** inflammation of the aorta

**Asymptomatic:** showing no symptoms

**Bartholin's glands:** of the female reproductive system

**Candidasis albican:** a genus of yeast–like fungi

**Coccidioidomycosis:** generalized fungus infection

**Dysuria:** painful or difficult urination

**Epididymis:** an oblong body attached to the upper part of each testicle

**Etiology:** the study or theory of the causation of any disease; the sum of knowledge regarding causes

**General paresis:** a chronic disease of the brain characterized by progressive loss of mental and physical power

**Gonococcic opthalmia:** severe inflammation of the eye caused by the organism of gonorrhea

**Histoplasmosis:** a disease caused by a fungus which attacks the cells of the spleen, lymph, and other glands

**Indolent granulomatous:** formation of multiple tumors causing little pain

**Infectious mononucleosis:** an active infectious disease characterized by a sudden onset with fever and inflammatory swelling of the lymph nodes, especially those of the cervical region

**Leucocytes:** white blood cells

**Moniliasis:** infection caused by parasitic fungi

**Morphologic:** pertaining to the science of the forms and structure of organized beings

**Primary optic atrophy:** degeneration of sight

**Proctitis:** inflammation of the rectum

**Salpingitis:** inflammation of the fallopian tube

**Serologic:** pertaining to serums and the study of serums. Used most commonly to mean a blood test for syphilis

**Skene's ducts:** the ducts of two glands just within female urethra

**Spirochete:** any cork-screw, spiral-shaped microbe; it usually refers to the pale, delicate, infecting organism of syphilis

**Stenosis:** narrowing or constriction for any reason of a body canal or duct

**Streptococci:** microbes or bacteria, sometimes called "strep" and associated with many illnesses

**Tabes dorsalis:** degeneration of locomotor functions of the body induced by syphilis

**Urethritis:** inflammation of the urethra or the mucous-lined tube that carries urine from the bladder to the outside of the body

## Questions for Study and Discussion

1. Why are close, intimate relations with people conducive to the transmission and survival of microorganisms?
2. Do you think the fear of venereal diseases will alter behavior and moral codes in today's youth?
3. Why are young people afraid to seek treatment for venereal disease?
4. Why is there reluctance to name a sexual contact if suspicious of venereal disease?
5. How have vaccines been helpful to the total health of an individual?
6. Why has there been an increase in venereal disease among teenagers?
7. What is mononucleosis? How is college living associated with its transmission?
8. Define hepatitis and its mode of transmission.
9. Explain epidemiology as associated with public health personnel today.

## References

*Basic Statistics on Venereal Disease Problems in the United States,* ed. 25. National Communicable Disease Center V.D. Fact Sheet, 1968.

Benenson, A. S. *Control of Communicable Diseases in Man.* New York: The American Public Health Association, 1970.

Harnett, A. L. *Health.* New York: Ronald Press, 1969.

*Journal of the American Medical Association,* vol. 210, no. 2, October 13, 1969.

Schwartz, William F. *Teacher's Handbook on Venereal Disease Education.* Washington, D.C.: The American Association for Health, Physical Education and Recreation, 1965.

Smartt, W. H., and Lighter, A. C. *Gonorrhea: The Silent Epidemic.* Los Angeles: Los Angeles County Health Department, n. d.

*Textbook of Medicine,* 12th ed. Philadelphia: W. B. Saunders Co., 1967.

*The Medical Clinics of North America,* vol. 48, no. 3, May, 1964.

# 4

# Chronic Disease

## General Concept

Chronic diseases such as cardiovascular diseases are the leading cause of death in the United States.

## Outcomes

The student should be able to:
1. Describe the present importance and incidence of chronic disease
2. Define various chronic diseases
3. Identify signs, symptoms, terminology, and treatment of various chronic illnesses
4. Use professional and educational resources available for prevention and control of disease
5. Select sound health habits that may serve as preventive measures from chronic disease

## The Diseases

All the diseases that man is subject to may be classified broadly into those which are acute, subacute, and chronic. An acute disease is one in which duration of the signs and symptoms will end before 30 days in either complete recovery or in a fatal termination. In a subacute disease, signs and symptoms will persist for longer than 30 days, but usually will have subsided prior to 6 months duration. In a chronic disease, signs and symptoms will be present for longer than 6 months duration. In a person who has a chronic disease, the signs and symptoms may be dormant for weeks, months, or years, and he may have no outward manifestation of the disease. This period of quiescence of the chronic disease may be interrupted by intermittent periods of time during which the signs and symptoms of the underlying disease may be manifested in an acute form. This is referred to as an "acute exacerbation of the underlying disease," and may persist for a varying period of time.

For example, an adult may have contracted rheumatic fever as a teenager. Following recovery from the acute attack of rheumatic fever, the person may have had no further symptoms for many years. Then following a particular infection of the throat by streptococcal organisms, the person may have an acute flareup of rheumatic fever once again. The acute attack may be treated and the person returned to a period of quiescence during which time he may experience none of the symptoms that he did during his acute attack. Another example would be an individual who has bronchial asthma and is sensitive to various weeds and flowers. So long as he does not become exposed to the offending weeds and/or flowers, the individual's symptoms of tightness in his chest, wheezing, and difficulty with breathing will not be present. As soon as he is exposed to the offending agents that he is sensitive to, however, the individual will immediately tighten up in his chest, and have considerable difficulty in breathing. Through medical treatment, the acute flareup or exacerbation is relieved and the person returns to a period of quiescence until such time as he is exposed to the offending agents once again.

In recent years chronic disease has become much more prevalent, the reason being that the population is living much longer. Usually in the natural history of disease, the disease has been uncovered initially in its acute form and, as such, its signs and symptoms have been initially described. Now that people are living much longer however, the disease may be present in a much milder form in which the signs and symptoms that are seen in the acute form may not be present. For example, when diabetes mellitus was recognized initially centuries ago, it was described as being a markedly debilitating and wasting disease in which the individual had a marked loss of weight despite the fact that he had a good

## Emotions and Asthma

Emotions have been found to influence asthma attacks. McDermott and Cobb of the Massachusetts General Hospital were able to find, with only a two-hour interview, that emotional factors definitely influenced the attacks of asthma in thirty-seven of fifty cases. More recent reports have been made which more strongly substantiate this analysis. For instance, one patient who was sensitive to roses developed asthma when presented with a paper rose. Another similar case occurred when a man who had severe asthma in one city moved to another city and was completely relieved until he received a letter recalling him to his former residence. A time-clock case was a man who regularly had an attack each afternoon at five. One day he failed to notice the time until seven o'clock, whereupon he immediately went into an attack which he had missed. Thus it is quite possible that asthma attacks are triggered when victims are emotionally stimulated.

Frank G. Slaughter, M.D., *Your Body and Your Mind* (New York: The New American Library, Inc., 1963), p. 77.

appetite and usually consumed large quantities of food. In addition, the individual had an intense thirst and produced large quantities of urine every 24 hours. This remained essentially the classical description of diabetes mellitus. The person who developed this disease did not live very long. It is now known that individuals in their fifties and sixties may become diabetic. The presenting symptoms of these individuals may be a heart attack, a stroke, diminution of vision, pain and coldness in a foot, or abdominal pain. When these symptoms are investigated, it is then found that the underlying cause is diabetes mellitus. Thus it is now known that there is a classical or juvenile type of diabetic and there is an adult type of diabetic. The underlying trouble in both is the abnormal handling of sugar or carbohydrates by the body due to the lack of available, effective insulin. The diagnosis, regulation, treatment, and control of these two forms of the same disease differs considerably.

In man, most of the diseases caused by microorganisms, viruses, fungi, parasites, rickettsial organisms, and protozoa will be present as acute forms of the diseases. There are exceptions, however, such as the spirochetal infection responsible for syphilis (see chap. 3). Another example of chronic infection is to be found in the parts of the United States that are warm and moist. Here the individual may be chronically tired, underweight, undernourished, and anemic, and yet have a more than adequate intake of food. In this case the person may be infected for many years with intestinal parasitic worms which are responsible for his symptoms. It is usually possible with the use of various medications to eliminate the intestinal parasites and restore the individual to normal health. He will remain healthy, however, only so long as he avoids the ways of life which led him to acquire the intestinal parasites.

All of the systems of the body as well as the tissues and organs are subject to chronic diseases. In a large percentage of cases, the presenting sign or symptom is usually very mild, and for this reason it is often overlooked for months or years. Very often the person who has the chronic disease has learned to live with the mild symptomatology for a long period of time and thus not seek help, mainly because he does not realize that anything is seriously wrong. For example, the person may be chronically tired and have no other symptoms. The underlying cause for this may be a mild deficiency of the thyroid, or it could be due to a chronic anemia which has been caused by a bleeding area within the intestinal tract. The latter may be a diverticulum or outpouching of the bowel. It may be a polyp, an ulcer, or a developing malignant lesion. Usually the person who has this symptom will live with it for months or years before other signs and symptoms have developed or before this symptom becomes so pronounced that he finally seeks medical help. There are a number of other mild symptoms which may also be present for a long period of time. Some of these are minimal elevation of temperature in the afternoon or evening, a gradual loss of appetite, intermittent bleeding from the rectum, gradual loss of weight, or the gradual loss of feeling in the feet or hands. These symptoms are all mild and do not by their very nature call attention to any specific disease or system in the body. It is primarily for these reasons that the underlying disease causing these symptoms is overlooked for so long a period of time.

This chapter concerns itself only with chronic diseases. Examples will be given of how chronic diseases can affect any and all tissues of the body.

## Allergy

One of the most common diseases of allergy is bronchial asthma. This may develop in early childhood or in later life. The substance called an allergen that will bring on an attack of bronchial asthma in an individual may be one or several, but is very specific for a given person. When the person comes in contact with the particular allergen that causes his particular bronchial asthma, he usually has considerable trouble in breathing. The more concentrated the exposure, the more severe the symptoms. The particular symptom that bothers the person is difficulty in breathing; while he can get air into his lungs, he has difficulty in getting it out because of the spasm of the muscles along the bronchial tree itself.

In between acute episodes, the person remains asymptomatic. There are numerous skin rashes which can be seen as a result of allergic conditions. These rashes are usually red and may be confined to certain portions of the body, or may be generalized. For example, the individual may develop a rash around the feet and ankles and nowhere else, and this may be related to the type of socks the person wears. The rash may develop with considerable itching in both armpits, and this could be related to the type of deodorant the person uses. A person may suddenly develop diffuse hives over the general body surface, and this may be brought on because he has ingested chocolate, tomato, or a particular type of seafood to which he is sensitive. All of these conditions will usually clear on their own with a minimum of treatment so long as the offending agent is removed.

There is a more serious form of this, however, wherein an anaphylactic shock can develop upon exposure to any particular allergen. In this condition of anaphylactic shock, the individual suddenly has a loss of blood pressure. His pulse becomes very weak; he becomes lightheaded and dizzy; his throat may tighten up and he may be unable to breathe. He may even suddenly collapse and expire. Fortunately, this condition is rare, but it does exist and is usually seen when a chemical substance, an antibiotic, or an iodated compound is administered to the person who is extremely sensitive to the particular allergen. Occasionally it may be the first exposure to this particular substance which produces the anaphylactic shock. Usually the person has had the particular substance or a variation thereof on several occasions before the one that causes the anaphylactic reaction.

## Respiratory System

This particular system has a variety of chronic diseases, and the primary symptom that they cause is shortness of breath. Emphysema is a good example. This develops only after many years of bronchial irritation. Smoking for example can cause bronchitis, and when this is continued for many years the chronic bronchitis which develops tends to predispose the individual to pulmonary infections. In addition, there is a gradual but steady loss of the elasticity of the lung substance itself, and as the elasticity decreases breathing becomes more difficult. When the disease has fully developed, the lung remains chronically infected. Breathing becomes progressively more difficult, and as it does the individual's activity is markedly restricted. In addition, there are a number of diseases which are labeled under the general term of pneumoconiosis. Fundamentally, these diseases are caused by the gradual but continued inhalation of foreign substances, whether these be metal, fiber, silica, or other agents into the lung. The lung will attempt to clear itself by coughing, but it will be unable to remove all of these agents. The ones that are left will become imbedded in the lung substance, and attempts will be made to wall these foreign substances off by providing a heavy coat of reactive tissue around them. As this process occurs, it begins to reduce the effective respiratory surface. Since the lung has such a large respiratory reserve, it will take many years before the reserve can be used up, but once it has been, the person will start to become short of breath.

At this point, continued inhalation and exposure to the offending substance will then begin to produce shortness of breath rather quickly. These diseases have been referred to as "chronic lungers" or the "black lung disease." In the past, tuberculosis was always considered to be a

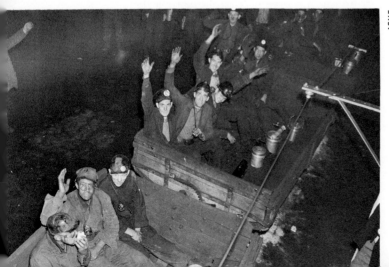

ACME

An occupational hazard for miners is the high incidence of "black lung" disease.

chronic disease. This was because the treatment was not definitive but only symptomatic. In addition, various types of surgery had to be done, thus the disease was not only debilitating but quite disfiguring. With the advent in recent years of specific drugs to effectively treat tubercular infections, the course of treatment has been greatly reduced and the person is no longer confined for years in a hospital or sanitarium. Thus the treatment will permit tuberculosis now to be classified under either an acute or subacute type of disease.

## Cardiovascular System

In the cardiovascular system there are numerous parts which are subject to chronic diseases. One would be the peripheral arteriole system. As the small arteries to the extremities gradually narrow, the person will begin to complain of coldness as well as the feeling of pain. Exposure of the affected part of the extremity to cold increases the individual's symptoms because it further enhances the arteriole insufficiency to this particular region. With the use of heat, particularly moist heat, this area of arteriole insufficiency will improve some and the color will very often become quite red, at least temporarily. Much of the pain will be relieved. Smoking will usually accentuate the symptoms of arteriole insufficiency. If the arteriole insufficiency is due to a type of disease which is causing the definite narrowing of the inside diameter of the artery, then the disease will reach a point at which amputation will have to be performed.

If the arteriole insufficiency is being aggravated by intermittent episodes of vasoconstriction so far as the artery is concerned, then the severing of the sympathetic nerve fibers which cause the vasoconstriction may help the individual. In the large arteries of the body, the wall may become more thin and begin to bulge out. This would be called an aneurysm. There are several sites in the large artery where this aneurysmal dilitation is prone to occur. One is immediately above the heart where the major vessel called the aorta arises. In this ascending part of the aorta the wall becomes thin because of some congenital defect as would be seen in Marfan's syndrome, or because of an infective infiltration and gradual destruction of these walls as would be seen by the spirochete responsible for syphilis. Once the dilitation starts, it gradually and steadily progresses.

Another site that is common for this type of dilitation is in the abdominal portion of the aorta below the level of the diaphragm. The rea-

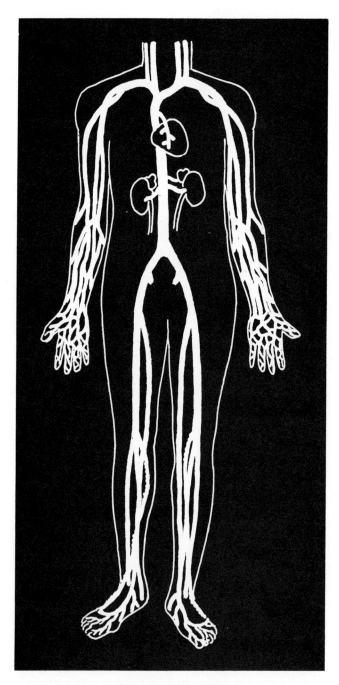

The circulatory system

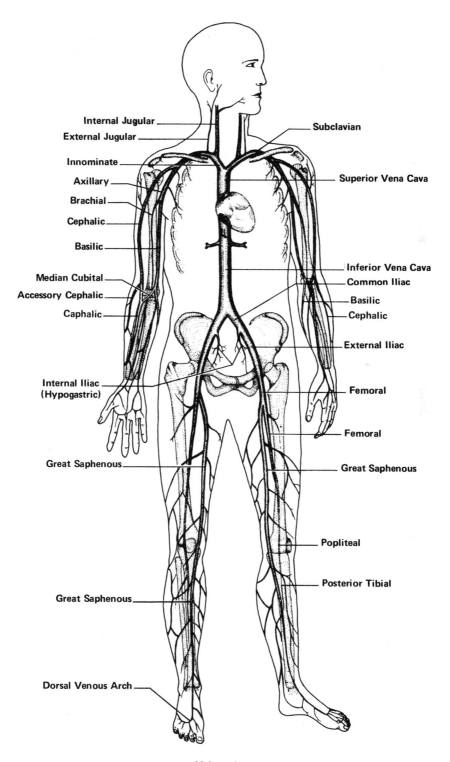

Internal Jugular

External Jugular

Innominate

Axillary

Brachial

Cephalic

Basilic

Median Cubital

Accessory Cephalic

Caphalic

Internal Iliac
(Hypogastric)

Great Saphenous

Great Saphenous

Dorsal Venous Arch

Subclavian

Superior Vena Cava

Inferior Vena Cava

Common Iliac

Basilic

Cephalic

External Iliac

Femoral

Femoral

Great Saphenous

Popliteal

Posterior Tibial

Major veins.

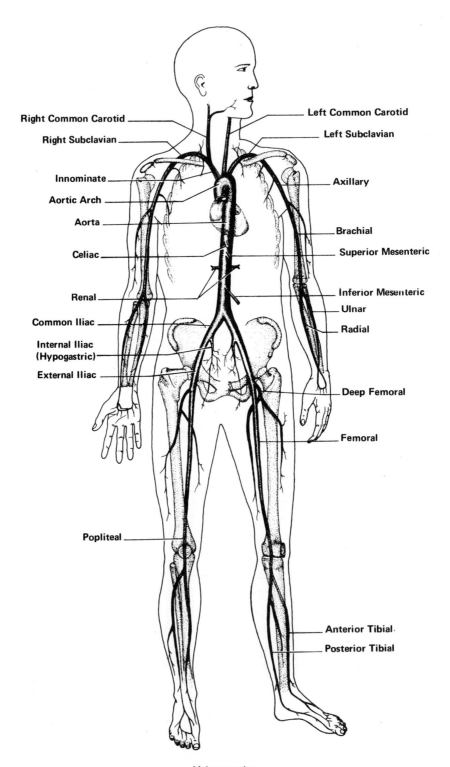

Right Common Carotid

Right Subclavian

Innominate

Aortic Arch

Aorta

Celiac

Renal

Common Iliac

Internal Iliac
(Hypogastric)

External Iliac

Popliteal

Left Common Carotid

Left Subclavian

Axillary

Brachial

Superior Mesenteric

Inferior Mesenteric

Ulnar

Radial

Deep Femoral

Femoral

Anterior Tibial

Posterior Tibial

Major arteries.

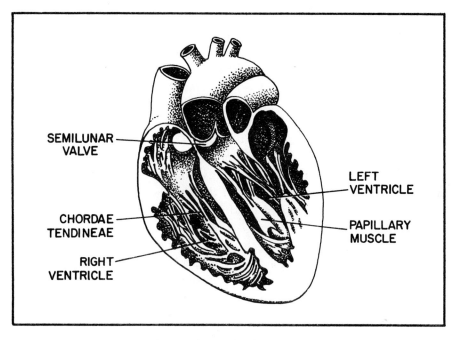

SEMILUNAR
VALVE

CHORDAE
TENDINEAE

RIGHT
VENTRICLE

LEFT
VENTRICLE

PAPILLARY
MUSCLE

Cross section of the human heart

son for its development is that the artery has been subjected to severe wear and tear through the age of the person, and the wall is becoming hard and has lost a lot of its elasticity. The presenting complaint or symptom of the person with the aneurysm varies depending not only on its location, but also upon any structure or structures that it may impinge upon. For example, in the ascending aorta, as the aneurysm increases in size and pulsates, the individual may complain of pain in the back due to the erosion of part of the vertebral column. It may also come forward and present as a pulsating mass in the upper portion of the center of the chest. Hoarseness may develop because of pressure on the pharyngeal nerve. Or the individual may experience difficulty in swallowing because of esophageal pressure. The aneurysm in the abdominal aorta located below the level of the diaphragm may be asymptomatic and is often discovered when the individual is examined for some other reason. The continued presence of an enlarging aneurysm presents a potentially serious threat to the individual's life.

Another source of chronic disease of the heart itself would be disturbance in the conducting system of the heart. An occasional beat out of time occurs in practically all individuals and by itself does not constitute any form of serious disease. In some individuals there is an abnormal type of anatomy and/or of the developmental conducting time differentials in the conducting tissue which permit the normal impulse to be conducted much more rapidly. Such a condition is seen in the Wolff-Parkinson-White syndrome. The presenting symptom is usually a rapidly beating heart which suddenly starts and which races for a few minutes to a day or longer before suddenly stopping. The individual who has this does not know when it will start nor when it will stop. It does not usually pose a serious threat to the individual unless there is associated myocardial damage or impairment of the circulation to the heart itself, which is further compromised by the decreased cardiac output during the rapid beating.

The most common type of chronic disease associated with the heart or cardiovascular system is that which involves the circulation to the heart muscle itself. This is called the coronary artery blood supply of the heart or myocardium. The coronary arteries are usually two in number and arise from the initial portion of the ascending aorta. These coronary arteries normally supply a very rich and extensive blood supply to the entire heart muscle so it can be well fed and oxygenated whether the individual is at rest or extremely active. As atherosclerotic disease begins to narrow the inside diameter of either one of the major coronary arteries or of any large branch the individual will begin to complain of chest pain when he starts to engage in activity. The less the narrowing the more activity the individual can perform before chest pain will start.

As narrowing progresses, however, the degree of activity necessary to bring on pain becomes much less. Rest usually will relieve the individual's chest pain and soreness, which is called angina pectoris. So long as the individual's condition remains at the anginal level there will be no permanent damage or destruction of myocardial tissue. However, once the coronary artery or a major branch thereof becomes completely blocked or occluded, then myocardial damage and muscle death will result. This condition is then called a coronary, a heart attack, a coronary thrombosis, a coronary occlusion, or myocardial infarction. Over the years all of these terms have gradually come to be synonymous so far as the average person is concerned. Once a person has recovered from a heart attack, he will have to be more careful to attempt to avoid the occurrence of a second. He may be symptom-free so far as his heart is concerned, angina pectoris may develop, symptoms of congestive heart failure, or disturbance in the conducting system of the heart itself.

## Research and Heart Disease

The American Heart Association recently sponsored scientific meetings to share the latest findings pertaining to cardiovascular diseases. Some of the research reported appears to be highly technical and often experimental. For example:

1. *Echo movies.* Dr. William Friedman announced results of a new machine that takes moving pictures by high frequency waves. These are transmitted as electrical impulses to a graph print-out. This enables physicians to diagnose without invading the organ with any instrument.

2. *Mapping Nerves.* Surgeons now have an electric probe to follow nerve pathways picking up electrical discharge and registering it on a screen thereby providing the surgeon with a precise map of the heart.

3. *Hopkins Test.* This is a simple method of injecting special radioactive materials into a vein and monitoring the condition of the left ventricle. This method aids in determining whether or not surgery is necessary.

4. *New Instruments.* The development of a new forceps at Stanford Medical Center enables the surgeon to clip tiny slices of the heart quickly without shock to the patient. This helps physicians find hidden abnormalities that can only be seen in fresh tissue.

5. *New Heart Cells.* The University of Chicago scientists are attempting to regenerate heart cells in the human body. They have succeeded in coaxing cells of human heart muscles to cluster together and beat under laboratory conditions. In the future, heart cells may be kept in a "bank" as blood is now.[1]

The many implications of transplants and heart surgery continue to be debated at length. Even cardiologists and other specialists are not in complete agreement in these controversial areas. For example, Dr. Denton Cooley of St. Lukes Hospital in Denton, Texas was a pioneer in placing the first artificial heart in a human being. The patient, Haskell Karp, died 32 hours later, and since this event in 1969, much publicity sur-

1. "Latest on Heart Problems and New Machines," *U.S. News and World Report,* Feb. 4, 1974, pp. 76–7.

rounding the litigations with the medical profession has arisen. Legal and moral issues have been disputed to the extent that continued research and experiments have been somewhat stifled. In contrast to the practice of major surgical procedures is a report by Dr. Henry Russek at the Texas Heart Institute in which he advocates the lessening of heart surgeries. Over 25,000 times a year, physicians open chests and implant a piece of one's own veins or arteries to carry blood around an obstruction. Believing these operations to be unnecessary, Dr. Russek advocates the use of drugs and other forms of medical care as better options for the treatment of angina (chest pains that are forerunners of heart attacks). He states, "More lives have been lost through by-pass surgery than saved by it."[2] Although over 600 hospitals in the United States perform these operations, the risk factors of any heart surgery are still high since complications such as heart attack, brain damage, hemmorhaging, and kidney failure are quite common. Alternatives to surgery include taking nitroglycerin to expand arteries, losing weight, quitting smoking, and relaxing. Also, drugs such as *propanerol* may be helpful since they slow down the heart and reduce its need for oxygen.

## Joints

There are numerous joints throughout the human body and these have a very special function. They normally permit the flexibility of a rigid, bony structure in such a manner that the individual has no pain and bone does not touch bone. Each joint is lined with very delicate membranes which are highly sensitive to pain because of the numerous nerve endings in them. When the smooth surfaces begin to change due to roughness or swelling, then pain will occur with movement of the joint and the individual begins to suffer from arthritis. Arthritis has several varieties. One is the type associated with advancing age and is due to gradual wear and tear. The smooth structures become rough and calcification begins to appear. The joint spaces become more narrow, and movement of the bones which make up the joint cause pain. This type of arthritis is associated with older age and may involve any joint, whether it be hands, feet, knees, ankles, hips, or any of the joints of the vertebral column. A second prominent type of arthritis is called rheumatoid and

2. "Overdoing Heart Surgery," *Time,* March 4, 1974, p. 60.

## *Alcohol and the Heart*

The recognition that ethyl alcohol may be associated with heart disease dates back more than 100 years. However, during the past fifteen years the view that alcohol is a direct myocardial toxin has been supported by several studies in animals and man:

1. The group of patients having myocardial problems of an unexplained nature includes an appreciable number of alcoholics.
2. After ingestion of alcohol in man, there is an accumulation of lipid in the heart.
3. Gradual cardiac failure has been discovered among alcoholics. When cessation of alcohol intake occurs, disappearance of cardiac abnormalities often follow.
4. An increased incidence of sudden death has been demonstrated in alcoholic dogs and humans.
5. Gould and coworkers have shown that small amounts of alcohol in coronary patients may depress myocardial functions appreciably and lead to a fall in cardiac output. These findings suggest that the common practice of administering alcohol to coronary patients as a "tonic" or as a "coronary artery dilator" may be unwise.

Brent Parker, M.D., "The Effects of Ethyl Alcohol on the Heart," *Journal of the American Medical Association*, May 6, 1974, pp. 741–2.

occurs when the smooth lining and membranes that make up a normal joint space become inflamed and swollen, and thus narrow the joint space. Movement of the bones making up this type of a joint also causes pain.

A special form of arthritis which has received much publicity through the ages is that called gout or "the disease of the rich." The afflicted individual is usually depicted as being overweight and wealthy, sitting around with his leg propped up and his foot wrapped to prevent anyone or anything from coming in contact with it, particularly the great toe. This particular type of arthritis was initially thought to be due to the ingestion of very rich type of foods. Underneath the heavy wrappings will be found a swollen, painful, red joint involving the great toe. While this is one of the major joints that seems to be always involved in gout, it is by no means the only one, since it is now known that the finger joints, for example, are almost always involved.

The cause of gout is now known to be an individual's inability to correctly metabolize proteins known as purines. Afflicted individuals metabolize purines down to the level of uric acid and permit this substance to accumulate in the body's tissues in much larger quantities than normal. This substance is deposited as crystals in and around various joints. This crystal deposition can gradually destroy a given joint. With today's knowledge of the basic cause of gout and the improved methods of treatment, it is hoped that the severe destructive disease process previously seen in chronic gouty arthritis can be in a large measure prevented in the future.

## Nervous Diseases and Mental Disorders

In man, the nervous system is composed of highly specialized tissue. It may be divided into the brain, spinal cord, and peripheral nerves. The brain itself has several subdivisions and these may be called the higher centers of the brain, the lower centers, and brain stem. The peripheral nerves are paired, that is, one for each side of the body, and they arise at multiple levels of the spinal cord. Their function is to act as insulated wires to carry impulses to and from the spinal cord. The spinal cord itself is made up of numerous columns or tracts, each of which is responsible for the carrying of specialized impulses from the peripheral nerves to the brain substance and from the brain substance back to the peripheral nerves. The impulses that the peripheral nerves bring to the spinal cord include the sensation of pain, touch, pressure, changes in temperature, as well as the carrying of the impulse from the spinal cord to cause movement of muscles. These impulses traverse the nerves without changing their anatomy or function.

The peripheral nerves are also called voluntary nerves because the individual person can acquire voluntary control over them. This is in contradistinction to the so-called involuntary nervous system or autonomic nervous system over which the individual has no control. The autonomic nervous system is a highly complex interlacing network of nerves which controls vital functions of the body, such as breathing, partial control of the heart rate and beat, control of the entire gastrointestinal tract, urinary bladder, and the reflex control of the pupil of the eye, as well as blinking. It is necessary that the system have such an auto-regulating mechanism in order that vital functions of the body such as the maintenance of respiration and the heart beat, may be performed while the individual is sleeping.

A form of chronic disease involving the peripheral nerves can be caused by certain poisons such as lead, as well as vitamin deficiencies. The onset of these diseases is usually spaced over a long period of time. A chronic disease which can involve not only the peripheral nerves but also the spinal cord, as well as parts of the brain substance, is to be found in multiple sclerosis. Here the basic trouble lies in the intermittent removal by an unknown cause of the insulating substance surrounding the nerves. This causes impairment in the normal nerve function. As a result, the individual's symptoms are quite varied. He may have trouble speaking clearly at times, or parts of one side of the body may become spastic or somewhat rigid, which makes movement difficult. He may complain of intermittent numbness and tingling of any portion of the body. The disease usually develops in younger individuals and undergoes numerous exacerbations and remissions. At no time during the course of the disease is there any impairment in the individual's mental power. Another form of chronic disease of the nervous system is to be found in paralysis agitans, or Parkinson's disease. Here the fundamental difficulty is to be found in specialized areas in the lower centers of the brain being without a substance known as dopamine. The disease progresses gradually over many years and is manifested by gradual increasing rigidity of the general musculature of the body together with the characteristic pill-rolling effect of the fingers. In these types of diseases the individual's mental function is not disturbed.

Today a common complaint in many individuals is that they are nervous and that they feel that their nerves are sick. What they actually mean is that the nerves themselves are not at fault, but that the emotional side of the individual has undergone stress or tension. Here the higher centers of the brain are involved, because it is in this area that the individual is able to formulate knowledgeable thought and it is here that the emotional control areas are located. Disorders of this nature are discussed at some detail in chapter 2.

## The Endocrine System

This is a highly complex interrelated system of many organs within the body. All of the glands that make up this system elaborate within themselves protein substances called hormones which act on other organs and tissues of the body to regulate their enzymatic functions. The overall system involves the pituitary gland, which is located in the brain and which acts as the master control gland. The other glands involved are the adrenals, thyroid, the parathyroid glands indirectly, the pancreas, and gonads, which include the ovaries and testes.

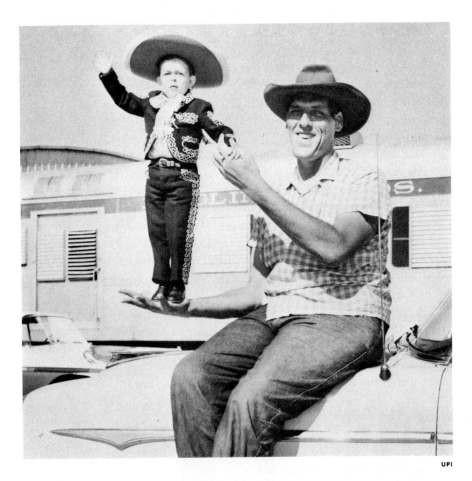

UPI

**When a hormone of the pituitary gland is produced in excess, abnormal growth results.**

The pituitary gland elaborates within its own substance numerous hormones. One of these is the growth hormone, which is responsible for the regulation of the normal growth pattern of a given individual. When this hormone is produced in excess, abnormal growth results. If this overproduction occurs before the growing areas of the bones are closed, then unusually tall individuals or so-called giants will be the result. If the overproduction occurs after the growing areas or lines of the bones have closed, then an individual with massive features will result, and this condition is called *acromegaly*. Associated with this condition would be headaches, high blood pressure, weakness and tiredness, the latter symptoms being very definitely out of keeping with the physical features of the person.

Most of the other hormones that the pituitary gland produces act directly upon another organ in the endocrine system and thus this particular type of hormone is called a trophic hormone and the gland involved is called a target gland. The function of these trophic hormones is to regulate the adequate amount of hormone to be released and made available to the body by the target gland. When the target gland produces too little of its own hormone, then the pituitary will increase the production of its specific trophic hormone until such time as the target gland produces a normal amount, at which time the overproduction of the trophic hormone will be reduced to normal. Thus tumors of the pituitary gland may cause dysfunction of the body by producing an excess of the trophic hormones which, in turn, overstimulate the target glands, causing the target glands to overproduce their own specific hormones. The afflicted person will often present marked weakness and fatigability; there may or may not be weight loss; menstrual irregularities are often present; unusual hair amount and distribution will be encountered as will obesity, impotence, and decreased libido.

If the pituitary gland is gradually destroyed by tumor or hemorrhage so that it is no longer able to function, then the target glands no longer can be regulated by the trophic hormones, and thus they will produce very little of their normal type of hormone. The person will gradually become thin with considerable weight loss, and apathetic, having low blood pressure; the skin becomes cold and dry; gonadal function ceases; furthermore, he may have various types of seizures due to low blood sugar level. In addition the individual may show unusual swelling of the extremities and undergo very definite psychological changes.

In the posterior region of the pituitary is produced a hormone which has to do with the regulation of the urinary output per day of an individual. Destruction of this area will cause the loss of the control of diuresis, and the individual will produce abnormally large amounts of dilute urine per day. The amount may range in excess of a gallon and a half or two gallons per day. This disease is called diabetes insipidus.

The thyroid gland may show overproduction of its normal hormone thyroxine due to a localized tumor, called an adenoma, within the thyroid substance. These tumor cells will not respond to the normal regulatory control from the pituitary gland. The individual becomes gradually agitated, irritable, emotionally upset, thin, and has a very warm, moist skin. On the other hand, if the thyroid tissue is damaged or removed, then it cannot produce a normal amount of thyroxine and no amount of stimulation by the pituitary trophic hormone will cause it to do so. Thus in the intrinsic disease of the thyroid gland itself additional forms of treatment are necessary since the body's regulatory mechanism has been made inoperable.

Parathyroid glands are small glands which normally number four, although there may be more; they are usually found imbedded in the thyroid tissue itself, although some may be within the chest cavity. The function of these glands is to regulate the calcium metabolism of the body in order to provide normal bone structure and to prevent tetany. Overproduction of the parathormone will cause calcium to be removed in excess quantity from the bones, which will, of course, weaken them and cause pain. In addition, the excess amount of calcium in the blood stream will cause calculi or stones to occur within the kidney system, which can cause kidney damage as well as severe pain. Inadequate production of the parathormone will cause an excess amount of calcium to be deposited in the bones and the patient will be very subject to tetanic-type seizures.

The pancreas normally produces the hormone insulin, which is responsible for the normal metabolic control of the sugar or carbohydrate metabolism of the body. Disease of this gland may be present in several forms. One is diabetes mellitus in which the gland is unable to manufacture any insulin on its own and thus is unable to regulate sugar metabolism. There are also associated abnormalities in the lipid or fat metabolism, and the individual will develop marked weight loss, intense thirst, increased appetite, and an overproduction of urine. This is a classical type of diabetes mellitus. Overproduction by the pancreas of insulin may cause the individual to be weak, hungry, and to have a strong tendency to become unconscious. He tries to overcome this by eating, particularly foods containing sugar, such as candy, as he finds these foods will temporarily make him feel good. He thus consumes not only his normal amount of food, but usually a considerable amount by snacks throughout the day. He usually winds up overweight. There is an adult type of diabetes mellitus which does not have the classical symptoms of the juvenile diabetic. Very often the adult begins to have difficulty with his vision or may develop anginal symptoms, or may begin to complain of headaches, and as these symptoms are being evaluated it is discovered that they are due to diabetes mellitus. In this type of diabetic, his pan-

---

### Are You a Hidden Diabetic?

It is estimated there are approximately 2 million known diabetics in this country, plus another 1,400,000 or more "hidden" diabetics—persons who have the disease in mild stages and are unaware that they have it. And there are about five-and-a-half million more persons who are potential diabetics—persons now alive who are likely to develop diabetes during their lifetime.

Diabetes is the seventh leading cause of death by disease in this country. A big reason diabetes remains a serious disease is the great number of "hidden" diabetics. The illness is fairly easy to detect and can be controlled if it is found early enough. But if it is overlooked or neglected it can lead to serious complications. That is why it is vital to find the unknown diabetics and encourage them to seek medical care.

Here is a list of the danger signs of diabetes: excessive thirst, unexplained loss of weight, intense itching, changes in vision, slow healing of cuts and bruises, excessive hunger, chronic skin infections, easy tiring, pain in the extremities.

If you have any of these symptoms, see your physician. It may not be diabetes but by means of a simple urine test your doctor can determine if further studies are needed to make sure. . . .

From "Are You a Hidden Diabetic?" *Health Tips* (San Francisco, Calif.: California Medical Association), November 1967. Reprinted by permission of the California Medical Association.

creas is still able to produce a normal amount of insulin, but for several reasons the insulin is made ineffective within the body and cannot be properly utilized. This type of diabetic can very often be regulated by diet and reduction of the usual accompanying overweight. Sometimes additional medication is necessary so that the insulin can be made once again effective.

The adrenal glands are usually two in number and are usually to be found in the area just above the upper part of each kidney. These glands produce several hormones which have to do with the regulation of the normal salt metabolism of the body, as well as being involved in partial regulation of the sugar metabolism. They are also involved in the regulation in part of the blood pressure, and the production of androgenic hormones. Abnormal production of the androgenic hormones in a child would give him the picture of sexual precocity with the secondary sexual characteristics of an adult. Excess production of the salt-regulating hormone, androsterone, will cause the individual to have high blood pressure together with loss of an essential electrolyte, potassium.

If the adrenal cortex is destroyed by disease, the individual will be very weak; his blood pressure will be very low; the skin will begin to darken; there will be weight loss, anorexia, nausea, vomiting, abdominal pain; and in many cases he will develop a craving for salt. A tumor of the medulla of the adrenals may cause marked elevation of the individual's blood pressure, and this may occur intermittently. The individual very often complains of severe associated headaches. Removal of this type of tumor can effect a cure so far as this type of hypertension is concerned.

## Gastrointestinal Tract

The gastrointestinal tract has the normal function and responsibility of taking in food and liquid and completely processing it so as to effectively remove all essential materials from it for the body's needs. It then discards that which is of no value to the body. The entire tract acts as a conveyor belt, with specific functions being performed by definite areas of the tract itself.

The major portion of the breakdown of food occurs within the small intestine and the absorption of all necessary and vital substances for the body's needs occurs in the terminal ileum, which is the last section of the small intestinal tract. The large bowel or colon takes the large amount of liquid residue and reabsorbs the bulk of the fluid back into the system, excreting the waste in solid form. Chronic diseases of the gastrointestinal tract can be exemplified by peptic ulcer, regional enteritis, and chronic ulcerative colitis. The most common symptom these diseases present is abdominal pain, with or without cramps.

Peptic ulcer usually involves the first part of the small bowel, known as the duodenum, or occasionally the lower end of the stomach in the region of the pyloric antrum. Regional enteritis involves primarily the terminal ileum. Chronic ulcerative colitis involves usually the sigmoid colon, descending colon, and part of the transverse colon. Regional enteritis can be a very serious and devastating disease so far as the individual is concerned. Here, intermittent sections of the terminal ileum become narrow and hard due to considerable swelling. No effective absorption occurs in these segments. These segments very easily may rupture and form a fistulus tract to an adjacent portion of the intestinal tract, or may in part remain open so that abdominal contents may be spilled into the peritoneal cavity. This causes a considerable amount of malabsorption of food, peritonitis, loss of blood, anemia, weight loss, severe abdominal cramps, and very often generalized frustration. It is a difficult disease to treat effectively because all of the affected segments cannot be successfully removed surgically. The individual experiences many exacerbations of his chronic disease.

In chronic ulcerated colitis, there is a loss of the mucosal surface and lining of large continuous sections of the colon. This causes considerable diarrhea, the contents of which contain large amounts of both mucus and blood. The individual is capable of losing large quantities of fluid and essential electrolytes by this method. The individual with a peptic ulcer may experience not only severe pain, but the ulcer may gradually perforate, causing peritonitis, or may erode into an adjacent artery, causing hemorrhage, which may be both acute or chronic. All three of these conditions are definitely influenced by the emotional makeup of the individual. When he is subjected to considerable pressure and tension— regardless of the source—the underlying disease becomes activated. It takes considerable patience, time, treatment, and understanding in order for the individual to live with his disease.

In the older individual in his sixties and seventies, absorption from the gastrointestinal tract is not accomplished as well as it was in his younger days. As a result, even though he takes in an apparent adequate quantity of food, he does not effectively absorb all that he should. Any reduction in his appetite would definitely render him more liable to malnutrition. Thus this individual requires added food supplements and vitamins in order to maintain good nutrition.

## Blood

The blood system in the body is responsible for providing normal quantities of red cells with adequate amounts of hemoglobin so that all cells in the body may be fed and oxygenated while the end product of metabolism, carbon dioxide, is removed from the cells. It is also responsible for supplying adequate numbers of various leucocytes so that the body may be afforded protection from various invaders. In addition, there are some 13 different essential substances needed to provide for adequate coagulation of the blood. Chronic diseases involving this system are many, and the universal complaint the individual has is weakness and tiredness.

A hemophiliac is a male who cannot clot normally because of the lack of a very specific substance known as factor 8. Hemophilia is transmitted by females but develops only in males. When this factor 8 is supplied to him, he is capable of clotting normally, and any hemorrhage that he may have can be controlled.

Anemia, a reduction in the number of red cells available to the body, can result from a chronic bleeding source, very often from the gastrointestinal tract. Others may develop as a result of gradual destruction or replacement of normal bone marrow. There are anemias such as sickle cell anemia that exist because of abnormal hemoglobin formation. This is inherited and persists throughout the individual's life. Chronic leukemia may involve either the myelocytes or lymphocytes, and the onset is usually very insidious. Occasionally the individual who already feels weak and tired becomes aware of a fullness on the left side of the abdomen which turns out to be an enlarged spleen. Very often the chronic form is discovered when the person is examined for some entirely different reason. These conditions are prone to develop in later life and may or may not at this time contribute to the individual's final demise. In chronic leukemia, the white cells, which normally number from 10,000 to 11,000, are found to number anywhere from 50,000 to 500,000. Despite this marked increase in the number of cells, the individual is much more susceptible to infection, since these cells are not normal.

In polycythemia vera, there is an overall increase in the red cells, white cells, and platelets in the circulatory system. The person has quite a red to violaceous color as far as the skin is concerned, yet is persistently weak and tired. Such an individual is in danger with a markedly increased count of forming spontaneous clots within any small blood vessels in his body. For this reason, he may have a variety of symptoms, depending upon where the clots may form.

Pernicious anemia develops because there is a lack of the intrinsic factor necessary for the normal maturation or development of red blood cells. This substance is normally found in the upper portion of the stomach and is absorbed in the terminal ileum. Thus, removal of the upper portion of the stomach, surgical removal of the terminal ileum, or severe regional enteritis that would involve virtually all of the terminal ileum could lead to the development of pernicious anemia. The serious complication of this disease is the gradual destruction of essential portions of the spinal cord.

## Liver

This is probably the largest organ in the body and has a multitude of functions. It stores sugar as glycogen which can be released as needed by the body so that it does not always depend upon the availability of food. It manufactures many necessary substances involved in the clotting mechanism of the body. It will break down and detoxify injurious substances that may enter the body. It is the prime source for the production of albumen, which is a necessary protein for the maintenance of normal osmotic pressure and which provides transport for many vital body substances.

In cirrhosis of the liver, part of the liver tissue is replaced by scar and fibrous tissue. As the amount of the scar and fibrous tissue increases, the normal flow of large quantities of blood through the liver is impaired. This leads to what is known as portal hypertension and creates a tremendous back pressure in the venous system in the abdominal cavity, and subsequently into the chest cavity. The veins become quite engorged and dilated because of this pressure; they may then rupture and bleed profusely, so that within a relatively short period of time the individual may lose three or four quarts of blood. In addition, the individual becomes quite edematous and this is difficult to control. Very often the cause for the development of this type of cirrhosis is poor nutrition coupled with a large and steady ethonolic intake.

## Muscular Dystrophy

These disorders involve essentially the voluntary muscles of the body. The disease is slow but steadily progressive in its development. There is a gradual loss of the structure of the muscle cells and its replacement with fibrous tissue. As a result, the individual muscles gradually become weaker and less effective. In such an individual the onset of a cold can pose a serious threat to his life because bronchitis will often develop in the wake of a cold. It is absolutely necessary that the individual be able to cough and to maintain the bronchial tree free from retained secretions and foreign substances. In the individual with muscular dystrophy, the muscles are unable to contract normally and thus he cannot effectively cough. For this reason the terminal end is very often bronchopneumonia.

## Kidney

Each individual has normally a pair of kidneys that are concerned with effective filtration and removal from the blood stream of substances to be eliminated in the urine. The kidneys have a wide built-in margin of safety, and a person can be perfectly normal as far as life and longevity are concerned having only one normal kidney. The filtering system of the kidney begins with the glomerulus and this part is vulnerable to attack by disease and degenerative changes. The gradual development of chronic glomerulonephritis leads to gradual elevation of blood pressure, anemia, impaired blood filtration with subsequent retention of excess quantities of urea causing azotemia. As the disease progresses, the azotemia increases, as does the anemia, and edema begins to develop. Blood pressure continues to go up, and the individual eventually develops uremia.

A chronic infectious disease of the urinary system is seen in chronic pyelonephritis, which may be present for many months or several years before being detected. Very often the only complaint is that the person feels tired or is subjected to intermittent headaches. If the disease is not vigorously treated and the infecting organism is not systematically and persistently removed, continued gradual destruction of kidney tissue will develop. This leads inevitably to the end condition of uremia, which is fatal.

## Summary

Chronic diseases may involve any and all tissues of the body. Symptoms are usually very slow to develop and very often the same symptom may be found in a multitude of diseases. Many forms of chronic disease are found accidentally when the individual is examined for some other reason. When the disease is uncovered, questioning the individual about previous symptoms will often reveal that symptoms such as weakness, tiredness, and intermittent headache have been present over such a long period of time that the individual has learned to live with them. The individual usually did not think that the complaint was sufficient enough to warrant medical aid. Often if an individual with such vague symptoms sought medical help, they may initially have gone unrecognized as being related to any form of serious disease.

There are a number of ways in which chronic diseases may be treated. A few of them lend themselves to specific and curative type of treatment. An example would be chronic pyelonephritis in which there had not been too extensive kidney damage prior to the onset of treatment. In addition, tumor of the medulla of the adrenal gland, called a pheochromocytoma, which is responsible for the hypertension in the individual, can be cured by surgical removal of the tumor.

The underlying disease may have to be treated by a form of suppression. This would be exemplified by the suppressive type of chemotherapy that is used in controlling a chronic form of leukemia. Other forms of chronic disease have to be treated symptomatically, primarily because the underlying cause is not known. Examples would be multiple sclerosis, muscular dystrophies, and some mental disorders.

The last form of treatment for chronic diseases is that of prevention. This is best exemplified by bronchial asthma, in which the individual is kept away from the causative allergen. Another form of prevention would apply to pneumoconiosis since, although these diseases are preventable, once they have developed they then can be only treated symptomatically.

The foregoing discussion has by no means been a complete one so far as all forms of chronic disease are concerned. It was intended to provide a panoramic view of the general topic of chronic diseases. The presentation was made complete enough to accomplish this objective, but is by no means intended to be a complete reference for all chronic diseases. It can now be appreciated that the same symptom may have many different underlying causes. There are many chronic diseases which can be held in fairly good check and permit the individual to live a reasonably normal life.

## Cancer

Although cancer today is not classified medically as a chronic disease, it still remains an insidious killer. It is the second leading cause of death for all ages in this country. More than 50 million people in the United States will fall victim to cancer, or one in every four persons each year.

Cancer may best be defined as uncontrolled, abnormal cell growth. Although cancer may be defined as one disease, actually it may be classified as a group of diseases for which there may be numerous causes. There are probably over 100 types of cancer, including such forms as lung cancer, cancer of the breast, uterus, colon, skin cancer, and leukemia.

Tumors are masses of cells resulting from uncontrolled growth and are either benign (harmless) or malignant. A benign tumor may be a wart or cyst, but still should be investigated by a physician upon its first appearance. Malignant tumors are not capsulated as are the benign ones, and therefore are cancerous. They multiply and grow in an uncapsulated fashion in their crab-like shape, destroying and crowding out functions of normal cell activity. If unchecked they may spread from one primary organ to a secondary location. The spreading from one area to another is called metastasis.

There are two basic forms of cancer: carcinomas and the sarcomas. Carcinomas are most common and originate from epithelial cells, which may be coverings or linings of tissues. Skin is composed of one kind of epithelium and when it becomes cancerous it is designated as skin carcinoma. Sarcomas occur less frequently and are a group of cancers arising from fibrous tissues, muscle, bone, and cartilage. Together they are both classified as solid tumors.

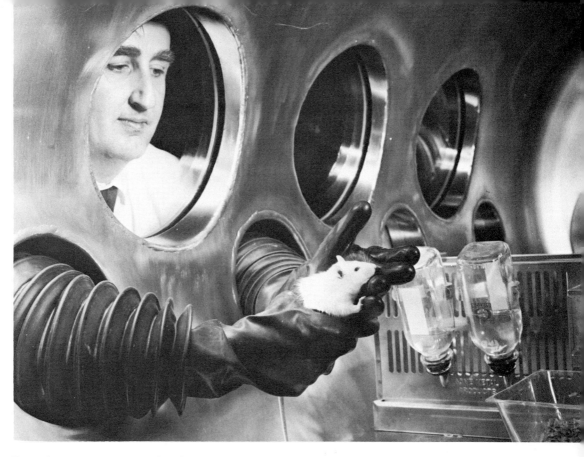

Researchers continue to probe the mysteries of cancer.

Since cancer is actually a group of many diseases, its causes are varied as well. Because there are so many types and possible causes of cancer, there has been a hindrance of scientific researcher's efforts to develop a sound means of eradication. Basically there are four groups of causes: chemical, physical, genetic, and viral.

Smog, burns, atmospheric pollution, and drugs may be contributing factors for chemical causes. Chemicals as a cause of cancer were first recognized by an English surgeon, Potts, in 1775, when he discovered frequent scrotal cancer of chimney sweeps due to soot exposure.[4]

Physical causes may be substances which emit carcinogenic radiations as they degenerate. One example of radiation as a causative factor of cancer would be indicated by an increased leukemia rate among

4. Richard Doll, *Prevention of Cancer: Pointers in Epidemiology* (London: Nuffield Provincial Hospitals Trust 1967), p. 62.

Hiroshima and Nagasaki survivors. Their incidence is five times higher than that of the remainder of the Japanese population.[5]

Heredity may be a consideration for encouraging cancerous growth, although valid studies have yet to reveal cancer can be inherited in humans. Heredity has been demonstrated as being significantly important in laboratory animals as mice are being bred that invariably contract or develop a specific cancer.

Animal studies continue to reveal more clues on the cancer riddle concerning viruses as a causative factor for some types of cancer. Early research was led by an Iowa physician, Richard Shope, who noted wild rabbits appearing in rural areas with skin warts. He later proved a virus could cause a solid tumor in a mammal. Shope died in 1966 of cancer and published a paper before his death stating that human cells are not that different from animal cells in regard to cell reaction to cancer-causing viruses.[6] Research continues in this area.

Recently there has been increased interest in new studies linking the affluent American diet to cancer of the colon and/or rectum. The last five years have seen a gradual steady increase in the number of Americans who contract these kinds of cancer. Some argue that linkage of diet to cancer is still largely statistical. However, there are marked differences and incidence of this kind of cancer. Dietary differences may account for the fact that the United States, Scotland, and Denmark have a high rate whereas Japan, Chile, and Israel do not. The spotlight appears to focus on beef and the influence of fat on the body after prolonged consumption.

Dr. John Berg of the National Cancer Institute conducted a comparative study of Japan and the United States. He discovered that Japanese immigrants in this country who developed a malignancy had a history of eating beef whereas their fellow immigrants did not. He also found that Argentina, Uruguay, and New Zealand have high beef consumption as well as a high incidence of cancer of the colon and/or rectum. Opponents of this diet theory argue that association does not always mean causation.

To prevent or reduce cancer of the colon and rectum, men, in particular should have regular examinations. After 40, one should have an

5. C. K. Wanebo, et al., "Breast Cancer After Exposure to Atomic Bombings of Hiroshima and Nagasaki," *New England Journal of Medicine* 279 (Sept. 26, 1968): 667–71.

6. Richard E. Shope, "Evolutionary Episodes in the Concept of Viral Oncogenesis," *Perspectives in Biology and Medicine* (Winter 1966), p. 273.

internal examination yearly, but many people avoid doing this because of the unpopular method of using the proctosigmoidoscope. This instrument, which has a light attached, is inserted rectally for diagnosis and is somewhat painful. Now scientists are experimenting with a more comfortable instrument called a colonscope. This instrument is a flexible rod made of optical fibers and flexible glass strands that guide light around corners and curves without the discomfort of the older method.[7]

Early detection and preventive measures appear to be of utmost importance in attempting to control cancer. Treatment today includes the utilization of surgery, radiation, laser beam, chemotherapy, and thermotherapy. New drugs are being tested and experimented with each day in search of a definite course of treatment. Today a cancer patient is considered cured if the disease does not recur within a five-year time span. The American Cancer Society spends billions of dollars each year for research and preventive measures for control of this disease.

Everyone should seek a yearly annual physical examination by a competent physician. Due to the increase in cancer of the cervix, all women should also have the pap smear test administered yearly. It is a simple, painless examination of vaginal fluid developed by Dr. George Papanicolaou, and serves as a diagnostic tool for cervical cancers.

Millions of women became aware of the importance of seeking routine pap smears and breast examinations when it was found that President Ford's wife Betty and Vice-President Rockefeller's wife Happy were both victims of breast cancer. Every woman should be familiar with breast self-examination which can be done simply in the privacy of one's own home. Mrs. Ford's and Mrs. Rockefeller's cancerous conditions generated public attention and created an opportunity to educate the American people of the need to erase the secretive, fearful nature of the disease and to seek immediate advice from one's physician in order to assure the feasibility of cure.

For many years it has been emphasized and proven that the best chance for beating cancer is early detection. Yet today many people still delay in reporting cancerous symptoms, often with fatal results. Common reasons for failure to see a physician include such ideas as: "It can't happen to me"; "There's no cure anyway"; "Ignorance is bliss"; and "I'm afraid to find out." Some people feel that current publicity may frighten people into an awareness of cancer thereby proving counter-

7. Jerry Bishop, "Cancer vs. What You Eat," *Science Digest* (March 1974):10–14.

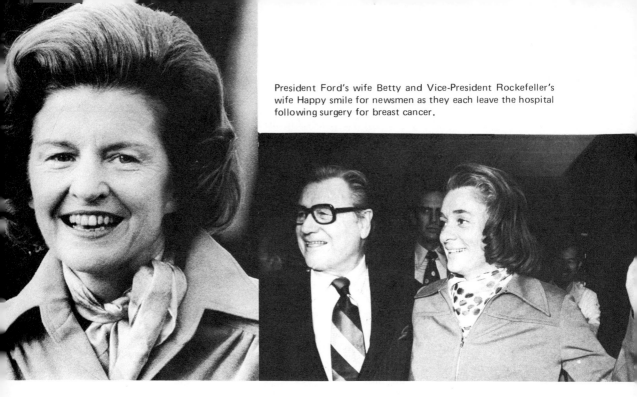

President Ford's wife Betty and Vice-President Rockefeller's wife Happy smile for newsmen as they each leave the hospital following surgery for breast cancer.

productive. The American Cancer Society changed the wording of seven *danger* signals to seven *warning* signals in hopes of reducing negative reactions on the part of the public. Studies on motivation reveal that, in terms of disseminating information, arousing a moderate amount of anxiety that is followed by a means of alleviating the anxiety is the most successful method.

Because of despair, social stigma, or fear, patients frequently fail to seek early treatment or notice early warning signals.

The American Cancer Society's cancer warning signals are:

1. Any sore that increases in size or does not heal.
2. Any lump or thickening that persists such as in the breast, groin, or under the armpits.
3. Any unusual bleeding or abnormal discharge.
4. A change in bowel habits or difficulty in passing urine.
5. Persistent indigestion.
6. Persistent cough or hoarseness and/or difficulty in swallowing.
7. Unintended weight loss.
8. Any change in color or size of wart, mole, or birthmark.
9. Persistent headache or difficulty in seeing.

# What Is a Pap Test?

This test is a simple but effective method of detecting cancer of the uterus at a very early stage. As is true of many parts of the body, cells are constantly being discarded by the wall of the uterus. These cells collect in the fluid film covering the surface of the vagina. In the Pap test or smear (developed by Dr. George Papanicolaou) a thin film of this fluid is spread on a glass slide and examined under the microscope. If cancer cells are present, they can be identified among the discarded normal cells. This method is so sensitive that it can reveal the presence of cancers so small that they can be found in no other way. Cancer is therefore detected at an early stage in its development, before it has had time to spread. At this stage treatment is effective and the danger is eliminated.

Fred Brown and Rudolf T. Kempton, *Sex Questions and Answers*, 2nd ed. (McGraw-Hill Book Company, 1970), p. 102. Reprinted by permission of the publisher.

Everyone should seek a yearly physical examination by a competent physician. Due to the increase in cancer of the cervix, all women should also have the pap smear test administered yearly. It is a simple, painless examination of vaginal fluid developed by Dr. George Papanicolaou, and serves as a diagnostic tool for cervical cancers.

It is estimated that 85 percent of human cancers may be controlled or even prevented if certain agents in the environment are evaluated and controlled. More lives can be saved if smokers begin to accept the fact that cigarette smoking is a causative factor in lung cancer. Occupational workers in mining and chemical research, for example, should insist on environmental protection devices and safety equipment to reduce their risks for cancer.

In the race for life, cancer always has a headstart. It need not win. It is delay, often based on fear, that ends in despair. "Through early diagnosis and early treatment and competent medical advice, the present survival ratio could be one in two."[7]

7. Benjamin A. Kogan, *Health: Man In A Changing Environment* (New York: Harcourt, Brace and World, 1970), p. 210.

## Questions for Study and Discussion

1. Why do heart disease and cancer remain at the top of the list of leading causes of death? Why have the "top ten" changed in the past fifty years?
2. Why are the leading causes of death only a part of the total health picture? For example, what factors other than mortality are important?
3. Where can you get reliable information, medical services, or other kinds of help for heart disease and cancer in your home community?
4. List the possibilities in the reduction of risk factors for both heart disease and cancer. Which of these do you now follow, and what more could you do?
5. Why does cancer lend itself so readily to the use of worthless remedies, unproven treatment, and quackery?
6. Why do college students smoke? Why is the habit difficult for some to break? Survey a sampling of students to discover their attitudes and opinions about smoking.
7. What are the effects of smoking on the respiratory system?

## References

Bishop, Jerry. "Cancer Vs. What You Eat," *Science Digest,* March, 1974:10–14.

"Fear Is Cancer's Friend," *Science Digest,* 74 (November, 1973):49–50.

Karvonen, M. J. and A. J. Barry. *Physical Activity and the Heart.* Springfield: Charles C Thomas Publishing, 1967.

Kogan, Benjamin A. *Health: Man In A Changing Environment.* New York: Harcourt, Brace and World, 1970.

Larson, Leonard, ed. *Health and Fitness in the Modern World.* Chicago: The Athletic Institute, 1960.

"Latest on Heart Problems and New Machines," *U.S. News and World Report,* 76 (February 4, 1974):76–7.

Minetree, Harry. *Cooley, The Career of a Great Surgeon.* Harpers Press, 1973.

"Overdoing Heart Surgery," *Time,* 103 (March 4, 1974):60.

Parker, Brent. "The Effects of Ethyl Alcohol on the Heart," *Journal of the American Medical Association* (May 6, 1974):741–42.

Staley, Seward, et. al. *Exercise and Fitness.* Chicago: The Athletic Institute, 1960.

# 5

# Physical Fitness

## General Concept

Regular physical activity can make significant contributions to human well-being.

## Outcomes

The student should be able to:
1. Identify the need for regular physical activity in modern society.
2. Describe the beneficial effects of regular, aerobic type, physical activity.
3. Identify the type, intensity, and duration of physical activities which will most benefit the cardio-respiratory systems.
4. Describe the role of exercise as both a risk factor and a part of preventive maintenance against cardiovascular disease.

## Hypokinetic Disease

Even the most casual observer must acknowledge that the necessity and opportunity for physical activity has been greatly reduced in the last century. Labor saving devices, industrial machinery, and the automo-

## 49 Million Americans Don't Exercise

Forty-five percent of all adult Americans (roughly 49 million of the 109 million adult men and women) do not engage in physical activity for the purpose of exercise. These sedentary Americans tend to be older, less well educated, and less affluent than those who do exercise.

Paradoxically, those who don't exercise are more inclined to believe they get enough exercise than those who do exercise. A recent national survey brought the following response to the question "which, if any, of these exercises are you doing now?"

| | % Total Public | % Men | % Women |
|---|---|---|---|
| None | 45 | 44 | 45 |
| Walking | 40 | 38 | 41 |
| Bicycling | 17 | 16 | 17 |
| Swimming | 13 | 16 | 10 |
| Calisthenics | 13 | 12 | 14 |
| Jogging | 6 | 8 | 3 |

"National Adult Physical Fitness Survey," *Newsletter:* President's Council on Physical Fitness & Sports, May, 1973.

bile have dramatically changed our work and exercise habits. Muscular effort has been carefully engineered out of our production and transportation systems and paradoxically we must plan physical activity and recreation. We have been chastised for being a nation of "spectators" when we do seek recreational activities.

The ravages of inactivity have not gone unnoticed. By mid-century the reduced physical capacity of his patients moved Han Kraus to say, "... we, as physicians, have come to accept as normal what even a century ago might have been looked upon as below-normal, abnormal, or even sick."[1] Kraus labeled the wide range of symptoms and ailments asso-

1. Hans Kraus, and Wilhelm Raab. *Hypokinetic Disease* (Springfield, Ill.: Charles C Thomas, Pub., 1961), p. 4.

ciated with inactivity as "hypokinetic disease," or literally diseases caused by lack of movement.

Foremost among the symptoms and ailments associated with inactivity are muscular-skeletal problems. Lack of activity causes shortening in the muscle and reduced flexibility. Combined with anxiety and stress these effects can result in muscular tension and pain. Medical authorities agree that much, if not most, of lower back pain, tension in the neck, and associated headaches could be relieved by regular exercise designed to work, stretch, and relax the muscles involved.

American school children traditionally score poorly on tests of upper arm strength, abdominal strength, and cardiorespiratory endurance. Some of the symptoms which later plague adult Americans are already developing including impaired muscular-skeletal flexibility. The habits of overeating and under-exercising associated with degenerative diseases have their origins in the early years of life. The medical profession has been shaken by the earlier and earlier appearance of coronary artery disease symptoms and even death in young adults. Autopsies during the Korean War yielded evidence of advanced atherosclerotic deposits on the arteries of young battle casualties. Heart disease may seem remote to you, the college student, but multiple associated risk factors have been identified in elementary-age-school children.

Medical science has made great strides in this century in eliminating many of the infectious diseases which have plagued man for thousands of years. Infectious diseases have fallen to a lower category, as the most prominent killers in modern society are degenerative diseases.

Countless authorities in medicine, physical education, health, and physiology ascribe to the concept that a sound preventive medicine approach would reduce the incidence of degenerative diseases such as obesity, high blood pressure, and coronary artery disease. Preventive medicine includes regular physical activity for the benefit of the heart and lungs as well as the muscles and joints. Positive prevention programs can contribute to reducing the staggering personal and economic losses of degenerative disease.

The pace of modern life and its time deadlines, pressures, and rapid communication has been linked to the rising level of degenerative disease. Anthropologists maintain that we are suppressing a biological function, the "fight or flight" mechanism, which has been habitual for thousands of years. The concept implies that the drive to release tension, aggression, nervousness, or fear through physical activity is as old as man. In primitive times the choice to run or fight was simple and the accompanying alarm reaction was defused by the subsequent physical action. Opportunities to defuse neuro-hormonal alarm reactions in modern society are relatively few. The sudden release of adrenaline and the accompanying increase in heart rate, blood pressure, breathing rate, and blood chemicals can be damaging to the organism if the imbalance is habitually repeated over a period of time. The inability to reduce such tension represents the classic example of psychosomatic illness.

The sense of well-being and physical relaxation associated with regular exercise is familiar to anyone who has maintained sufficient activity to increase physical fitness. Although the immediate reactions to vigorous activity are similar to the alarm reaction described above, the post-exercise effect is one of reduced tension in the muscles, mild to moderate fatigue, and finally a sense of invigoration. With a few isolated exceptions, this is one of the least understood or documented effects of physical activity, but one which probably ranks highest in satisfaction among habitual exercisers.

## Physical Fitness and Its Effects

The satisfaction from making a good tennis shot in a hard fought game, the invigorating swim in the early morning, and the sociability of a familiar foursome on the golf course all contribute to human well-being. Do they all contribute equally, however, to physical fitness? What is physical fitness anyway? Although the term may appear to be obvious, physical fitness is not a simple term to define. Both health and fitness infer more than an absence of illness or infirmity. Being physically fit means that the individual has sufficient strength, flexibility, and general endurance to carry on daily tasks without undue fatigue. It means being able to meet the extra demands of living also, such as meeting emergencies, and engaging in sports, games, or recreational activities of a vigorous nature without becoming prematurely fatigued. There can be many facets to physical fitness but the one which has overriding implications for health and well-being is the capacity for the cardio-respiratory systems to meet the demands of vigorous work and play. It is evident that not all sports, games, or physical activity contribute significantly to cardio-respiratory fitness. Activities which tax the heart and lungs are the major contributors to phyical fitness, while less vigorous activities may contribute primarily to the social and mental well-being of the individual.

Activities which are vigorous enough to enhance physical fitness produce *training effects,* which represent adaptations of the body to the demands of physical activity. Training effects can be characterized as beneficial to the 1) neuromuscular and muscular-skeletal, or 2) cardiorespiratory systems.

## Neuromuscular and Muscular-Skeletal Effects

Repeated performance of sports skill or activity results in greater efficiency in performing the task. Greater efficiency is synonymous with greater skill and results in easier performance of the task and more enjoyment from the activity. As learning progresses and skill improves, the effect becomes relatively permanent and hence the accomplished skier can expect good retention after several months without practice.

Muscles become stronger and develop greater endurance when subjected to frequent use. The increase in muscular strength and endurance results in less effort and fatigue to engage in the same physical activity. Combined with increased skill these effects mean that the active person can derive more enjoyment from sports, games, and recreational activities.

The active person also tends to have greater joint flexibility and is less likely to suffer from tension and pain in the active joints. This is particularly important as the individual ages and joint deterioration and muscle tension increase. The training effect is usually localized, thus concentration is encouraged to engage in whole body activities such as swimming, hiking, and tennis.

## Cardiorespiratory Effects

Activities which contribute significantly to cardiorespiratory fitness are the most important in terms of general health. The capacity and efficiency of the heart and lungs increase with habitual exercise. The well-exercised heart beats slower and stronger both at rest and during activity. The increased efficiency has resulted in the label "loafers heart" being attached to a well-conditioned heart. Additional blood vessels are opened in exercised muscles and in the heart this is referred to as collateral circulation.

The respiratory system develops greater capacity and efficiency with regular exercise. Combined with the increased capacity of the circulatory system, greater respiratory capacity leads to the ability to take in and deliver greater amounts of oxygen to the tissues. This is a major difference between the physically fit individual and the nonexerciser. There are many other training effects which add to the greater capacity of the physically fit person but they are omitted here for the sake of brevity.

Unfortunately the beneficial effects of physical fitness are fleeting and reversible. Discontinuance of exercise results in a gradual return to a preprogram level of capacity. It is not likely that a residual effect accrues from activity. Athletic experience in high school or college can do little to offset the ravages of thirty or forty years of sedentary living which so often follows.

## Exercise and Our No. 1 Killer

Year after year in this country the toll from all forms of cardiovascular disease rolls on consistently and unabated at 55 percent of all deaths or approximately 1.2 million persons per year. Cancer is a very distant second and would actually be third if deaths from heart attack and stroke were separated. This epidemic is of such proportions that it is estimated 27 million Americans have some form of cardiovascular disease. The cost in economic terms is a staggering 20 billion dollars annually in lost wages, production, and health care.

### Risk Factors and Exercise

Heart disease is unusual in the sense that it has no single cause which has been definitely identified. It has, rather, a number of risk factors which are associated with it and they tend to multiply geometrically. The disease attacks the coronary arteries primarily and the most effective diagnostic technique is a multistage treadmill exercise test with constant ECG monitoring. Such a test will give indications of narrowed or clogged arteries when the heart is under the stress of physical activity. Although medical scientists will place varying emphasis on the risk factors, most would agree that the following are important in assessing the risk profile: obesity, cholesterol, blood pressure, exercise, smoking, heredity, and stress anxiety. All of these factors are remedial with the exception of heredity and its impact can be reduced by controlling the other factors.

*Obesity* (over fat) is not heart disease but it is highly related to coronary artery disease, high blood pressure, and early death. It has long been established that physical activity can aid in the prevention and rehabilitation of obesity through increased caloric expenditure. The combination of dieting (reduced caloric intake) and exercise (increased caloric output) is the most rapid and effective means of combating obesity. Recent studies indicate that physical activity must be frequent (4 to 5 days per week), at least moderate, and of 30 minutes to one hour duration to be effective in reducing body fat significantly.

Blood *cholesterol* levels normally range between 150–300 mg/ 100ml, with an average in this country of approximately 200 mg. The upper end of this "normal" range is misleading however, because the Framingham Heart Study indicated that when the cholesterol level reaches 265 mg. the risk of coronary artery disease is five times greater than for individuals with an average (220 mg.) or lower level. There is controversy regarding the effectiveness of a low cholesterol diet in controlling blood fats. Diet will lower the cholesterol level but will not drastically reduce an abnormally high level to the average range. The extent to which physical activity can lower cholesterol appears to be inconclusive despite some evidence that it does reduce blood fat levels. It appears that frequent, vigorous, activity of some duration will produce significant reduction of cholesterol levels but this may not be within the reach of most individuals. A combination of dietary control and exercise may be the most effective approach as it is with the control of body fat.

*Hypertension* or high blood pressure is another key factor in coronary artery disease and the most prevalent form of cardiovascular disease. Numerous studies in recent years have reported decreased systolic and diastolic blood pressure after a period of physical training. Low level aerobic activity combined with diet and weight control is a most effective means of reducing blood pressure.

Rosenman and Friedman have identified the behavior pattern of the coronary prone individual and they label him a *"Type A."* This person is characterized by personality traits such as: aggressiveness, ambition, drive, competitiveness, and a profound sense of time urgency. In short, a profile that is alarmingly like the sterotype of the successful American. The pace of modern urban life and occupation may have less effect on the risk associated with a Type A profile than the personality that generates such high levels of stress and anxiety. To date there is scant evidence that physical activity influences anxiety as cause and effect relationships are always difficult to distinguish in such study. The reduced muscular tension and sense of "well-being" that occurs after exercise, however, is familiar to most habitual actives.

For more than two decades there has been a large and growing body of evidence linking *sedentary occupations* with higher incidence of coronary artery disease. The classic London bus drivers versus conductors study found that the more active ticket takers (double-decked buses) have significantly lower incidence of coronary artery disease. This result has been confirmed in various localities and occupations where work can be classified from sedentary to active. Postal employees, railroad personnel, farmers, and other industrial groups have been compared with similar results. It should be noted that a certain amount of natural selection may have taken place wherein the more healthy, energetic, and genetically advantaged individual chooses the more active occupation.

Several more recent investigations have sought to answer the natural selection factor. The Framingham study reports that the risk of death from heart attack, should it occur, is sharply reduced by regular physical activity regardless of occupation. The "Irish Brothers" study sought a link between dietary habits and heart disease comparing Irish brothers who had stayed in Ireland versus those who had moved to this country. Despite a diet higher in caloric content and cholesterol, the brothers who had remained in Ireland had a lower incidence of coronary disease. Their superior cardiovascular health was maintained by a much higher level of physical activity and an almost total lack of "hurry." Residents of the Israeli kibbutz have a two to four times greater incidence of coronary disease in the sedentary worker category. The unique aspect of kibbutzum living includes a uniform mode of life regardless of occupation (i.e., the standard of living, diet, income, and medical care are consistent).

Despite the impressive role of physical activity in maintaining cardiovascular health, it must be combined with other preventive approaches if the toll from cardiovascular disease is to be reduced. Preventive medicine includes changing dietary habits, stopping smoking, taking medication when appropriate, and actively reducing the daily tensions.

## Exercise For College Students

The most frequent question for exercise specialists is, "What kind of exercise and how much?" Nearly everyone would also like to know some sweet little exercise which removes the "roll" from around the tummy. Although there are frequently specialized reasons for exercising such as strengthening the legs for skiing or trimming the thighs to look good in a bathing suit, the major contributor to cardiovascular health and well-being is aerobic-type activity. Fortunately aerobic or heart-lung exercise will also help to reduce body fat and strengthen and trim muscles as well as produce beneficial effects to the heart and lungs.

## The Kind of Exercise

In 1968, Dr. Kenneth Cooper authored a best selling paperback entitled *Aerobics* in which he tried to answer the questions of what kind of exercise, for how long, and at what intensity. Aerobic activity refers to those activities which can be carried on for prolonged periods but are also demanding enough to produce beneficial changes to the cardio-respiratory system. These endurance type activities include: walking, jogging, cycling, swimming, hiking, climbing, and other continuous activities. Stationary cycling, running-in-place, and rope skipping represent indoor activities which are aerobic but also require a high level of motivation. Some recreational activities and games do not offer sufficient cardiovascular exertion to be beneficial such as golf, bowling, or weight lifting. College students are usually healthy and vigorous enough to derive aerobic benefits from more vigorous games such as tennis, handball, or basketball. In looking ahead to the choice and selection of activities which will be first, of interest and second, feasible, the college student should consider the problems of arranging a game of basketball in the adult years, or finding handball courts available. Some persons may elect to jog or swim for physical health and play golf for relaxation and sociability. If one can combine the benefits of an aerobic activity with something the person enjoys immensly both needs are met in a single activity session. There is a wide selection of aerobic activities and an individual may need to sample several before selecting one or more activities that can become habitual. The individual who is "turned off" by some aerobic activities unfortunately rejects all activities of this nature. College students are in an excellent position to sample activities before selecting favorites.

## Frequency, Duration, and Intensity of Exercise

Since physical fitness is so fleeting, it is necessary for exercise to be habitual by making it a part of the normal weekly schedule. *A minimum of three times per week* is recommended in order to reap the potential benefits of exercise. The length of time to engage in physical activity depends upon the intensity, for example fifteen minutes of jogging is as beneficial as thirty minutes or more of walking. A vigorous swimming session will be more demanding and beneficial than a like amount of leisurely cycling but the intensity could be reversed if so desired. The *intensity* of the activity is determined by the percentage of maximal capacity that is taxed by the task. A handy means of assessing the intensity of activity of a task is to take the exercise heart rate and compare it with an estimated maximum for that age range. Most college students will have a maximum heart rate in the range of 175–195 beats per minute. With middle aged and older adults this range will be considerably lower perhaps between 150–175. It is not necessary to reach maximum levels to produce beneficial training effects and this is one of the major advantages of aerobic activity. Aerobic activity will result in an initial increase in the early minutes of activity but a steady state is reached within a few minutes and the heart rate levels off. Some sports and games require brief bursts of intense activity at or near maximum heart rate and can actually be ill-advised for some adults with poor cardiovascular fitness. *A training effect* can be accomplished with 60–80 percent of maximum heart rate and for most individuals this will mean a heart rate in the range of 120–160. The exercise heart rate can be attained readily by counting the pulse at the carotid artery (neck) for ten seconds *immediately* as exercise ends. This count is then multiplied by six to estimate the exercising heart rate.

The recommended *duration* of activity would be as little as *15 minutes* on the high end of the intensity scale to *45 minutes* or more on the lower end of the scale. As little as *45 minutes per week* could be sufficient time to produce desirable results from an exercise program provided sufficient intensity is attained during that time.

## Precautions and Principles

Most college students can begin an exercise program with little concern about cardiac risk. Middle-aged adults are cautioned however, to have a physical examination and preferably a multi-stage ECG treadmill or bike test to assess the potential for asymptomatic coronary disease. The same advice could apply to those college students with known cardiac problems or multiple heart disease risk factors.

The exercise program should be started gradually not only for safety

# A Smorgasbord of Physical Activity

Dr. Kenneth Cooper has attached point values to common physical activities according to duration and intensity. He recommends a minimum of 30 points per week to produce beneficial cardiorespiratory changes and offers a wide range of options to meet the minimum requirements.

## WEEKLY PROGRAMS

I. The "Streaker": Quickest Way to Go (45 minutes)

| Exercise | Distance | Time | Frequency | Points/ Session | Weekly Total |
|---|---|---|---|---|---|
| Running | 2.0 mi. | 16 min./ or less | M W F | 10 | 30 |

II. The "Weekend Golfer"

| Exercise | Distance | Time | Frequency | Points/ Session | Weekly Total |
|---|---|---|---|---|---|
| Golf | 18 holes | No Carts | 3 times | 3 | 9 |
| Swimming | 40 laps (1000 yds) | 25 min. | 3 times | 8 | 24 |
| | | | | | 33 |

III. The "Shy One": Done Indoors and/or Walking Doesn't Look Like Exercise.

| Exercise | Distance | Time | Frequency | Points/ Session | Weekly Total |
|---|---|---|---|---|---|
| Stationary Running | | 10 min. | 6 times | 2 ½ | 15 |
| Walking | 3.0 mi. | 43:30 or less | 5 times | 3 | 15 |
| | | | | | 30 |

IV. The "Smorgasbord"

| Exercise | Distance | Time | Frequency | Points/ Session | Weekly Total |
|---|---|---|---|---|---|
| Cycling | 5.0 mi. | 15 min. | M | 5 | 5 |
| Tennis | 3 sets | 60 min. | T-W | 4 ½ | 9 |
| Handball | | 50 min. | Th | 7 ½ | 7 ½ |
| Swimming | 40 laps (1000 yds) | 25 min. | F | 8 + | 8 + |
| | | | | | 30 |

Source: Kenneth H. Cooper, *The New Aerobics*. (New York: M. Evans Co., 1970).

sake but to reduce soreness in the early sessions. There is no hurry to attain physical fitness and the results can accrue from less than maximum effort. Each session should include three distinct segments beginning with a 5–10 minute *warm-up period* of calisthenics, stretching, and mild exercise to stimulate circulation. The aerobic *activity* portion of the session will last 15–45 minutes or more as desired and should be followed by 3–5 minutes of *cooling off* to give the heart an opportunity to adjust gradually to the change of pace.

A few comments are in order regarding the consumer aspects of physical fitness. It should be obvious that active participation on the part of the individual is necessary to produce the sustained cardiac load necessary to produce significant health benefits. Passive involvement with equipment does not produce this effect, and the same can be said about "spot reducing." The American Medical Association has repeatedly voiced opposition to claims of spot reduction or passive physical fitness equipment. Fat is metabolized from throughout the body when it is mobilized as fuel and is not drawn from any specific area. It is, however, stored in greater abundance in certain areas of the body (e.g. abdominal, hips, and thighs). Hence proportional loss in those areas will be more marked and it is very evident that the individual has reduced body fat. Consumer protection agencies have been increasingly more aggressive in challenging the claims or ads of weight reduction salons. The "wrapping" technique is one such approach which has been cited as a misleading claim regarding weight control.

## Future Patterns of Exercise

Many major corporations have become so concerned with the cardiovascular health and fitness of key executives and employees that fitness and recreational facilities have been developed for both employees and their families. This is only one of several national trends toward a more active population. The increased interest in lifetime sports (tennis, golf, and handball), the "back to nature" movement (camping, hiking, and skiing), and the effects of more costly fuel (bicycling and walking) are examples of such trends. Nearly half of the adult population does not exercise but this percentage may shrink in the future as more individuals cycle to school or work, join employee fitness programs, or make use of increasing leisure time by pursuing lifetime sports or outdoor recreation with families. The potential benefits to the individual and the society

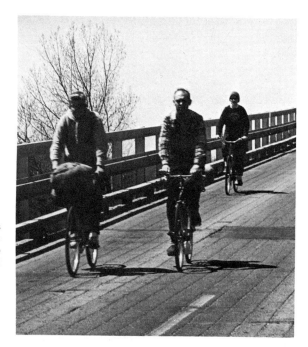

Bicycling on a regular daily basis provides excellent exercise, but local legislation is needed to provide safe, scenic, unpolluted cycling paths.

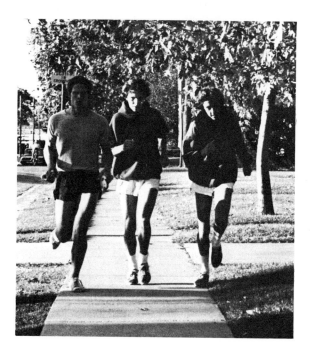

Jogging is a convenient exercise to continue throughout one's life as it requires no special equipment or facility.

make the prospects of such a trend welcome. As so often happens, college students appear to be among the first to have adopted a more active life-style.

## Questions for Study and Discussion

1. What are hypokinetic diseases and why have they become so prevalent in modern society?
2. Why do some experts believe that the death toll from cardiovascular disease could be reduced appreciably?
3. What beneficial effects does exercise have on the heart and blood vessels?
4. What are the seven major risk factors of coronary artery disease?
5. Which of the coronary disease risk factors are significantly affected by physical activity?
6. Why do physicians assume that most low back pain and neck-tension headaches could be relieved by regular physical activity?
7. What is aerobic exercise and why is it recommended for college students and adults?
8. What is the minimum frequency and duration necessary if aerobic activity is to significantly affect health?
9. Each activity session should consist of three distinct phases; what are they and why?
10. How can physical activity make contributions to mental and emotional well-being?

## References

Astrand, Per-Olaf and Rodahl, Kaare. *Textbook of Work Physiology.* New York: McGraw-Hill Book Company, 1970.

Boyer, John L. "Effects of Chronic Exercise on Cardiovascular Function." *Physical Fitness Research Digest* 2 (July, 1972):1–6.

Brunner, D. R. and Manelis, G. "Physical Activity at Work and Ischemic Heart Disease." *Coronary Heart Disease and Physical Fitness.* Baltimore: University Park Press, 1971.

Clark, H. Harrison. "Exercise and Blood Cholesterol." *Physical Fitness Research Digest.* 2 (July, 1972):6–15.

Cooper, Kenneth H. "Guidelines in the Management of the Exercising Patient." *JAMA.* 211 (1970):1663–1667.

Cooper, Kenneth H. *Aerobics.* New York: M. Evans and Co., 1970.

*Exercise Testing and Training of Apparently Healthy Individuals: A Handbook for Physicians.* New York: American Heart Association, 1972.

Fox, Samuel M. and Boyer, John L. "Physical Activity and Coronary Heart Disease." *Physical Fitness Research Digest.* 2 (April, 1972): 1–13.

Fox, Samuel M. and Boyer, John L. "Mechanisms by Which Physical Activity May Reduce the Occurrence or Severity of Coronary Heart Disease." *Physical Fitness Research Digest.* 2 (October, 1972):1–14.

Kannel, William B. "The Framingham Study and Chronic Disease Prevention." *Hospital Practice.* 5 (March, 1970):78–94.

Kraus, Hans and Raab, Wilhelm. *Hypokinetic Disease.* Springfield, Ill.: Charles C Thomas, Publishers, 1961.

Morris, J. N., et al, "Coronary Heart-Disease and Physical Activity of Work." *Lancet.* 2 (1953):1053–1057, 1111–1120.

"National Adult Physical Fitness Survey." *Newsletter:* President's Council on Physical Fitness and Sports, May, 1973.

*Physicians Handbook for Evaluation of Cardiovascular and Physical Fitness.* Nashville: Tennessee Heart Association, 1972.

Rosenman, Ray H. and Friedman, Meyer, "Observations on the Pathogenesis of Coronary Heart Disease." *Nutrition News.* 34 (October, 1971):9–14.

Stone, William J. "Physical Activity and Our No. 1 Killer." *Arizona JOHPER.* 17 (Fall, 1973):17, 23.

# 6

# Drugs:
# Use and Abuse

## General Concept

Drugs have the capacity to modify mood and behavior and in doing so can be both a benefit and detriment to man.

## Outcomes

The student should be able to:
1. Trace the historical significance of drug usage
2. Explain the nature of the impact that drugs have in present-day society
3. Define the various terminology employed in the discussion of use and abuse of drugs
4. Explain the various means by which drugs are classified
5. Describe the actions and resulting complications of drugs that are commonly abused
6. Explain the various means and difficulties in controlling drug abuse
7. Describe the motivational and social forces underlying drug abuse
8. List what he considers to be usable alternatives to the drug experience

9. Discuss the question of the morality of man seeking to artificially stimulate and/or relax himself in today's society
10. Express an opinion on the existence of a relationship between respect for one's mind, body, and future, and drug abuse.

## A Chemical Way of Life?

## Historical Perspective

It has been said that we are a society in a drug-induced state, following a way of life that will lead us to physical and moral decay. We ingest pills to pep us up and pills to calm us down; pills to help us sleep and pills to keep us awake; pills designed to offset the effects of other pills. Many individuals seek to escape a painful reality by consuming chemicals that modify mood and behavior.

Although it is true that we ingest chemicals in large quantities today, it is equally true that we have been doing so for centuries. Naturally, the choice of drug differs, but man has always energetically sought out substances and means for altering his conscious state. The use of such substances as opium, hemp plant, and fermented fruits has been documented for many years. In the United States chloroform and nitrous oxide (laughing gas) were favorites during the early nineteenth century; after the Civil War, dependence upon morphine and distilled spirits became a serious problem.

The fact that drug abuse existed in the past does not lessen the gravity of our present situation, though we do seem to view the problem as a recent phenomenon.

## The Place of Drugs in Present-day Society

With increased dissemination of information about drug abuse through all media, one tends to forget the many benefits that have been and continue to be derived through chemicals. Most drugs that are abused have legitimate medical purposes; the same drug that can relieve suffering when employed under controlled dosage can create suffering when abused. There is nothing inherent in a chemical to create a pattern of abuse. For example, barbiturate sedatives and tranquilizers have been put to invaluable use in treating the mentally disturbed. Under certain circumstances these drugs may help to relieve the tension found in an anxiety-ridden individual and thus allow him to function more effectively. But these same drugs are abused when large amounts are ingested in uncontrolled circumstances. So, although one person may be released from a mental hospital because of a drug, another may be admitted to the same institution because of drug abuse.

Unfortunately, there is a paucity of scientific information as to the underlying reasons for abuse of drugs. Even a complete understanding as to the way in which drugs affect the mind is lacking. Because the drug usage question is so entangled with one's attitudes, emotions, and values, very few individuals can be truly objective when discussing the "drug problem in America." Confusion, myths, misinformation, and outright ignorance abound. Extremists on all sides of the drug abuse issue stand ready to espouse their views. Many adults in our society are quick to indict the younger generation for pursuing the kicks of a drugged and euphoric state, yet it is an ironic fact that these same adults do not consider their ingestion of amphetamines, barbiturates, and alcohol as being problems of drug abuse as well.

## Useful Definitions

A broad objective definition of a drug becomes difficult to determine since there exists a variety of drugs used for as many reasons. The term *drug* will not have the same meaning for a practicing physician as it will for a junior high school student. For our purposes, we will define a drug as "any chemical that modifies one's state of mood or behavior." This definition implies that drugs are psychoactive, since the mind is the organizer of mood and behavioral patterns.

**Use** and **abuse** are terms that are often used interchangeably and add to the communication difficulty when speaking of the drug problem. For example, a drug abuser most certainly is a drug user, but is a drug user necessarily a drug abuser? It is also difficult to gain widespread acceptance for a definition of *abuse*. Certainly any such definition must employ a value judgment, a judgment that has found some agreement among professionals interested in preserving the social structure. It is then helpful to define *abuse* operationally as the excessive use of a substance producing some change in the user which is detrimental to either the individual or society or both.

Unfortunately, this kind of semantic confusion pervades much of the discussion of the drug problem. One is often in error when he speaks in generalities about drugs. It is more useful to be specific by naming the chemical, the nature of the dependence, and other pertinent information. The result will be increased clarity and more accurate communication.

**Drug habituation** was a term formerly used by the World Health Organization's Expert Committee on Addiction-producing Drugs. The term has since been discarded by the committee because of its confusion with the term *addiction*. The former was originally intended to describe a pattern of repetitive drug use that did not necessarily include concomitant physical dependence. Habituation described a condition in which the use of drugs was related to one's psychic needs.

**Drug addiction** is a term that has been applied to the overwhelming compulsion (more than desire) to continue taking a substance. This craving is usually accompanied by a physical dependence which causes persistent use of the substance. Sudden withdrawal of the drug will result in the appearance of certain physical symptoms known as the *abstinence* or *withdrawal syndrome*. The World Health Organization no longer uses this term since the general nature of the definition does not deal with the drug problem from the standpoint of specific drugs.

**Drug dependence** is the term presently used by the World Health Organization. The Expert Committee recommended substituting drug dependence for drug habituation and drug addiction and defined the former as follows:

**Drug dependence** is a state of psychic or physical dependence, or both, on a drug, arising in a person following administration of that drug on a periodic or continuing basis. The characteristics of such a state will vary with the agent involved, and these characteristics must always be made clear by designating the particular type of drug dependence in each specific case; for example, drug dependence of morphine type, or amphetamine type, etc.

**Physical dependence** results when certain drugs are used over a protracted period of time. This type of dependence is marked by the appearance of the abstinence syndrome when the drug is withdrawn. For example, the abstinence syndrome involving heroin dependence includes a group of physical symptoms such as nausea, abdominal cramps, perspiration, chills, and tremor. The severity of the symptoms has come to be used as an indicator of the degree of physical dependence. The abstinence syndrome occurs only when the drug, or a drug similar in action, is withdrawn or is not used in sufficient quantities.

**Psychic dependence** refers to a strong desire or craving to experience the effects produced by a drug or drugs. The psychological need is of such intensity that the individual finds it necessary to return to the drugs continually. The drug-induced state becomes the normal and preferred one. When this occurs, the psychologically dependent drug abuser may begin to turn away from those things (goals, values, relationships) he once considered important in his life.

Physical and psychological dependence may occur together. However, it is possible for one to be physically dependent and not psychologically dependent. Conversely, one can be psychologically dependent and not physically dependent. Indeed, many drugs create psychic dependence with no possibility of physical dependence occurring. For the purpose of this chapter, the term **addict** will refer to someone who has become physically and/or psychologically dependent upon a drug.

**Tolerance** refers to the increasing need for stronger dosages of a drug in order to achieve the effects found earlier from a lesser dosage. The body gradually resists the chemical effects of the drug and, thus, an increase in dosage is required in order to attain the desired effect. The phenomenon of tolerance does not occur for all drugs or to the same extent with various drugs. **Cross-tolerance** develops when there is a tolerance to the effects of a drug other than the one originally taken; this second drug does, however, share similar pharmacological properties with the original.

**Set** and **setting** are terms often used together although they have distinct meanings which are significant. **Set** refers to the mood, personality, past experience and concommitant expectations of the individual. It is helpful to think of this as a "mind set." **Setting** refers to the immediate environment of the person when taking the drug. This includes physical environment as well as presence or absence of others. That these are powerful phenomena is evidenced by experiments in which subjects claim they experienced subjective effects such as euphoria after taking a placebo (i.e. a sugar pill).

## Classifying Drugs

Drugs can be classified in numerous ways. One general classification would pertain to the chemical affinity of a substance for certain organs or tissues of the body. Other means of classification involve the measuring of the substance's effect on perception, consciousness, and mood, and, finally, medical use of the substance. One often finds drugs being classified as either *stimulants* or *depressants*. A *stimulant* has the capacity to increase or step up body processes because of the substance's action on the cells of the central nervous system. *Depressants* decrease or slow down body functions because the chemical composition of the substance alters the cellular function by decreasing the activity of a cell.

## Drugs of Abuse

There is a wide range of substances which have been or are at present being abused. In general, chemicals of abuse can be placed into five categories: (1) narcotics, (2) sedatives, (3) tranquilizers, (4) stimulants, and (5) hallucinogens.[1]

*Narcotics* are medically defined as any drugs that produce sleep or stupor while, at the same time, they relieve pain. *Sedatives* are defined as substances that allay activity, excitement, or overt anxiety. *Tranquilizers* (ataroxics) have the principal effect of acting as a depressant on the central nervous system, thereby relieving anxiety, tension, and sometimes relaxing the muscles. *Stimulants* are drugs that excite or stimulate some organ or part of the body to greater function or activity. *Hallucinogen* is derived from the Latin word *hallucinari,* which means "to wander mentally." Hallucinogens produce pseudo-hallucinations or episodes of hearing, seeing, or feeling things that are not in the realm of physical reality (although some might argue that this becomes a question of metaphysics).

With these categories in mind, we can proceed to a specific discussion of commonly abused drugs.

**Opium.** This is a gummy substance derived from unripe seed pods of a poppy plant. Because the effects of opium are narcotic, it has been used both medicinally as well as for pleasure. Tolerance to the drug's effects develops as well as withdrawl symptoms when the opium dependent individual finds himself without the drug. In this country, opium is abused to a very small extent, the greatest abuse occurring in China and Southeast Asia.

**Morphine.** This drug is an alkaloid in opium. Morphine is used beneficially in medicine because of its analgesic (pain-relieving) properties. A state of euphoria is produced when the drug is taken in sufficient quantities, thereby relieving worry and anxiety. Although physical dependence does develop after a few weeks of usage, psychic dependence may or may not be a concomitant problem. When the dosage is increased, death from respiratory failure becomes an imminent possibility. The abuse of morphine has declined since the advent of heroin. The two

1. Smith, Kline and French, *Drug Abuse: Escape to Nowhere* (Philadelphia: 1967), p. 27.

have similar effects, although heroin is said to produce a state of greater euphoria.

**Heroin.**   This is a semisynthetic derived from morphine, and as such is much more potent analgesically. Ironically, heroin was developed in an effort to find a substance that could be as medically beneficial as morphine but would not result in physical and psychic dependence. At first it was thought that such a drug had been found, since heroin counteracted the withdrawal symptoms associated with morphine. Unfortunately, authorities learned too late that heroin had greater dependence-producing qualities than morphine. Thus, heroin became the foremost drug associated with drug dependence.

Psychic and physical dependence of the worst order are found among those who have become "hooked." Tolerance develops rapidly. Since heroin has no legal use whatsoever, the abuser often resorts to criminal acts in order to satisfy an increasingly expensive habit. Prostitution, the selling of drugs ("pushing"), and theft are the usual means for financing the insatiable need. It is not uncommon for the heroin user to need 60 to 70 dollars a day to maintain his habit. At this point the frantic user may voluntarily undergo the withdrawal syndrome in order to reverse the tolerance effect. He may do this "cold turkey" (not using any drugs to ease the physical symptoms), or he may commit himself to a hospital for detoxification. Once back on the street, however, he will usually start the pattern of use all over again. Only a very small percentage of heroin users do not return to the drug.

Heroin can be administered in several ways. The user may begin his habit by sniffing the white, crystalline powder. More commonly, he will inject the drug subcutaneously ("skin-popping") or intravenously ("main-lining"). The latter method is the ultimate to those who are hooked, since the effects are felt much more quickly; the sensation of the initial "rush" is highly desired.

The effects of the drug are narcotic and produce a semistate of wakefulness ("nod") in which the individual experiences a euphoric unconcern with the world of reality. As this drug-induced state becomes a constantly desired goal, the pain, both psychic and physical, of being without heroin is unbearable.

At one time the vast majority of heroin users were found in the lower socio-economic inner-urban areas. One can understand that the drug-induced escape from the painful reality of life in these areas may require little temptation. However, heroin use did not remain solely an inner

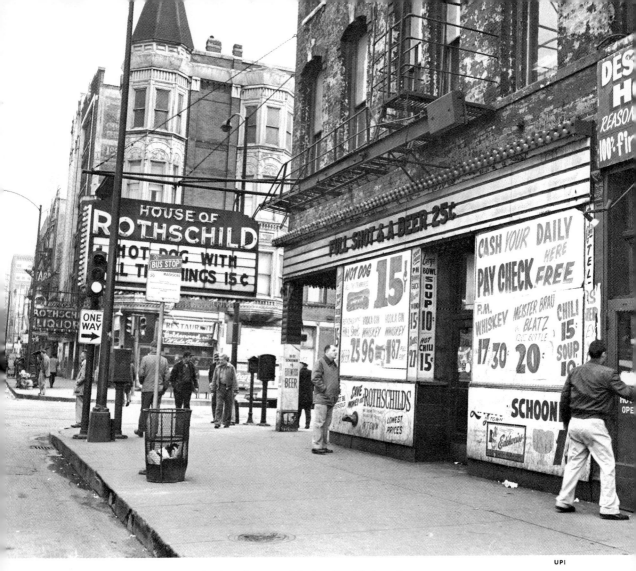

The inner city, is a breeding ground for heroin addiction.

city problem but alarmed many by moving into middle-class suburbs and the military. Within the past year, some evidence has suggested that the heroin problem is declining. It is more accurate to say that the rate of increase for heroin use is decreasing.

The hard-core heroin-dependent individual's life span is much shorter than the average. Heroin itself does not produce organic damage, but the life-style and associated medical problems often result in disease and death: hepatitis from unclean needles, collapsed veins, abscesses, malnutrition (heroin suppresses appetite), and death from overdosage are all possible consequences of continued abuse of this drug.

**Methadone.** This is a synthetic narcotic which acts like morphine. It is an analgesic which is used medically to treat heroin- and morphine-abstinence symptoms. There are several advantages to using methadone for this purpose. Once it is substituted for heroin or morphine, the withdrawal symptoms will become those of methadone. Since methadone withdrawl symptoms are less severe, the addict will lose some of his anxiety and find the withdrawl experience more bearable. This type of treatment is usually administered in a clinical setting, accompanied by psychotherapy. Another advantage is that the effects of the drug are achieved just as well when taken orally as when taken by injection. The drug, therefore, is most commonly administered by mixing it with orange juice.

Since a high percentage of addicts return to heroin or morphine after being detoxified in this way, many authorities recommend indefinite maintenance therapy utilizing methadone. In this way the heroin or morphine addict becomes dependent upon methadone. The individual is given a controlled dosage daily as an outpatient, and since the effects of methadone are not as intense as heroin or morphine, he may hold a job and generally function in society. Other groups argue, however, that since psychic dependence, physical dependence, and tolerance develop with continued methadone use, the individual cannot truly live a normal life, since he still remains an addict. Whether the methadone addict can return to a drug-free life by obtaining gradually decreasing dosage remains to be proved. Undoubtedly, something must be done to counteract the psychic dependence.

**Demerol** (meperidine). This drug is a synthetic which is dissimilar to morphine in its chemical structure but has a similar effect. In medicines it is used as an analgesic and sedative. It does not, however, create as much physical dependence. The lack of side effects such as depression of respiration makes the drug more medically efficacious.

Psychic and physical dependence do occur, and tolerance after continued usage does develop, although at a slower rate than with either morphine or heroin. Although withdrawal symptoms also occur, they are much less severe than those associated with morphine or heroin.

The addict often finds Demerol to be a poor substitute, since its effects are not so intense. Abuse occurs most frequently among those in the medical profession who take the drug for its analgesic and sedative effects to cope with the stress and pressure of their work. Although there are no statistics available, the rate of abuse is probably not high.

**Codeine** (methylmorphine). This narcotic is found in the same plant as opium; however, it is usually extracted from morphine. The effects of codeine are similar to those of morphine but much milder.

Since it is chiefly effective as a cough suppressant, this drug is commonly found in cough medicine. It produces only a mild form of physical dependence, although psychic dependence may be much more intense. Tolerance does develop with continued use, but since the effects are mild, the withdrawal symptoms are also mild.

Abuse of codeine is most likely to occur when the drug is taken in pill form; in this way a stronger dosage may be ingested.

## Sedatives

Sedatives, in general, are depressant in their action and are used medically to promote sleep and to relieve anxiety and tension.

**Barbiturates.** These are the most widely used sedatives. Since they can produce sleep when used in sufficient strength, they are also called *hypnotics.* When taken in smaller doses, these drugs are effective in relieving tension and anxiety. Other medical purposes include use as a preoperative anesthetic, a source of relief for minor pain and high blood pressure, and a treatment for mental disturbances.

When abused, the drug is usually administered orally or intravenously. When taken in sufficient dosage, providing sleep does not occur, barbiturates can produce euphoria, confusion, and a release of inhibitions—a state similar to alcohol intoxication. Because of the confused and disoriented state, the barbiturate-intoxicated individual may ingest an overdose which can be fatal. This is especially true when a long-acting barbiturate is the user's choice.

Chronic abuse of barbiturates will result in the development of tolerance, psychic dependence, and physical dependence. In some cases, physical dependence to barbiturates can be more dangerous than physical dependence to narcotics. Sudden withdrawl of barbiturates carries the added danger of convulsions and the lack of muscular coordination. Convulsions, occurring with no medical supervision, can be fatal. It is not likely, however, that physical dependence will develop unless there is continued misuse by ingesting dosages greater than those used for therapeutic purposes.

In many instances the person who depends on barbiturates to induce sleep will, in turn, rely on a drug with antagonistic action (amphetamine) to get through the day. Thus, a cyclic form of dependence develops.

Barbiturates are sometimes used in combination with alcohol. This practice is dangerous since alcohol *potentiates* (makes more powerful) the effect of the drug; the result could be death due to respiratory failure.

There is much about a barbiturate addict that resembles the chronic alcoholic. He may become a detriment to himself, his family, and society for all the same reasons associated with alcoholism.

Approximately 30 to 40 commercial preparations of barbiturates are now marketed via prescription. The street names vary from terms such as "yellow-jackets" (nembutal) to "red-birds" (seconal).

If the drug culture of the 1960s could be termed the "speed generation," then the drug culture of the 1970s would be the "downer generation." That is, use of amphetamine type drugs is less favored now than the depressants, particularly barbiturates and alcohol.

**Tranquilizers.**   This term is applied to a large group of synthetic drugs that have a depressant action on the central nervous system. They are used medically to repress anxiety and tension but do not have a hypnotic-sedative effect. Tranquilizers are employed in the treatment of severe emotional disturbances; "minor" tranquilizers are used in treating milder forms of emotional disorders.

When tranquilizers are abused, the minor group is generally chosen. Even with these, psychic dependence, physical dependence, and tolerance can develop; withdrawal symptoms similar to those of barbiturates have been noted. By and large, however, tranquilizers have not been abused to any great extent by youth. More typically tranquilizers are chosen by the housewife or white-collar worker to allay tension or bolster confidence. Through continual use it is possible to stay mildly intoxicated a good portion of the time.

**Methaqualone.**   This chemical is a nonbarbiturate sedative that has recently gained widespread favor and in so doing has created overdosage and addiction problems on a new front. It has been used medically to promote sleep and to sedate. It is marketed under various brand names as Quaalude, Sopor, or Parest, but it is more often known on the street as "luding, Sopors, or Soapers."[2]

2. National Clearinghouse For Drug Abuse Information, Clearinghouse Report Series, Series 18, No. 1, "Methaqualone," October, 1973, p. 1.

Unfortunately, the almost instantaneous popularity of methaqualone was based in part on the mistaken belief that it was safe and non-addictive. Subsequent reports by the scientific community indicate that the drug is both dangerous and addictive. Overdosage can result in coma, delirium, and muscle spasms leading to convulsions. The user does, however, receive one break not afforded the users of many other drugs; methaqualone is not as yet manufactured underground and thus the pills on the street are pure, legally manufactured, and free of adulterants or impurities.[3]

## Stimulants

Amphetamines and methamphetamines are the stimulant drugs of primary consideration. Called stimulants because of their capacity to stimulate the central system, these drugs are used medically to treat mild depression and control appetite. Other legitimate uses involve counteracting fatigue and controlling narcolepsy.

Drugs of the amphetamine family do not produce physical dependence. Thus, unlike the case of narcotic and barbiturate dependence, an abuser of this drug will not experience withdrawal symptoms once the chemical is removed; tolerance, however, does develop. Often, the abuser will make the transition from "popping pills" to injecting intravenously because of increased tolerance. There seems to be a great potential for amphetamines to produce psychic dependence. Indeed, psychic dependence is the only real hold that this drug has. For example if one uses this substance to counteract fatigue in performing a task (cramming for exams or driving for a prolonged period), he may come to rely on this aid more and more. Because the fatigue itself is only masked and thereby accumulates, the chronic amphetamine user will eventually collapse in a state of exhaustion often accompanied by malnutrition.

Amphetamine-type drugs are abused as well for the euphoria they produce. Occasionally, the user who seeks an extra "kick" will mix the amphetamine-type with other drugs to create a "chemical potluck"; this sense of experimentation may heighten the psychic thrill for the chronic abuser.

In some individuals, amphetamines produce an acute form of psychosis. This is usually a paranoid reaction accompanied by auditory

3. *Ibid.* pp. 4, 5.

and visual hallucinations as well as anxiety. Such an episode is most likely to occur in those who have been taking the drug for protracted periods, although it has happened after a single dose.

**Methedrine** (meth-speed). This drug, which employs a methamphetamine substance, is usually the choice of habitual amphetamine abusers. It produces euphoria, hyperexcitability, violent and irrational reactions, and active psychosis when taken in massive dosage. It is usually injected intravenously, since the abuser desires the immediate onrush of euphoria, which has been likened to an intense and lengthy sexual orgasm.

The abuse of methedrine becomes a habit fraught with considerable hazards. Continued "highs" for days on end carry great risks: the abuser may suffer acute psychosis, a feeling of omnipotence often resulting in self-destructive acts; he may contract disease from unsterile needles; or, he may suffer health problems associated with undernourishment and loss of weight. "Speed Kills" was a slogan found on lapel but-

### The Great Banana Hoax

Three physicians with the Neuropsychiatric Institute of the University of California at Los Angeles reported that bananas do not contain any psychedelic properties. The smoking of dried scrapings from the inner portion of a banana peel called bananadine "mellow yellow" was thought to produce a "high" and visual hallucinations. Yet after a recent study no "trips" were reported; instead, the most common reactions seemed to be feelings of nausea, sore throats, dizziness and coughing spasms during and after the smoking of banana scrapings.

Chemical analyses of scrapings of banana peels and several samples of mellow yellow revealed only inert carboniferous material. Therefore all claims that this substance contains psychedelic or hallucinogenic properties are fraudulent. The only active ingredient in the banana appears to be the psychic suggestibility of the smoker in a proper setting.

Oliver E. Byrd, "The Great Banana Hoax," in *Medical Readings on Drug Abuse* by Oliver E. Byrd (Reading, Mass.: Addison-Wesley Publishing Co., Inc., 1970), pp. 188–9.

tons circulated in the Haight-Ashbury section of San Francisco some years ago. Unfortunately, this warning has not been heeded, and methedrine, when abused, continues to take its toll.

**Cocaine.**   This substance appears as a processed white powder extracted from the coca bush of South America. Although at one time cocaine was used in medicine because of its anesthetic properties, it is rarely used today.

The stimulant effects of cocaine are similar to those of amphetamines—excitability, euphoria, masking of fatigue, and anxiety. Ingestion occurs either by sniffing the powder or by injecting it with needle and syringe. At times cocaine is mixed with heroin when the antagonistic action of the two drugs is desired.

Since physical dependence and tolerance do not develop, psychic dependence is the primary factor in continued use. Cocaine has become more popular in the mid-seventies with those who can afford it. It has become a problem to such an extent that many concerned individuals are calling for an end to its manufacture.

## Hallucinogens

Because this group of drugs may be of diverse chemical structures, they produce auditory and/or visual illusions in varying duration and degree. They do not produce hallucinations in a true sense since the user is aware that the auditory and visual distortions are the result of the chemical within the body.

**LSD** (d-lysergic acid diethylamide tartrate 25).   This synthetic pseudo-hallucinogen is one of the most powerful drugs known to man. Lysergic acid is derived from a fungus (ergot) which is found in certain grasses, especially rye. It was first developed in 1938 by Dr. Albert Hoffman, who was experimenting with various substances in order to find a drug effective in combating migraine headaches.

There is a wide variance in the effects of LSD caused by such factors as dosage, mental state of the individual at the time of ingestion, and the setting in which he uses the drug. The effects are not predictable, since a pleasant experience may be followed by an extremely unpleasant one. The first effects of the drug are felt after about 45 minutes. Initially, the first reaction is one of anxiety, which is probably due to some apprehension on the part of the user. Immediate physiological changes due to the drug's influence are of little or no consequence. The psychic effects, however, usually last for several hours, but some have been recorded as lasting for several days. Occasionally, after the effects have worn off, they will return at a later time—perhaps even days or weeks later. This reoccurrence of the LSD experience is most frequent among chronic abusers.[4]

The effects one feels when under the influence of LSD are similar to those produced by other hallucinogens, but on a grander scale. These include: euphoria, feelings of anxiety or panic, intensification of the senses (colors are more vivid, sounds are magnified), distortions in perception of time and space, a feeling of merging with the external world, various hallucinations, impairment of the thought processes. It is theorized that these effects result from a breakdown of the brain. There is a loss of the orderly, selective perception and analysis of incoming sensory data. The consciousness is bombarded by a wide variety of external stimuli and subconscious material at random, which are both unstructured and startling.[5]

For some abusers the LSD experience produces terror and panic. This is especially true when the person has not been prepared for the experience or is alone when under the drug's influence.

If the precise effects of LSD on the brain are poorly understood, the "bad trip" is even less well understood. Researchers Ungerleider, Fisher, Fuller, and Caldwell compared 25 patients who had been hospitalized for psychotic reactions from LSD with 25 persons who had not been hospitalized, but who took LSD regularly. These investigators found that 12 percent of the hospitalized patients and 4 percent of the nonhospitalized patients were psychotic; 24 percent of the hospitalized and 48 percent of the others were diagnosed as having character disorders; 24 percent of the hospitalized and 16 percent of the nonhospitalized were found to be borderline psychotics. These investigators concluded that there is no single factor that prevents an adverse reaction to LSD.[6] Drs. Ungerleider and Fisher also claim that the values of LSD have not been sufficiently tested under well-controlled research conditions. The legitimate

4. Richard R. Lingeman, *Drugs from A to Z: A Dictionary* (New York: McGraw-Hill, 1969), p. 130.

5. *Ibid.*, pp. 131–34.

6. J. Thomas Ungerleider, Duke D. Fisher, Marielle Fuller, and Alex Caldwell, "The Bad Trip—The Etiology of the Adverse LSD Reaction," *American Journal of Psychiatry* (May 1968), 124:1483–90.

use of LSD as an adjuvant in psychiatry, in treating alcoholics and homosexuals, and in "death therapy" has been explored. To date, however, there is no unanimous agreement as to the efficacy of this chemical for such purposes.

There have been widely publicized reports of LSD's causing brain damage and damage to chromosomes that will affect future generations. Some research studies, for example, have found electroencephalographic (brain-wave patterns) readings of chronic LSD users to be similar to those of epileptic patients. Genetic studies of animals have revealed cases of chromosome breakage; among the offspring of animals that have been given LSD, birth defects have been noted. At this point, conclusive evidence pointing in any one direction is lacking. Too frequently the situation is further clouded by sensationalized reports of damage caused by LSD. A few years ago, for example, a reputable government official reported that a group of LSD users became blinded from staring at the sun while on a "trip." This story was later proved to be untrue.

Since LSD does not result in physical dependence, there is no abstinence syndrome. Tolerance occurs rapidly but diminishes just as rapidly; however, cross-tolerance to several other hallucinogens does de-

---

### Interviewing a User

The following is a conversation one of the authors had with a nineteen-year-old drug user:

*Q.* How long have you been using drugs, Roy?
*A.* Three or four years—four, I guess.
*Q.* What kinds?
*A.* Grass, acid, downers, speed.
*Q.* Heroin?
*A.* Just chipping, acid and grass mostly.
*Q.* How many acid trips have you taken?
*A.* I don't know, at least 300 I'd guess—a lot anyway.
*Q.* Any bad trips among them?
*A.* Yes, three.
*Q.* And you still went back for more?
*A.* Sure. You have to look at bummers just as something that can happen. I mean, it's a growing experience.

velop. Psychic dependence becomes a problem for some, although the intensity of this dependence may not be as great as with some other drugs. For the most part, LSD is not the kind of drug that is illicitly used on a daily basis, because of the intensity and duration of the experience.

In a clinical setting the drug has been used as a therapeutic aid in treating chronic alcoholics, severely emotionally disturbed patients, homosexuals, and autistic children. When used for these purposes, LSD has been reported to be beneficial. Other authorities, however, are skeptical of its efficacy. At present the number of research projects involving LSD usage have been drastically cut back, probably due to adverse publicity.

**Peyote.** This hallucinogen is derived from a portion of a cactus plant called *peyotl,* which is indigenous to Mexico. The button-shaped growths of the plant are the actual source of the drug. Ingestion takes place after the growths have been dried in the sun.

Use of this drug causes hallucinations and intensification of color and sound, but to lesser intensity than produced by LSD. Physical dependence does not follow continued use, but psychic dependence may be induced. Tolerance occurs to a limited degree.

---

It's possible to control them. By that I mean if you don't get greedy and drop too much at once, know where you are, etc., you'll be ok.

Q. Any problems when you're down? Any flashbacks?

A. No flashbacks, but I do have trouble concentrating at times and movements that people make are disconcerting. I mean sometimes it's hard to concentrate on what someone is saying when they're moving their hands and arms.

Q. Do you plan to continue to use LSD?

A. I don't think so. Well, maybe just once in a great while as a refresher about what is really important in life.

Q. Do you have a job, going to college or anything?

A. No, nothing now.

Q. How do you provide for yourself?

A. I manage. I don't need much to get by.

Peyote is used legally by North American Indians as a sacrament in the religious rites of the Native American Church of North America. Illicit use of the drug is not as frequent as abuse of some other hallucinogens, a fact attributed to the relative mildness of its hallucinogenic properties and to its lack of availability.

**Mescaline.** This substance is one of the alkaloids found in the peyote plant. It is very likely that this alkaloid produced the hallucinogenic action of the peyote buttons; dependence and tolerance, too, develop just as with the use of peyote. In synthetic form, however, mescaline does not produce as many unpleasant side effects as peyote and is therefore more favored by drug abusers.

**STP.** These initials have come to mean more than the motor oil additive. STP belongs to a family of chemicals called the *amines* that include the hormones epinephrine and norepinephrine, two of the body's substances that affect the mind-body relationship. The Federal Bureau of Drug Abuse Control classifies this chemical as a derivative of mescaline.

Users of STP claim that the drug produces a heightened sensation of energy and that the hallucinogenic action is more intense and longer-lasting than that of LSD. Localized epidemics of psychotic breaks have been reported resulting from the use of STP.

**DMT** (N-dimethyltryptamine). This hallucinogen is sometimes referred to as the "business man's lunch," because its effects come about quickly and last for only upward to an hour. Although physical dependence does not develop, tolerance and psychic dependence will develop with continued use. The abuse of this particular drug is said to be increasing at present.

**Marijuana.** Although legally defined as a narcotic, marijuana is more hallucinogenic in its effects. It is derived from the Indian hemp plant (*Cannabis sativa*), the same plant used at one time in the manufacturing of rope. The leaves, stalk, and flowering top of the female plant are cleaned, dried, and shredded before being employed for their hallucinogenic effect. The drug is then usually smoked in cigarette form or by means of a pipe.

The potency of *Cannabis sativa* varies from place to place, depending on climate, soil, and the degree of cultivation it receives. The variety found in Middle and Far Eastern countries is of a much greater strength than the North American variety. In the eastern part of the world, marijuana is known as *hashish, charas, ghanja,* and *bhang.* Described as hav-

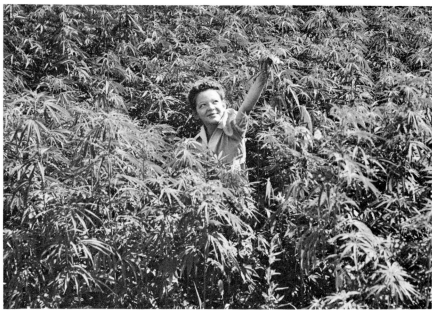

A field of the hemp plant (Cannabis sativa).

ing 8 to 10 times the potency found in our home-grown variety, hashish is principally composed of the resin found in the plant's flowering tops. The resin contains the hallucinogenic-activating ingredient (tetrahydro-cannabinol) in concentration.

Authorities agree that physical dependence and concomitant withdrawal symptoms are not associated with marijuana use. However, as with any drug, psychic dependence is possible. The tolerance phenomenon occurs only to a slight extent.

After ingestion, fairly immediate physiological changes such as dizziness, conjunctivitis, hunger, increased heart rate, lack of muscular coordination, and tightness in the chest may occur. There is no concrete evidence to support a view as to physiological alterations caused by long-term abuse of marijuana.

Subjectively, the user may experience a sense of well-being, euphoria, hilarity, spatial and time distortion, fragmentation of thoughts, anxiety, and hallucinations. The latter occur when the more potent variety (hashish) is used.

Several studies have indicated that the magnitude or even the presence of any effects at all seems to depend on one's expectations, mood, and the setting. This is especially true for the neophyte, since one must learn certain techniques in order to achieve the greatest return in effects. For example, in a laboratory setting the user may experience little or no effects; he may even experience dysphoria. At a party, with its psychedelic atmosphere and spirit of camaraderie, the sought-after effects may be attained. The suggestive influence produced by group expectations as to behavior may play a part in producing these effects.

Psychotic breaks due to a "bad trip" with marijuana have been reported but are rare in this country. Reports of this nature from other countries, where there is continued use of the more potent form of the drug, occur with greater frequency.

No other drug, with the exception of alcohol during the Prohibition Era, has been so widely used in defiance of the law as has marijuana. Some authorities estimate that 20 million persons either have used or are at present using the drug.

The stringent legal controls placed on marijuana sale, possession, and use date back to the Marijuana Tax Act of 1937. Under federal statutes, mere possession of the drug is a felony. Conviction can mean a prison sentence, loss of civil rights, and a criminal record that can return to haunt even the one-time experimenter. Similarly, many states classify possession of marijuana as a felony. Responsible people and organizations throughout the country have gone on record requesting the easing of these penalties. These people argue that the law is not realistic and, since the penalty is so severe, it is not being enforced. There are also those who advocate immediate legalization of marijuana. To them, it is a harmless intoxicant which is actually healthier to use than alcohol.

All the evidence on marijuana is not in. It has only been within the last few years that the activating principle (THC) has been synthesized for the purposes of research. Now answers are needed to important questions. What physiological and mental alterations, if any, develop in the chronic user? Why do some users go on to other more dangerous drugs, while other users do not? If marijuana becomes legal, will it be legal for everyone, and in all the varieties of the drug? What are the possibilities of marijuana dependence becoming a problem similar in magnitude to present alcohol dependence? Why do some chronic abusers of marijuana begin to focus on the drug to the extent that they turn inward, disregarding prior personal goals as well as society in general?

Consideration of legalizing marijuana is irresponsible until there is a compendium of supportive evidence. However, because of their dire consequences, a reevaluation of the present marijuana laws is in order.

**Solvents.** These include volatile substances such as glue, gasoline, paint thinner, and lighter fluid which are used for their intoxicating effects. Of these, model airplane glue is abused to the greatest extent; the substance is placed in a bag or handkerchief and the fumes are inhaled. After a number of whiffs, the individual experiences a euphoric feeling akin to the effects of alcohol. Similarly, he may exhibit a staggering gait and slurred speech, both of which are associated with alcohol intoxication. The period of intoxication is followed by drowsiness, stupor, and, in some cases, loss of consciousness.

Physical dependence does not develop. While complete information is lacking, one can assume that tolerance does develop to a slight extent; the same can be said of psychic dependence. Possible, although unsubstantiated, medical problems associated with solvent inhalation include damage to liver, heart, blood and the nervous system. Development of psychotic behavior has also been exhibited following solvent inhalation.[7]

## Controlling Drug Abuse

Attempts by society to control the abuse of drugs bring us back to our original definition of drug abuse. It is explicit in this definition that substances are abused when they become detrimental to the individual and to society.

## Federal and State Statutes

Much federal legislation, dating back to the turn of the century, has formed the primary basis of control over drugs. By and large, state legislation has been modeled after federal enactments, although state laws do vary considerably.

The U.S. Congress passed legislation under Public Law 91–513, The Comprehensive Drug Abuse Prevention and Control Act of 1970, which served to increase some penalties for selling, while reducing other penalties for simple possession. Generally, greater discretionary powers are given to the courts. This act, along with the Drug Abuse Control

7. Smith, Kline and French, *Drug Abuse,* p. 43.

Amendment of 1965 and the Dangerous Drug Penalty Amendment of 1968, established machinery to control the dispersal and usage of depressant and stimulant drugs. Any drug having a potential for abuse is included under these regulations. Determination of whether or not a drug has potential for abuse is the task of an advisory committee to the Food and Drug Administration. For example, hallucinogenic drugs have been included under these regulations as being potentially abusive. As a result, possession of these drugs for the first offender constitutes a misdemeanor; conviction can carry a prison sentence up to one year and a fine of not more than $1,000.

In many cases individual states have more stringent regulations and penalties than those at the federal level. In some states, for example, marijuana is legally defined as a narcotic; possession is therefore considered a felony which, upon conviction, can carry a prison sentence of 2-10 years. More startling is the fact that in some states, for selling any dangerous drug, one can receive the death penalty.

In 1968 the Federal Bureau of Narcotics was removed from the Treasury Department, and the Bureau of Drug Abuse Control was removed from the Department of Health, Education, and Welfare. This action resulted in the formation of the Bureau of Narcotics and Dangerous Drugs within the Justice Department. Effective May 1, 1971, the Comprehensive Prevention and Control Act further clarified the function of the Bureau of Narcotics and Dangerous Drugs. This apparent strengthening of a law enforcement approach to drug control was continued under the Nixon administration.

To be sure, regulations designed to promote abstinence have had some impact in the past. Many concerned individuals, however, agree that the drug problem is multifaceted; it is much more than simply a medical and legal problem. Demands for immediate and total abstinence through legislation have never been nor ever will be the ultimate solution to the drug abuse problem.

## Toward a Solution

In order to understand the effects of drugs, it is necessary to understand the psychology of the individual who uses them. Progress is made in those quarters where the chronic abuser is considered to be emotionally troubled rather than a criminal. Abusers of drugs do not fit into the mold or stereotype in which they are often placed. The real problem therefore,

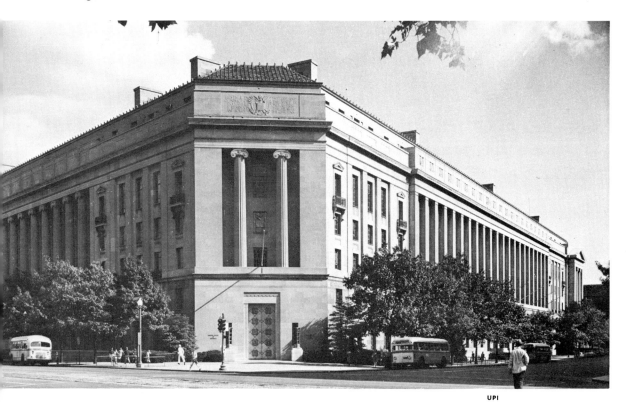

UPI

Justice Department Building in Washington, D.C.

is not drugs but the people who use drugs. Use of drugs involves problems of a personal, social, and intellectual nature. It is the individual with motives for using drugs who is the real key to understanding the drug problem. Thus, there is an immediate need for scientific inquiry into all facets of the drug problem, but with a priority for investigation into the psychology of the user himself.[8]

## Drugs and the College Student

One must accept the fact that drug usage satisfies some needs, whether the need is to satisfy one's curiosity or to escape reality. It is Dr. Helen Nowlis' contention that in order to understand drug usage on the college

8. *Ibid.,* p. 43.

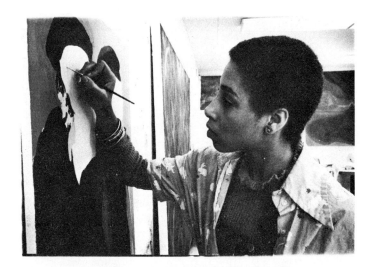

Finding satisfaction in reality through creative channels can deter young people away from escape through drug abuse.

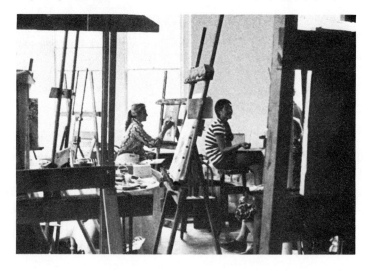

campus it is necessary to look at the student and the demands of the world he lives in. She offers the following general observations:

1. All college students are at one or another stage in growth from childhood to adulthood. This growth process involves both the unlearning of modes of behavior which were appropriate and rewarded in childhood and the learning of new modes in accordance with society's definition of the adult role, a definition that is neither clear nor consistent. Neither meaningful identity nor

a set of values to live by are easily bestowed. The irony of the appeal of LSD is that, in one way or another, it can be perceived as offering a promise of help in all of these difficult tasks. What LSD is said to offer is inviting for the weary traveler, inviting in direct proportion to the degree of weariness.

2. Other reasons why students use drugs are, for the most part, the same reasons that adults use drugs such as alcohol, tranquilizers, amphetamines, barbiturates, aspirin, nicotine, and caffeine. All of these are used by a variety of people for a variety of reasons. Some adults try these drugs, some react badly or do not find what they are seeking and never try again; some use them to escape; some are as dependent, psychologically or in some cases physically, as they would be in their dependence on an opiate. The main difference is that these substances are socially acceptable and are fairly easily available.

3. More young people than most adults would care to admit are weary of chasing the same carrot at the end of the same stick for 14 to 16 years. They dream of getting out of the "rat race" just for a while. For some, this may be accomplished by dropping out with the assistance of marijuana or LSD.

4. The response of society to student drug use may foster further use when the response is based on assumptions which seem contradictory or hypocritical to the student.

5. The more one inquires into all aspects of the drug problem, the more one is impressed with the importance of availability. Since infancy the student has learned to open his mouth on command and swallow whatever was popped in to cure what ailed him, and he has watched his parents do the same.

6. Another important aspect of current society is its attitude toward risk. Students have grown up in an atmosphere which takes risks for granted and assumes that there is little that can be done without risk. Thus, an adequate description of risks involved in drug use may serve as an effective deterrent to some but have no effect or even the opposite effect on others.

7. Students feel the need for deep and meaningful experience in an increasingly secular society. They want a personally meaningful part in a world which seems so full of aggression, discrimination, poverty, famine, alcoholism, divorce, and hypocrisy that the individual seems superfluous. They want a "frontier" in which to find adventure, challenge, and an opportunity to prove themselves at a time when the only frontiers available for the many would seem to be the technological jungle or the world within. Some of them are rejecting the jungle and withdrawing into the inner world.[9]

## Designs for Progress

There is a need for society to understand that the real problem of drug abuse involves people more than drugs, to understand that the problem

9. Helen Nowlis, *Drugs on the College Campus* (Garden City: Doubleday, 1969), pp. 18–19.

## Most Frequently Used Drugs
## at Five Major Universities

During the fall semester of the 1970–71 academic year, a drug use questionnaire was administered to undergraduate students enrolled in health education classes at five universities. This questionnaire was designed to measure drug use behavior and certain social values related to drug usage. . . .

The universities participating in this study were:

1. Arizona State University, Tempe, Arizona.
2. Pennsylvania State University, University Park, Pennsylvania.
3. Northern Colorado University, Greeley, Colorado.
4. New York State University, Geneseo, New York.
5. University of Tennessee, Knoxville, Tennessee.

A review of the data indicates that alcohol is the most widely used mood modifying drug. The percentages ranged from 78% at Pennsylvania State University to 92% at New York State University at Geneseo. . . .

Marijuana ranked second to alcohol as a drug most frequently used to alter mood and perception. The percentage of students who had used marijuana at least once ranged from 49% at Arizona State University to 28% at New York State University at Geneseo. . . .

The majority of those using marijuana are either one time users or have used the drug less than eleven times. For example, 56% of the marijuana users at Arizona State University

is complex and multidimensional.[10] There is the need to realize that the drug abuse problem has been sensationalized and that the important scientific questions are only now being asked. The drug abuser must be

10. *Ibid.*, pp. 22–24.

have used the drug less than eleven times; however, 32% of the users consider themselves weekend and party users. This same pattern is reflected at the other universities involved in this study. . . .

Concerning marijuana and certain social values, the students questioned indicated they considered their present state laws relative to marijuana possession too harsh. Tennessee was somewhat conservative, but a majority (57%) expressed displeasure with the law, while 70% of the Penn. State University students considered the law too harsh for marijuana possession.

When we asked marijuana users if they turned others on to drugs, 40% of the users at the University of Tennessee said they did, while only 26% at Northern Colorado University were concerned with encouraging others to use marijuana.

Do marijuana users tend to abuse their drug more than alcohol users? The answer is yes if you utilize daily use as the criterion for abuse. At Northern Colorado University 4% of the alcohol users were daily users, while at the same university 13% of the marijuana users were daily users. At Arizona State University 5% of the alcohol users were daily imbibers, while 10% of the marijuana users "lit up" daily. . . . Paradoxically, the two eastern universities reversed this trend with alcohol users abusing their drug more than marijuana users. . . .

Jack V. Toohey, "An Analysis of Drug Use Behavior at Five American Universities" in *Student Guide to Personal Health* by Betty J. Bachmann, Thomas L. Dezelsky, and Jack V. Toohey (Dubuque, Ia.: Kendall/Hunt Publishing Company, 1971), pp. 122–3. Reprinted by permission of the authors.

investigated in his own native habitat. There is a need for education, since prevention is the key word for the drug abuse problem. This education must involve learning how to "turn on" without a chemical aid. It must involve learning how to cope with one's frustrations and how to escape from the "rat race" without dropping out of the human race by totally turning inward.

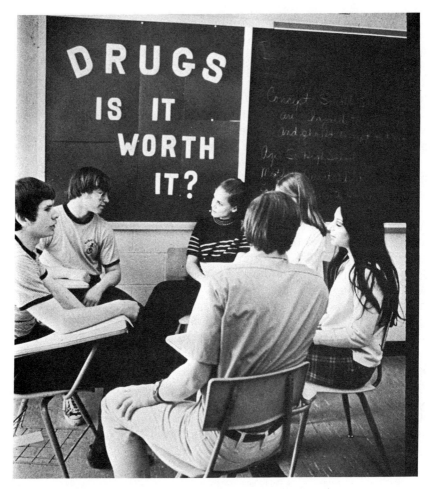

Society needs to understand that the real problem of drug abuse involves people more than drugs.

## Questions for Study and Discussion

1. What effect, if any, has the advancement in medical science had on the abuse of drugs?
2. Why should a chronic abuser of drugs be considered emotionally troubled, rather than a criminal?
3. Is there any relationship between criminal activity and the use of marijuana?

4. Is there any one personality type that is most inclined to experiment with drugs?
5. Why are there individual differences in regard to hypersensitivity to drugs?
6. Is there a difference in meaning between the terms "experimenter" and "user" when used in reference to drug taking?
7. Why has there been little success in completely rehabilitating the heroin user?
8. Compare the United States and British systems as to their effectiveness in controlling their drug abuse situations.
9. What methods are currently being employed in the treatment of those persons physically dependent upon narcotics?
10. Compare the methods of treatment of the government hospitals at Lexington, Kentucky, and Fort Worth, Texas, to such private organizations as Synanon and Daytop Village.

## References

Cohen, Sidney. *The Drug Dilemma,* New York: McGraw-Hill, 1969.

Commonwealth of Pennsylvania, Division of Public Health Education, Division of Drug Control. *Teachers' Resource Guide on Drug Abuse.* Harrisburg, 1968.

Ebin, David (Ed.). *The Drug Experience.* New York: Grove Press, 1961.

Hyde, Margaret O. *Mind Drugs.* New York: McGraw-Hill, 1969.

Jones, Kenneth L.; Shainberg, Louis W.; Byer, Curtis O. *Drugs and Alcohol.* New York: Harper and Row, 1969.

*Journal of the American Medical Association,* "Dependence on Amphetamines and Other Stimulant Drugs," vol. 197, Sept. 19, 1966.

Lingeman, Richard R. *Drugs from A to Z: A Dictionary.* New York: McGraw-Hill, 1969.

Nowlis, Helen H. *Drugs on the College Campus.* Garden City: Doubleday, 1969.

Smith, Kline and French Laboratories. *Drug Abuse: Escape to Nowhere, A Guide for Educators.* Philadelphia: 1967.

# 7

# Alcohol: Your Decision

## General Concept

Alcoholic beverages may alter behavior and produce certain physiological effects upon the body, dependent upon strength and frequency of consumption.

## Outcomes

The student should be able to:
1. Explain the psychological and physiological effects of alcohol
2. Explain how alcoholic beverages may manifest mood alterations and inability to control behavior
3. Realize that alcoholic beverages may produce unpredictable behavior
4. Avoid regular usage of alcoholic beverages if it appears to lead to dependency, disease, or undesirable social patterns
5. Explain the signs and symptoms of alcoholism
6. Identify misconceptions associated with alcoholism
7. Explain treatments and preventive programs for alcoholism.

## Decision to Drink

Have you ever attended a fraternity party where booze flowed abundantly, where students were intentionally gulping drinks to escape aca-

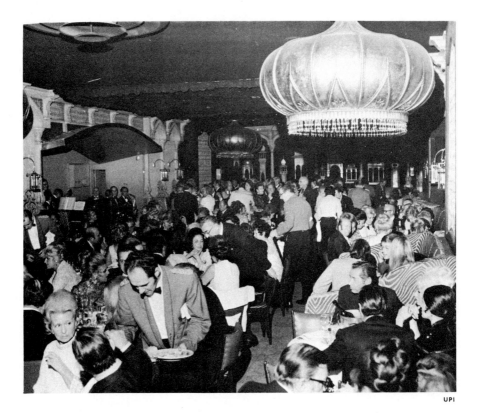

UPI

Approximately 70 percent of adult Americans drink, and 40 percent are regular drinkers.

demic pressures, or where individuals were merely attempting to relax and become sociable through the use of alcohol?

On any given Friday or Saturday evening, students seem to migrate to parties, apartments, drive-in movies or a local bar. The catalyst that will initiate the guaranteed pleasurable experience will be some type of alcoholic beverage consumed throughout the evening.

Some students drink because their friends or dates encourage them to. Others drink out of curiosity, to rebel against legal ages for drinking, to appear mature, to appear sophisticated, to relax, to become slightly euphoric—and some simply drink to get drunk. Surprisingly, most young people have decided whether or not to drink prior to arriving on a college campus. In fact, the proportion of high school students who drink has doubled from 39 percent in 1969 to 74 percent in 1972. There is now

## Teen-agers' Drinking Habits

92% of American high school students have at least
sampled alcohol.
23% use alcohol occasionally.
9% class themselves as drinkers.
6% say they are frequent users.

These are the results of a survey of American high school
students as reported by Dr. George Maddox in his book *The
Domesticated Drug.*

A further interesting fact is that as many as 80% of teens
in the Northeast use alcohol while as few as 25% in the South
use it.

Since many young people attempt to mimic adults, their
ultimate outlook on alcohol is largely influenced by the conduct and attitude of their elders; by and large the latter tend
to view alcohol as a recreational beverage rather than as a
drug. Furthermore, Maddox believes that teenagers' values
are affected greatly by the advertising media which try to
identify the fundamental values of the young with alcohol.
One of the strongest influences, however, is peer pressure;
one drinks to be included.

According to Maddox, only three human conditions tie up
more medical resources than alcohol-related problems—
heart disease, cancer, and mental illness.

Excerpt from "Study Reveals Drinking Habits of Teen-agers," *Today's Health,* November 1970,
p. 72, published by the American Medical Association. Reprinted by permission of the
publisher.

an increase in arrests of young people for intoxication.[1] In contrast, however, few students are aware of, or understand the traditional American
custom of social drinking or the problems of the alcoholic.

It is estimated that between 70 and 75 percent of our population
does engage in drinking, whether it be an occasional sip of champagne

1. "Rising Toll of Alcoholism," *U.S. News,* October 29, 1973, p. 45.

at a wedding, to a regular evening cocktail session. Some people drink daily while others, frequently students, restrict themselves to weekend drinking patterns. Those who abstain on campuses may do so because of violation of college regulations or because they cannot afford the practice. Administrators on some campuses have permitted alcoholic beverages to be sold in the student unions if not in violation of state laws. Some authorities feel that eighteen should be the legal age for drinking, but in most states it is illegal to drink before the age of twenty-one.

At The Pennsylvania State University, a sample survey of drinking practices was conducted by random interview in an attempt to make a videotape on alcohol. The majority of students interviewed did not hesitate to admit that they drank regularly at all social events and were minors. Many students feel that present drinking laws are outdated and seldom enforced, except if they are caught in an automobile accident or if they are making an illegal purchase of an alcoholic beverage.

College students usually find a friend of legal age to make the purchase for them to avoid entanglement with law enforcement. It is not uncommon to find one fraternity brother purchasing for his entire house. While drinking on campus or in fraternity houses may not be acceptable university policies, students continue to do so because everyone else does—and the laws are seldom enforced. Once driving is involved, however, police rarely hesitate in making proper arrests.

Each individual must decide for himself which direction he intends to follow regarding alcohol. One cannot wait until he is offered a drink or a cocktail to weigh the facts and decide.

There are three alternatives for the adult of legal age today. He may (1) choose to abstain, (2) choose to become a social drinker, or (3) become an alcoholic. Those who become alcoholics never *choose* this alternative, but according to statistics one in fifteen Americans will become an alcoholic once he has selected the social drinking pattern. (One-third of the population abstain, two-thirds drink socially.)

## Historical Significance

For more than 3,000 years, human beings have consumed some type of ethyl alcohol ($C_2H_5OH$). Where the practice first began is unknown to man, but some authorities think that the discovery of alcohol took place when early cavemen left their dwellings to go hunting, left behind

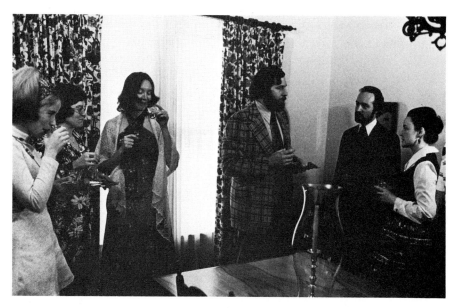

One in fifteen Americans will become an alcoholic once he has selected the social drinking pattern.

a bowl of grapes, and returned to see and smell a changed appearance in the grapes due to the then unknown process of fermentation. The Cro-magnon might have tasted it, noticed the unusual tang, and gulped it down. Thereafter, having experienced the first "high" or state of inebriation, he probably spread the news to his friends.

Although we cannot trace the discovery of alcohol, the impact that alcohol has had upon the history of mankind is phenomenal. As a sage commented in 1690: "You say man learned first to build a fire, and then to ferment his liquor. Had he but reversed the process, we should have no need of flint and tinder to this day."[2]

References to alcohol are found in ancient Babylonian tablets, Hebrew scripts, and Egyptian carvings. Archeologists recently discovered the ruins of a huge winery 2,600 years old in Gideon, near Jerusalem, which had a storage capacity of 30,000 gallons of wine as well as stone presses for grapes.

During the period 500 to 1400 A.D., Europe became known as the winegrowing center of the world. Poets, artists, and monks were all in-

2. Morris Chafetz, *Liquor, the Servant of Man* (London: Phoenix House, 1967), p. 12.

spired by the influence of alcohol. In Greece and Egypt, alcohol was said to be a gift of the gods. At some ancient drinking parties, people would drink for days during any given festival period. Legend has it that one drinking festival lasted a full year without interruption after a successful year of grape production. Ancient drinkers consumed wine at festivals but also used it as a substitute for water, as a seal of agreement, and in battle and war, as well as for social hospitality.

At the close of the eighteenth century, the Industrial Revolution stimulated workers to turn to drink and England became famous for her gin and ales. Spain, Italy, and France battled for prestige and economic prosperity in their continued production of fine wines. Germany produced some wines but was later to become famous for her tasty beer and ales. Today West Germany still observes ancient drinking customs. Each year in the fall Munich establishes a festival grounds area for a spirited 16-day beer bust called the "Oktoberfest." (For more than 300 years Munich used brewery horses to deliver beer to nearby inns and taverns, but studies recently revealed that the horses were becoming ill and losing their glossy coats due to air pollution in Munich. Now they only appear in colorful decor delivering beer during the Oktoberfest.)

When the Puritans arrived in the United States, they brought with them their liquor, a reputation for enjoyment, and excessive drinking habits. They drank hard cider, applejack, and imported Jamaican rum. Later they manufactured rum in New England, and it soon played a significant role in the American Revolution. It expanded commerce, built the slave trade, and enriched the cities.[3]

Later, as the frontiersman moved West, he realized that he could not afford rum and soon began to make his own whiskey from corn and rye. Wines were ignored and the Americanized bourbon soon became the most sought-after beverage.

The adventurous frontiersman, stricken with anxiety, troubled with uncertainty, distressed with hardship, soon began gulping drinks. Saloons appeared in various towns where hard liquor, easy women, and gambling became a popular way to relax. Drinking and violence were closely related, and eventually the prohibitionists were successful in abolishing alcohol with the Eighteenth Amendment.

3. *Ibid.,* p. 30.

Just as drinking laws are ignored today in many places, so may we visualize the drinkers in a frenzied era of the "Roaring Twenties." In 1921, Monahan wrote in *Dry America:*

To believe that Prohibition will stand is, in my view, to believe that the Republic has lost her way and is without the guiding light of her noblest traditions. Every hour since the adoption of the Eighteenth Amendment has borne witness to the monstrous folly and unintelligence of the act. But what the American *people have done,* the American *people can undo.*

The undoing of this amendment took thirteen years.

To avoid the stigma attached to drinking in a saloon atmosphere, advertising, films, and magazines soon painted a new picture of drinking America. Drinking became a respectable pastime once again. The "cocktail hour" appeared; beautiful restaurants and cocktail lounges were built, and the states once again controlled drinking regulations.

Today, whether you chug 12 beers at a fraternity party, attend a sophisticated cocktail hour in suburbia, occasionally sip champagne at a wedding reception, or patronize a local Playboy Club or tavern, alcohol has once again renewed its force in our American culture.

## $C_2H_5OH$

What is an alcoholic beverage? Two types of alcohol are methyl and ethyl. Methyl alcohol is used for commercial purposes in the manufacture of such items as perfume, shaving lotion, and rubbing alcohol. Ethyl alcohol, or "beverage alcohol," is the active ingredient present in beer, wine, and distilled liquors. Ethyl alcohol is a liquid which is odorless, has no color, and can readily be mixed with water.

The three families of ethyl alcohol consist of beer, wine, and distilled liquors. Interpretation of the measurement of alcohol frequently is confusing because of the way in which it is advertised. For example, if a bourbon is advertised at "86 proof," there is 43 percent alcoholic content, the remaining 57 percent consisting of flavored water. Interpretation of percentage of alcohol is always translated at one-half the advertised proof. Since distillers want to promote strong liquors, they do not advertise by percentage, for fear customers will think their product weak. Beer and wine, however, are measured by percentage of alcohol by volume.

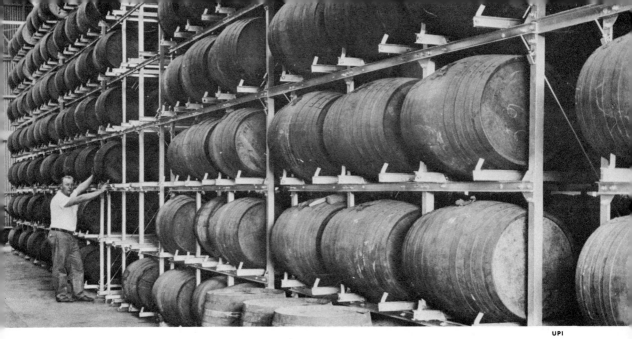

The aging process of two hundred and fifty thousand gallons of rum.

Beer usually contains 4-7 percent alcohol, simple fermented wines 12-14 percent, up to 21 percent in fortified wines, and hard liquors from 40-50 percent alcohol. Although all ethyl alcohol produces similar effects, methods of production differ.

Beer and ales are produced by the process of brewing, using corn, barley, or wheat. These grains are soaked in water to cause them to sprout. A chemical action transforms the starch in the grain into sugar. When dry, the sprouted grain is mashed into a fine powder called *malt*. Malt is added to grain and placed in vats of hot water where hops and yeast are added. Fermentation begins and when the alcoholic content reaches 3-5 percent, it is beer. If fermentation continues up to 6 or 8 percent alcohol, it is called ale.

Wines are processed through fermentation in which the action of the yeast cells on fruits or grapes changes the sugar content into alcohol and carbon dioxide gas. Fermentation usually stops when alcohol content reaches 14 percent.

Hard liquor such as whiskey, rum, brandy, and gin are derived from the process of distillation. The level of alcoholic content is determined by distilling. The more the liquid is distilled, the less water will be present. Hard liquor is made from grain and vegetables and the fermenting process changes starch to sugar and sugar to alcohol. When the alcohol boils at 173° and the water at 212°F., they rise and steam, passing through coiled pipes, resulting in an alcohol-water combination such as distilled whiskey.

## Effects of Alcohol

The primary effect of alcohol on the brain is that it serves as a depressant or a narcotic. Although it is a popular misconception that alcohol is a stimulant, it is actually a means of depressing the highest areas of the brain, such as intelligence, judgment, and our behavioral control centers. Although many individuals appear to loosen up after a few drinks and may appear stimulated, they have actually sedated or depressed their inhibitions.

As the amount of alcohol in the blood increases, more areas of the brain are affected. If enough alcohol is consumed, death can result if the respiratory and circulatory centers become depressed.

Alcohol is a unique substance in that it is absorbed immediately into the blood stream, without the digestive process. It is usually absorbed directly through the walls of the stomach if the stomach is empty. Food in the stomach will retard absorption rate. The degree of intoxication or rate of absorption varies among individuals.

Body weight and tolerance level may affect intoxication because of the amount of alcohol in the blood. Often a small, light person will become intoxicated more quickly than a large, heavy person since the percentage of alcohol in his blood compared to the large heavy person is greater, assuming that each consumes the same number and type of drinks. If the larger person seldom has a drink, however, and the smaller person is a heavy drinker, the smaller person will have increased his tolerance level, thereby retarding his intoxication. For example, in identical circumstances, a big man weighing 200 pounds would have to take twice as much alcohol as a woman weighing 100 pounds for both to reach the same concentration in their blood.[4]

---

4. "Alcohol and Alcoholism—A Police Handbook," prepared by the Correctional Association of New York and The International Association of Chiefs of Police, pp. 9–11.

In the majority of the states, drivers are considered legally inebriated if the alcohol concentration in their blood exceeds 0.15 percent. Generally speaking, the percentage of alcohol in the blood will produce the following effects:

0.1 percent—noticeable breath odor

0.15 percent—legal intoxication

0.2 percent—awkward, clumsy movements

0.3 percent—staggering, hesitant walk

0.4 percent—helplessness

0.5 percent—fatality (death likely to occur)

In some states tightening up intoxication laws, 0.1 percent is the standard set for legal intoxication. The breathalyzer is now replacing the balloon and Hargometer tests once used for detection by law enforcement personnel.

Since alcohol first alters the behavioral control centers of the brain, it will also retard muscular control and the sense organs. Alcohol does, however, affect other parts of the body:

1. Small blood vessels become dilated in the skin.
2. As a result of dilation, the skin becomes red and the person feels warm.
3. Coordination is retarded.
4. Over 90 percent of alcohol absorbed into the body is disposed of by oxidation to carbon dioxide and water, which could result in eventual damage to the liver.
5. Reaction time and speech are retarded.
6. A person may experience double vision and color blindness.
7. Hearing is impaired, so drinkers at a party begin talking louder without being aware of it.
8. Because of the sedated effect, one may become dizzy or fall asleep.
9. Two minutes after consuming a drink, alcohol is directly in the blood stream.
10. About 2 percent of the alcohol is released through breath, urination, and sweat.

Each individual should be aware of his own absorption rate and the number of drinks he is able to consume without serious negative results. The average person should be able to oxidize one-half to an ounce of whiskey per hour. This might be compared to six or twelve ounces of beer per hour. A rule of thumb to remember when driving is to wait an hour per drink before attempting to handle the wheel.

Contrary to what advertising might have you believe, a drink does not make you appear more attractive. Because the intelligence and self-critical faculties are the first to be affected, the drinking individual is not realistically aware how he may appear to others.

Terhune categorizes intoxication by the following behavior degrees:

First degree: A smile, slight relaxation, a sense of well-being.

Second degree: Loss of intelligent behavior, impaired judgment, loud boastful, tells off-color stories. Typical at cocktail parties.

Third degree: Noisy, irritable, poor manners, may fight or weep, inconsiderate, vulgar sexual advances and exhibitionist tendencies. May result in nausea or sleep.

Fourth degree: An inability to stand or walk, irregular breathing, unconsciousness, loss of sphinetic control.[5]

Alcohol causes a "hangover." A hangover is a feeling of nausea, gastritis, headache, anxiety, or fatigue. It may be only one condition or a combination of these factors. When a person indulges in heavy drinking during an evening, there is the possibility of a hangover the next morning. The drinker may have overexhausted his muscles and body processes, just as he had temporarily lost an element of his reasoning powers. He has exerted the body beyond its means. Therefore, even if the drinker does not feel the other conditions, he will be fatigued the next day—a type of hangover.

The hangover, while unpleasant, is rarely dangerous. Unfortunately, there is no scientific evidence to support various home remedies proposed for curing hangovers. Such theories as "drink coffee," "have a hair of the dog," "eat a piece of bread," "try Alka-Seltzer," are unfounded. For general treatment, physicians usually prescribe aspirin, bed rest, and ingestion of solid foods as soon as possible.[6]

Other physical effects may occur besides oxidation, tolerance levels, and absorption processes. Obesity may eventually be an end result of continuous drinking, since alcohol has a high caloric content which makes for extra calories in the diet. Yet alcohol is not a complete food, since it fails to meet the requirements of a nutrient (it does not contain vitamins, minerals, or amino acid). Alcoholics or regular heavy drinkers may

5. William Terhune, *The Safe Way to Drink* (New York: William Morrow, 1968), pp. 31–32.

6. National Institute of Mental Health, "Alcohol and Alcoholism," Public Health Service Publication no. 1640, U. S. Department of Health, Education and Welfare.

---

### The Congeners in Drinks

It has been discovered that the congeners in drinks, the chemicals of various sorts that become incorporated into alcoholic beverages during their manufacture, play a disputed role in causing hangovers. Hangovers are blamed on both alcohol and congeners, the substances sometimes formed during fermentation. But congeners have been particularly implicated by a few studies, and as those done by Dr. Henry B. Murphree of the Neuropsychiatric Institute. One group of volunteers had drinks heavily spiked with congeners. He found that these people exhibited more hangover symptoms than did those members of the control group who were given similar drinks with fewer congeners. Therefore, as a cautionary measure for party goers, bourbon whiskey (.246) and brandy (cognac) (.212) contain a high percentage of congeners, while gin (.0039) and vodka (.0026) have the lowest percentage.

Walter Modell and Alfred Lansing and editors, *Drugs*, Life Science Library (New York: Time-Life Books, A Division of Time, Inc., 1969), p. 39.

---

frequently fail to eat well-balanced meals because they reduce their appetites by drinking. Over a long period of time, this may lead to malnutrition.

## Social Implications

Why do people drink if they are aware of the limited physical benefits of alcohol? If the majority of the adult population chooses the social drinking pattern, there must be reasons to justify this decision.

Many find alcohol to be an ego booster, assistance for sociability, or a means to simple enjoyment. Some individuals feel that alcohol may relax them for increased and prolonged sexual activity. Other individuals may drink to escape from problems—to relieve their personal tensions and frustrations. In contrast, one must also be aware that drinking may be a factor in employment, reputation, marriage and the family, and certainly may cause accidents while one is driving under the influence of

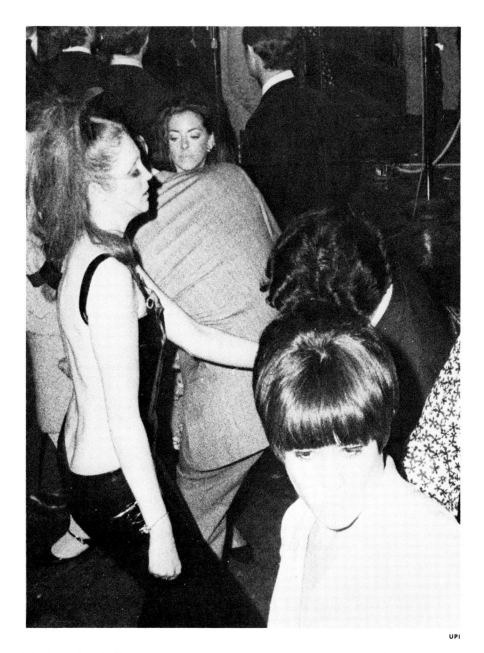

UPI

Behavior and sociability with the usage of alcohol has been altered and justified over the years.

an alcoholic beverage. It can drain one's income as well as decrease one's productivity in society.

Behavior and sociability with the usage of alcohol has been altered and justified over the years. There is greater acceptance of women drinking and men drinking in the presence of women. Cultural practices have also influenced certain people to drink. More drinking is being done in homes and clubs than ever before.

What can be the results of social drinking concerning mood alteration or behavioral changes? Chafetz believes that:

... most people *will* really *not,* under the influence of liquor, *do anything they wouldn't do without it.* The virgin who succumbs because she drank too deeply was tired of waiting *before* her first drink; that man who wanted to see what the inside of a prostitute's house looks like had his bulging eyes *before* the first swallow; the venereal disease sufferer was not too choosy an *individual* before drinking . . .[7]

It is interesting to note that social drinking has been a sign of hospitality through the ages, although drunkenness is considered to be in poor taste. Society now tends to overlook questionable behavior, however, if one is drinking in a public drinking establishment.

Cavin conducted a study of "bar behavior" patterns and collected participant-observation data from over 100 different bars in San Francisco. In reference to general behavior while drinking she concluded:

What goes on in the bar is localized in time and place, and one need not anticipate being held accountable for one's conduct at some later time or in some other setting. As a result, behavior which is either permissible or constitutes no more than normal trouble in the bar encompasses a broad range of activities that are often open to sanction in other, more serious public settings.[8]

Trends of social drinking and behavior continue to change and appear to be more liberal at this time. Since Americans are confronted with more leisure time, the frequency of drinking patterns will probably increase. It is up to every individual who decides to drink socially to be aware of his physical limitations and of his own alteration in behavioral

7. Morris Chafetz, *Liquor, the Servant of Man,* p. 90.

8. Sherry Cavan, *Liquor License* (Chicago: Aldine Publishing Co., 1966), p. 67.

patterns. It has been said that we never see ourselves as others see us. Obviously, if drinking occurs, one is unlikely to visualize how his behavior and actions appear to those around him.

## Alcoholism

The word *alcoholic* was once associated only with skid-row bums, with anyone who drank heavily, or with emotionally unstable individuals who did not appear to have the will power to stop drinking. Today the alcoholic and the problem drinker are closely related and alcoholism is recognized as an illness.

Because of the lack of accurate reports regarding the number of alcoholics in this country, one can only estimate the extent of this illness. It is generally accepted that one in fifteen Americans who drink will become alcoholics, but it is difficult to differentiate statistically the degree of the drinking problem.

Senator Harold E. Hughes, a Democrat from Iowa, a former alcoholic and current head of a special Senate subcommittee on alcoholism recently stated, "It is incredible that we cannot face realistically the alcoholism epidemic in this country which costs us more lives each year than the Vietnam War." Other political leaders agree and the government has legislated funds for rehabilitation and educational programs for informing the public about the nature of alcoholism as a disease. Studies reveal that there are about ten times as many alcoholics in this country as there are drug addicts, yet the mass media and federal government have been concentrating only upon the other abusive drug issues of narcotics and marijuana.

As the number of Americans with a drinking problem has continued to rise, federal spending for treatment and prevention of alcoholism has increased since 1970 to 86 million dollars a year. Alcoholics Anonymous has grown from 4,775 groups in 1958 to more than 10,000 groups in 1973. The National Commission on Marihuana and Drug Abuse recently stated: "Alcohol dependence is without question the most serious drug problem in this country today. Altogether alcoholism is said to cost society around 15 billion dollars annually.[9]

Government, business, labor, and social groups have been slow to encourage positive attempts in handling the high rise and increasing incidence.

9. "Rising Toll of Alcoholism" *U.S. News,* (Oct. 29, 1973):45–8.

What is the difference between a heavy drinker and an alcoholic? One may generalize by saying that a heavy drinker has control over himself and his drinking. An alcoholic, once striken with alcoholism, no longer has control over himself or his drinking and it eventually damages his home, his family and community life, and his occupation.

Mark Keller of the Center of Alcohol Studies at Rutgers University defines alcoholism:

Alcoholism is a chronic disease, or disorder of behavior, characterized by the repeated drinking of alcoholic beverages to an extent that exceeds customary dietary use or ordinary compliance with the social drinking customs of the community, and which interferes with the drinker's health, interpersonal relations or economic functioning.[10]

In 1956 the American Medical Association voted that alcoholism was a disease and must be regarded as a medical problem. Since that time courts have upheld cases wherein the individual was unable to control his actions due to alcoholism. Thus, the courts are beginning to rule that chronic alcoholism is not a crime. Society has been slow in accepting alcoholism as a disease, since it feels that many alcoholics use the disease theory as an alibi for continued drinking that could be controlled. The AMA continues to encourage physicians and hospitals to treat alcoholism as a chronic disease, but many hospitals still reject the care and treatment of alcoholics, thus reinforcing the misconception that alcoholism is a problem of character rather than a chronic disease.

The term *alcoholic* does not refer to the person who drinks heavily and regularly. The heavy drinker chooses to drink and has a choice as to what degree. The alcoholic's loss of the ability to *choose* is the nature of his disease.

## Skid Row Myth

At one time it was commonly believed that only the poor were alcoholics, men likely to be found in a community's skid row—an area of poverty and unemployment.

However, more than 70 percent of all alcoholics are living in suburban homes, are active in community affairs, have families, are college graduates, and are church members. Alcoholics may be executives of

10. National Institute of Mental Health, "Alcohol and Alcoholism."

corporations, doctors, lawyers, teachers, housewives, farmers, sales clerks, or secretaries.

Many alcoholics are hidden from the public eye. A housewife may drink all day to escape from her problems until the disease has progressed beyond her control and she is forced to seek help. It is difficult to estimate the number of women alcoholics however, since a housewife is able to conceal her disease so that it may not be noticeable to those outside the family.

In all, approximately nine million persons are alcoholics. Some estimate that of this figure approximately 25 percent are women and five percent are persons aged ten through nineteen. These alcoholics pose serious problems for over 36 million families.[11]

A man who holds a job may find his disease affecting his work and will eventually be identified by his employers. Today most estimates conclude that there are six male alcoholics to every female alcoholic. Others feel that these figures are misleading, since many women will seek help before the disease progresses to any real danger point.

Dr. H. J. Johnson, who has researched businessmen and drinking habits, reports that businessmen who drink thirty-five or more drinks per week will suffer from health problems. Lunchtime drinking, which is encouraged, will slow down afternoon *productivity*. For some, cocktails at lunch becomes a habit like drinking coffee. Industry needs to recognize dangers of potential alcoholism in businessmen. Even conventions frequently have reputations for being a justified business excuse for a wild week of drinking escapades.[12]

Many myths and misconceptions surround us daily concerning the problems of the alcoholic. For example, the National Council of Alcoholism and Alcoholics Anonymous are trying to dispel the following: (1) "Alcoholics are hopeless drunks." True, there is no known cure for this disease but just like diabetes, it can be *arrested*. (2) "Alcohol is the cause of alcoholism." If this were true, then everyone who drank would be an alcoholic. Alcohol by itself is not the only single causative factor. Some people develop cancer, others do not. Why is still unknown to man. (3) "Alcoholics can use willpower and recover." One cannot convince himself he does not have cancer or diabetes and the same is true of alcoholism. Recovery from any serious illness necessitates professional

11. "Rising Toll of Alcoholism," *U.S. News,* Oct. 29, 1973, p. 46.

12. H. J. Johnson, "Business Drinking," *U.S. News,* March 13, 1972, pp. 70–71.

assistance. (4) "Alcoholism is a self-inflicted moral problem." This is not exactly true, unless we also believe that the heavy person inflicts his heart attack, or the person who fails to rest properly has caused a self-inflicted cold to occur.[13]

## Causes of Alcoholism

For every disease there is a causative agent. Alcoholism has been categorized as a chronic disease because: (1) it is known to kill people; (2) it is known to shorten the life span; (3) it has certain symptoms and progressive stages of damage; and (4) it is a disease combining physical and emotional factors.

To date, no one has found a *single* causative agent for alcoholism. This has also been true of other chronic diseases such as heart disease and cancer.

One theory proposes that alcoholism is due to *physiological* factors. Supporters of this theory advocate that chemicals in alcoholic beverages affect certain individuals due to their hormonal make-up, metabolic defects, or genetic defects. Although alcoholism occurs frequently in families of alcoholics and may have a hereditary factor, Bleuber discards this theory. He found that alcoholism may occur in the children of devout abstainers.[14] This appears to add to the belief that alcoholism is related more to environment than to genetic factors.

Research is still underway to link alcoholism to physical causes. Scientists are questioning if alcoholics metabolize alcohol through different enzymatic processes than nonalcoholics. Until this is proved or disproved, of course, further studies and investigations will be needed.

Although we do not know if the cause is of physical origin, we do known that alcoholism has harmful physical effects, affecting the liver, and the nervous system, and often giving rise to malnutrition. Alcoholics often have a chronic inflammation of the lining of the stomach called gastritis. Their livers may become swollen and yellow with fat, which may lead to cirrhosis of the liver. The brain may be damaged in alcoholics, which may result in delirium tremens, a type of neuropathy. Vitamin deficiency diseases may occur as well.

13. Manfred Bleuber, "Familial and Personal Background of Chronic Alcoholics," in Oskar Diethelm, *Etiology of Chronic Alcoholism* (Springfield, Ill.: Charles C Thomas, 1955).

14. National Council on Alcoholism, "The Modern Approach to Alcoholism" (1965).

## Reflections on Drinking

I started drinking when I was fourteen and stopped when I was twenty-eight. Twelve of those fourteen years were filled with excitement and fun. The last two were brutal.

I might have escaped those last two years if I had recognized the symptoms of my illness earlier. I had every symptom of alcoholism when I was sixteen; as the illness progressed they only intensified. And progress it did—alcoholism is a cumulative disease.

Why did it take me so long to recognize my symptoms? In large part because I had the same misconceptions about liquor and stereotypes of the alcoholic that most people have, whether they're drinkers or nondrinkers.

Along with most, I believed that the alcoholic enjoys getting drunk. Since I didn't, it followed that I wasn't an alcoholic. In reality, one of the surest indications that a man has a drinking problem is his deadly fear of getting drunk.

I have known thousands of alcoholics, and, like me, most of them loathe drunken behavior. What we really want is to drink more than anybody else and remain sober.

Anonymous, *The Drinking Game and How to Beat It,* Benco edition (New York: The Benjamin Company, Inc., 1970), p. 5. Reprinted by permission of the publisher.

Psychological factors have been suggested as the cause of alcoholism. Psychologists and psychiatrists seem to think that there are certain ingredients that create the personality make-up of the potential alcoholic. They usually describe these characteristics as including social maladjustments, emotional instability, and neurotic tendencies. Freud believed that excessive drinkers were attempting to repress unconscious homosexual instincts.[15] Researchers also indicate studies revealing that alcoholics frequently have experienced a broken home situation, or have been deprived of love and a feeling of acceptance in their childhood. But here again, there are many individuals with the same environmental

15. Morris Chafetz, "Practical and Theoretical Consideration in the Psychotherapy of Alcoholism," *Quarterly Journal Study of Alcohol* 20:281 (1959).

problems and backgrounds who do *not* become alcoholics, and further research is necessary on the psychological theories as well.

M. E. Chafetz, Director of the Alcoholic Clinic at the Massachusetts General Hospital, classified patients into reactive and addictive alcoholics. Reactive or neurotic drinkers have pre-illness personality structures—they are usually faced with some external stress. Their lives are one of acceptable family relationships, with educational goals met, and they are considered successful. Then a crisis occurs and the drinker escapes by drinking and regressing to behavior just as does an addicted alcoholic. Psychotherapy helps this type of neurotic alcoholic.

On the other hand, Chafetz identifies the alcoholic addict who has a different type of pre-alcoholic personality structure: difficulty in achieving goals, poor employment history, family and school relationships that don't last. The need to drink arises gradually for this individual; he can't adjust in society. (The neurotic or reactive alcoholic has adjusted as an individual but suddenly feels a situation forces him to alcoholism.) Thus, we know only that alcoholism can occur in any personality and that each individual must be treated as an individual, since problems and underlying causes, thus far at least, appear to be of an individual nature.[16]

Environment does appear to be of significance, however, in that—as research generally agrees—there is a low incidence of alcoholism associated with certain feelings and patterns of behavior such as:

1. Parents who teach their children to drink moderately
2. Parents who serve as an example of social drinking
3. Families who only drink with a meal due to ethnic background
4. Lack of moralism or preaching against drinking
5. Abstinence being accepted equally with social drinking
6. Those who *use* alcohol wisely and moderately and do not abuse this practice in any way

## Warning Signs of Alcoholism

Although it is impossible to determine at exactly what point controlled social drinking becomes uncontrolled alcoholism, there are general pro-

16. Morris Chafetz, "The Nature and Treatment of Alcoholism," in *Manual on Alcoholism for Social Workers,* published by North Carolina Department of Mental Health, pp. 18–19 (June 1965).

gressive signs and symptoms of the disease. These have been outlined by
Alcoholics Anonymous as:

1. You begin to drink moderately, following no particular drinking
pattern.
2. You begin having blackouts. The next day you have no recollection
of what you did or said while drinking. This is not to be confused with *passing out.*
3. You begin *gulping* drinks instead of sipping them and you are bel-
ligerent to your friends if they question your drinking patterns.
——DANGER LINE (about 2 years later)——
4. You consistently *drink more than you had intended to.*
5. You begin making up *excuses* why you drink.
6. You begin having *eye-openers* by taking a drink in the morning to
meet the day's responsibilities.
7. You begin to *drink alone*—solitary drinking which affects job, home
and family.
8. You are *anti-social* when you drink, and you can't control your
behavior.
——SERIOUS DANGER POINT (5-10 years later) ——
9. You begin going on *benders* and are now classified as a true alcoholic.
10. You feel deep *remorse* and *resentment.* Sober moments are terrible.
11. You experience nameless anxiety, and you *sneak* and *protect* your
liquor supply.
12. You realize *drinking has you licked,* and you admit you cannot control your drinking.
13. You seek help or go under. The bottle has proven false and left you
without love, life, employment, or a future.

If a person fails to go beyond step 1, he will *not* become an alcoholic.
Alcoholism may progress to step 13 in anywhere from 5 to 25 years.

Although one may not be classified as an alcoholic, there are still
many who have this potential and are often classified as *problem drinkers.*

The National Institute on Alcohol Abuse and Alcoholism says that
problem drinkers may not be full-fledged alcoholics but may have potential if they have symptoms such as:

• Drinking to get drunk frequently.
• Going to work intoxicated.
• Requiring medical attention because of drinking.
• Getting into trouble with the law while drinking.
• Doing something while drunk which one would never do sober.[17]

17. "Rising Toll of Alcoholism." *U.S. News,* October 29, 1973, p. 48.

## Treatment

Alcoholism has no cure, but it can be arrested and controlled if the individual seeks help. The alcoholic must decide for himself which method of recovery he will use. He may ask himself:

Should I go to my family physician?
Should I join Alcoholics Anonymous?
Should I try to reduce my intake of alcohol?
Should I seek help from a psychiatrist?
Should I commit myself to a sanitarium?
Should I ask my clergyman for assistance?
Should I use substitute drugs or tranquilizers?

The choice of any of these methods will depend upon the degree of alcoholism of the individual. Some may be admitted to general hospitals for therapy. Others may be helped to stop drinking by use of drugs such as Temposil and Antabuse. A psychiatrist may help an individual stop drinking by solving an underlying personal problem. Alcoholics Anonymous (A.A.) has helped many alcoholics. Most communities have such organizations whose members are alcoholics who meet on a voluntary basis. Their purpose is simply to stay sober and help each other stay sober. There are over 7,000 local chapters throughout the country. In the A.A. approach, the alcoholic must admit that he has no power or control over alcohol.

Many new experimental treatment approaches have evolved recently in an attempt to bring the problem of alcoholism under control. Half-way houses are springing up in most cities across the country. Here alcoholics and drug addicts live and work together in an effort to solve their problems. Frequently these programs are supported by federal grants and supervised by ex-alcoholics. In other cities, alcoholics are treated from hospital out-patient clinics each day but are able to live at home. Other approaches have been using conditioned response techniques in allowing alcoholics to try to return to a level of acceptable social drinking patterns. Most experts do not feel this results in a permanent recovery program over a long period of time.

More recent use of the drug *propranolol*, used to curb heart problems, is being reported. It is now being used to keep alcoholics from reaching for another drink.

Dr. Jack Mendelson of Boston City Hospital conducted tests and concluded that *propranolol* appears to block behavior and psychic effects of alcohol. He believes it has advantages over antabuse, which is a negative reinforcement, causing a patient to become ill. *Propranolol* acts as a neutralizing agent. Most people drink to achieve mood alteration. *Propranolol* has the effect of reducing anxiety which plays a major role in desire to drink.[18]

Less accepted in treatment approaches has been the unique approach by millionaire Patrick Frawley of Papermate Pen and Schick razor fame. A former alcoholic, he has established a chain of hospitals across the country based on a theory of retention of body fluids. He believes victims whose ancestors originate from wet or very dry climates are more susceptible to alcoholism. Examples cited were Eskimos, Indians, Irish, Scots and Africans. All are groups which seem to lose fluids rapidly and tend to gulp alcohol. Therefore treatment is given by keeping the patients suitably moist.[19]

Insurance companies such as Blue Cross and Blue Shield are now beginning to include some coverage for treatment of alcoholism in their health insurance policies. Also due to federal grants of 1970, most community mental health centers all over the country are providing treatment for alcoholics on an out-patient basis.

Regardless of treatment, most specialists concur that "once an alcoholic, always an alcoholic" and that an alcoholic will never be able to drink on a social basis. Because of this, *no one should ever insist* that someone accept a drink. Hostesses should always serve non-alcoholic beverages as well as cocktails.

## Prevention

Some authorities suggest that the incidence of alcoholism could be removed completely by enacting law enforcement to abolish liquor. In the past, however, legislative control was not the answer. Others suggest making price adjustments on the sale of alcoholic beverages so that drinking would be prohibitively expensive. Church authorities suggest attempting to remove social problems that could lead to excessive drinking. Educators feel that by means of mandatory alcohol education in the

18. "Psyching the Alcoholic." *Newsweek*, Aug. 21, 1972, p. 62.

19. *The Nation*, December, 1973, p. 614.

schools, students will learn to make intelligent decisions about drinking and become aware of the danger signals of alcoholism. Others, such as psychiatrists, claim that Americans should be taught how and when to drink safely so as not to abuse alcohol.

## Trends

Currently there is a slow, steady movement to emphasize positive solutions to alcoholism, rather than punishment. Until the last 20 years alcoholics were often locked up and placed in jails, but we are making gradual progress toward a disease concept of alcoholism. The Labor Department is now providing aid to its 2,200 offices to assist in helping unemployed alcoholics (along with narcotic addicts). Employees have been directed to treat alcoholics as handicapped and they have made them eligible for job-training programs.

A number of industries, instead of firing employees who are alcoholics, are introducing programs for dealing with problem drinkers. Some offer counseling and referral services. The National Council on Alcoholism has found more alcoholism among executives than among rank and file workers.) Controlling alcoholism will require a national, federal program to lend assistance and funds to state and local agencies, industries, and the schools for better educative means concerning alcohol.

If an individual abstains from alcoholic beverages, of course, he will have no problem. A teetotaler should not be ridiculed for his decision—nor is it wise for a teetotaler to ridicule or demoralize a drinker. But the decision to drink or not to drink is made due to a complexity of forces—parental attitudes, attitudes of one's peers, one's community, and the church, and the financial circumstances that will permit one to spend money on alcoholic beverages.

### Questions for Study and Discussion

1. How does alcohol alter *your* behavior and moods?
2. How do you feel toward a person who drinks, one who is a social drinker, and the alcoholic?
3. Why is there excessive drinking at fraternity parties and peer pressure to do so?
4. Do coeds know how to handle liquor?
5. What trends and social stigmas do you predict in the future for alcoholics?
6. How can we prevent alcoholism?

## References

Blakeslee, Alton. "Alcoholism, A Sickness That Can Be Beaten." Public Affairs Committee, no. 118 A, 1966.

Bleuber, Manfred. "Familial and Personal Background of Chronic Alcoholics," in Diethelm, Oskar, *Etiology of Chronic Alcoholism.* Springfield, Ill.: Charles C Thomas, 1955.

Block, Marvin. *Alcoholism Its Facets and Phases.* New York: John Day Co., 1965.

Cavan, Sherry. *Liquor License: An Ethnography of Bar Behavior.* Chicago: Aldine, 1966.

Chafetz, Morris. *Liquor the Servant of Man.* London: Phoenix House, 1967.

Chafetz, Morris E. "Practical and Theoretical Considerations in the Psychotherapy of Alcoholism. *Quarterly Journal Study of Alcohol* 20 (1959):281.

Johnson, J. "Business Drinking." *U.S. News.* March 13, 1972, p. 70.

Keller, Mark, "How Alcohol Affects the Body." New Brunswick, N.J.: Rutgers University, Center of Alcohol Studies, 1955.

Kent, Patricia. *An American Woman and Alcohol.* New York: Holt, Rinehart and Winston, 1967.

Linden, Arthur. "Some Random Thoughts on Alcohol Education." *Journal of School Health* volume 29 (January, 1959).

"Moistly Sober." *The Nation.* December 10, 1973.

Monahan, Michael. *Dry America.* New York: Nicholas L. Brown, 1921.

Plaut, Thomas. *Alcohol Problems.* New York: Oxford University Press, 1967.

"Psyching the Alcoholic." *Newsweek.* 80 (August 21, 1972):62.

Riddle, Paul. "Teenage Drinking . . . Impulse or Invitation." *Minnesota Journal of Education.* December, 1968, p. 968.

Terhune, William B. *The Safe Way to Drink.* New York: William Morrow, 1968.

Trice, Harrison. *Alcoholism in America.* New York: McGraw Hill, 1966.

*U.S. News.* March 13, 1972, p. 70.

# 8

# Consumer Health

## General Concept

Every consumer should be informed and seek reliable advice concerning health products and services.

## Outcomes

The student should be able to:
1. Explain the dangers of self-medication and of the techniques employed by quacks
2. Seek reliable products and services
3. Identify ways of consumer protection
4. Protect himself against health quackery and medical imposters
5. Avoid self-medication, and falsely advertised, dangerous products
6. Identify various professional health specialists
7. Explain the basic principles of health insurance

The American public still refuses to recognize that in our daily living, we are victims of deceptive and fraudulent products and practices. Because of our fears, our gullibility, and our ignorance, Americans today waste billions of their health dollars on quacks and nostrums. It is ironic that the typical educated American may buy the best clothes, select his car after comparing prices, take years to choose the right home for his

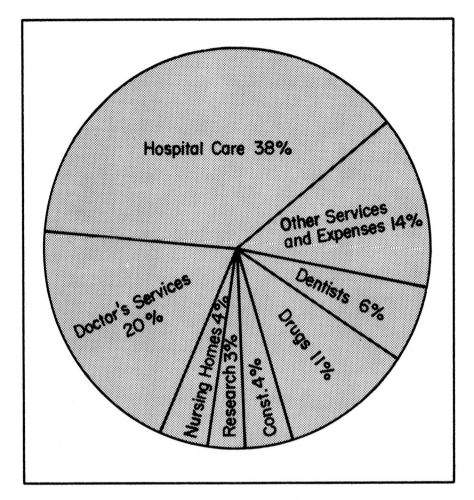

How the medical dollar is spent.

family, and eat only the food that he enjoys, regardless of price. However, when it comes to spending money on his health—his life—he may
haphazardly select his medical services. Due to the mass media, flexible
laws, and an uninformed public, the quack of today enjoys a lucrative
market for his fraudulent services and products.

Today, people are still buying baldness cures, bust developers, cancer cures, and wrinkle removers—because they have hope! With hope
there is always a chance that a product may work. But besides wasting
their money because of such false hope, many individuals are also en-

dangering their health. These ridiculous treatments and products cost more than money, because *precious time* is being lost. In most diseases, early diagnosis and prompt treatment may arrest or cure the malady. But with prolonged lack of responsible medical attention, an ailment may advance and progress, even to the point of death.

For example, if an individual has cancer and seeks the services of a chiropractor, thinking that he is a medical doctor or a licensed general practitioner, he is only delaying the time till he seeks reliable medical attention, which he urgently needs.

## Quacks and Nostrums

What is a quack? What is a nostrum? What is health quackery? Times have changed, and the quack is no longer a shifty-eyed, middleaged gentleman in a high silk hat with a smooth line. A quack of today looks like any other person or the professional that he is trying to imitate.

A quack is a braggadocio, an imitator or imposter of medical skills, who claims he can diagnose, treat, and cure a disease through his services or his product. Quacks do not have approved medical knowledge and often use worthless machines in an attempt to identify a malady. We call these cure-all drugs (or machines that have accompanying broad sweeping claims)—nostrums.

A quack tries to inspire confidence in his patients, convince them that he is a medical authority and expert. Frequently, quacks use convincing medical and scientific terms to impress the individual who seeks his services. The medical quack may have a beautiful, luxurious, office (why not? he has a fat bank account) and may even wear professional attire and have huge, complex, new machines in his office to assist him in diagnosis—as well as to impress patients.

Some individuals may avoid a medical quack but still fall prey to nostrums such as cold remedies, arthritis cures, cough remedies, and reducing techniques. Some of us prefer self-medication to a reliable physician because of fear, cost, lack of time, or worry. Health problems should be diagnosed by a knowledgeable physician. We take our disabled automobiles to a mechanic, our alterations to a dressmaker, our teeth to the dentist, our children to the schools, our dream house plans to a contractor, but we either seek the services of a quack for our health or try to diagnose our own health problems.

Health swindles cheat the individual. Older people, in particular, are frequently victims of quacks. A national survey has indicated that arthritic patients were spending over 250 million dollars a year on misrepresented remedies.[1] Some medicines on the open market do have limited value, but if health problems persist, one should consult his physician.

The quack of today is a sophisticated salesman posing as a medical authority, a man who speaks of "subclinical deficiencies," "vitalized food"

---

### A Chiropractic Advertisement

STOMACH

BOWEL

GALL BLADDER

Disorders such as indigestion, gas, bloat, constipation, abdominal pain, backache, burning, belching, biliousness, vomiting, headache, dizziness, fatigue, heartburn, palpitation, colitis, ulcers, bleeding, insomnia, and nervousness may be warning symptoms of some serious condition which can be prevented by proper examination, diagnosis and treatment. Great suffering, loss of time from work, hospitalization and surgery can be avoided by special treatment and care. Don't delay, call for an appointment or come in today . . . Treatments are non-surgical and painless.

Special Attention to Stomach and Bowel Disorders

*Phoenix Gazette*, October 18, 1971.

---

and "aging before your time." Quackery is widespread. It appears in bestseller diet books, and in most commercial magazines. Tragedy may befall the person who is gullible and believes that nostrums or quacks will cure his ailment.

1. "Your Money and Your Life," Food and Drug Administration Catalog of Fakes and Swindles in the Health Field, U.S. Department of Health, Education and Welfare, no. 19 (Oct. 1963).

The quack often falsely assumes a fictitious name and the title of "Doctor." He may have a printing company print up fraudulent degrees or certificates to place in his office. Occasionally a physician may turn to quackery for financial gain. The American Medical Association's Department of Investigation now screens applications for state licensers. Such intensive screening is a major deterrent to those who are attempting to become medical imposters.

Many imposters have fantastic abilities, even genius, but somehow they find it impossible to channel their natural gifts within the ethical structure of society. Some medical imposters show up casually in a community and stay there as the doctor. In Groveton, Texas, a man arrived in town and helped a small boy with a wound who came into a drug store. While sitting at a soda fountain he posed as a new doctor, "Doc Brown." After helping the child, several others received his services. He stayed in town, but months later was identified when a computer balked at filling a drug order for him because of a conflict in name and credentials. "Doc Brown" turned out to be a convicted bank robber who had acquired his medical skills at a hospital in Tennessee as an x-ray laboratory aide.

Most M.D. imposters have picked up some rudimentary medical information which permits them to "get by" in handling typical routine complaints.[2] Some advertise "new services," "new products," or a new nostrum. Everyone likes to inquire about "new" services or a "new" product. Quacks often claim that they have made a great medical discovery and that this treatment has won recognition abroad. Some say that the medical profession will fail to accept their treatment because it is envious of their discoveries. Chiropractors are the typical cultists who seek to attract patients through advertising and testimonials.

## Phony Marriage Counselors

Since statistics reveal that currently in the United States approximately one in three marriages ends in divorce, it is not surprising that imposters also pose as medical or professional counselors for patients with marital difficulties in order to deceive the public and achieve financial success. Many call themselves therapists and have made fake marriage counseling into a big business. Most charge high therapeutic fees and are involved with phony abortion referral services, instant divorces, prostitution, and nonprofessional counseling services. Many phony counselors actually ruin marriages. Few states have laws concerning procedures for prosecuting suspected quack marriage counselors, and many such counselors are causing physical and emotional harm as well as draining couples financially.

The quack counselor's major source of new customers appears to be the classified telephone directory. Ethical professionals do not advertise beyond a plain phone listing.

Phony marriage advisers are successful because so many Americans are emotionally troubled concerning their marriages and there are so few qualified professionals available to help them. Qualified professionals do not tell disturbed couples what to do, but rather guide the couple into deeper insight of themselves and open the paths of communication so that they may solve their own problems.

Here are some points to remember in spotting a quack marriage counselor:

1. He advertises in yellow pages in an obvious manner.
2. He offers quick solutions.
3. He charges high and excessive fees.
4. He makes a hasty diagnosis.
5. He fails to have credentials available in office.
6. His actions may be intimate or obscene.
7. He will fail to refer you to someone else, such as clergyman, lawyer, or physician.[2]

Many of these quacks are also initiating programs for group sessions, using sensitivity procedures for eradicating marital hang-ups. There is now national focus on sensitivity programs but again this type of therapy should only be directed and used by competent, trained, professional personnel.

## Mechanical Quackery

Many quacks use costly, worthless, machines in order to diagnose a disease. Dinshan Ghadiali, a native of India, claimed he had 15 degrees including an honorary M.D. (an *honorary* medical degree?). Ghadiali founded the Spectocrome in 1920, in which he diagnosed diseases by

2. Jack Kaplan, "Frauds Who Prey on Shaky Marriages," *Today's Health,* June, 1969, pp. 18–19.

means of colored lights. He was not prosecuted until 1947, and then only had to pay a $20,000 fine. Ghadiali's case appeared in court after he misdiagnosed a diabetic patient who died. Ghadiali, then 75, never went on trial for the death of the patient, however. When his probation period ended, he returned again to quackery.

Ruth Drown, a famous chiropractor from Los Angeles, claimed she had a machine that could diagnose an ailment with a sample of the patient's blood. For giving absent treatments she was fined $1,000.

Another area of mechanical quackery lies in reducing machines. One cannot shake off fat—reducing machines merely redistribute the fat through time-consuming, painful, wasted hours of hope and effort. Yet millions of Americans in their quest for the body beautiful are flocking to health clubs and health spas where they spend astronomical amounts in hopes of removing fat with some type of machine.

## Advertising and Labeling

Advertising plays an influential role in an individual's decision to purchase health products. It is true that not all advertising is false, but it is also true that much advertising does use false statements, exaggerates, or leaves an implied false impression. A recent investigation by the government into advertising promotions concerning the dry cereals and their nutritional values revealed misrepresentation. Companies had advertised for years nutrients that were present in the cereals but few contained extraordinary quantities of nutrients. Advertisements may be read in papers or magazines, viewed on television, heard on the radio, or demonstrated by a door-to-door salesman. The person-to-person contact is supposedly the most effective means of promoting a product, therefore many quacks employ this technique rather than pay for costly ads in magazines or on the radio.

Typical of health advertisements quacks usually use are:
1. A tricky layout
2. Large, bold headlines
3. Repetition of catchy statements
4. Use of words such as "plan," "method," or "system"

When a plan is offered such as for reducing weight, generally these plans involve:
1. The product the advertiser is selling
2. Exercise
3. Diet

The product of the advertiser, of course, has no weight reduction properties whatsoever.[3]

The health lecturers who advertise on television or radio may use a "free presentation" as a come-on for a paid series of lectures, a course of instruction, or a series of books they have published. Generally the cost of an advertised product is less than ten dollars. If an individual is gullible for a quack product at this price, he probably will feel it too time-consuming to investigate or press legal charges against the service or product. The individual rationalizes he has been had and is simply minus his ten dollars.

Because advertising has a significant effect upon the behavior patterns of the consumer, too many products fool the American public every day, insulting their intelligence as well as robbing their pocketbooks.

Hopefully over the next few years, new and more effective labels will appear on more items. No amount of research and law-passing can protect everyone from harm unless labels are carefully read and followed. The problem confronting many consumers is the confusing label or the label that withholds important information. Unfortunately, some consumers do not read any labels and believe if an item is marketed, it is safe—a false assumption.

Examples of new labeling have affected food items and the cosmetic industry. Effective in 1974 is the law requiring packaged foods to list nutritional values such as calories, protein, and fat content.[4]

Laws should probably be passed requiring the disposal of medicines after a specified time so that they don't become at best useless and at worst dangerous. The Food and Drug Administration may soon require more information on dangers of certain medications. It is now up to the individual consumer to take the extra time, at point of purchase, to obtain products with the new labels.

Unlike drugs that doctors prescribe, nonprescription antacids have not earned the complete approval of the federal government for safety and effectiveness. In the future, advertisements or labels that boast relief for "nervous headaches" or "nervous emotional disturbances" may have to be changed. Drug makers may only use for another two years

3. "Facts You Should Know About Health Quackery" (Educational Division, Better Business Bureau, 1957), p. 6.
4. Peter Weaver, "Toward More Effective Labeling," *Todays Health,* Feb., 1974.

"upset stomach" or "plain indigestion" ads unless they can prove that their product is related to stomach acidity. Aspirin has long been a stomach irritant and is included in such drugs as Alka-Selzer.[5] In the future such combination drugs for headache, stomachache, and indigestion may not be permitted unless specific labeling is given.

## Alcoholism

There is no easy remedy or cure for the alcoholic. There is no drug on the market that can overcome the alcoholic's addiction to alcohol. Recovery is only possible when the individual has the desire to seek reliable help either through a physician, a clergyman, or the efforts of Alcoholics Anonymous.

## Anemia

Self-medication can be dangerous for the anemic individual, especially if there is evidence of pernicious anemia. "Not a single vitamin-supplement on the market in usual doses can be depended on to prevent or cure iron-deficiency anemia."[6] Yet such products are advertised to cure tired blood (what is "tired blood" anyway?) and iron deficiency. A physician may take a blood sample to determine whether one needs to take a prescribed medication for iron-deficiency. Symptoms of tiredness may be due to many different causes.

## Arthritis

Arthritis is an age-old disease of which there are many forms. It generally affects the older portion of the population and is simply an inflammation of the joints. With rheumatoid arthritis, quacks offer hope for those who are suffering because:

    1. It is a disease in which discomfort comes and goes. Since the pain is not consistent, the quack and his remedy soon claim that the miracle or wonder of the product caused the momentary relief.

    2. Arthritis is a long-term illness. Because of this, patients will try *anything*—based upon hope—when the ailment persists. The truth is,

5. "Pills and Potions for Indigestion," *Changing Times*, Feb. 1974, p. 39.
6. The Medicine Show (New York: Simon and Schuster, 1961), p. 84.

there is no positive cure to this date, since the exact causes of arthritis are unknown.[7]

Quacks continue to sell and advertise immune milk, copper bracelets, wonder mittens, zinc disks worn in the heels of shoes, or vibrating devices. Arthritis victims should be aware of false promises of a positive cure advertised for arthritis.

## Baldness Cures

Since hair is not like a flower or plant, its growth is not altered by external application. Male baldness is an inherited characteristic that usually occurs early in adulthood. *Nothing can be done about baldness* unless the bald individual chooses to wear a wig or a toupee.[8] Manipulation of the scalp, ointments, or hair restorers are often advertised in newspapers. The quack announces his arrival in town via a local paper and offers to give "free" consultation in confidence. The privacy of his hotel room is the setting and the gimmick is to purchase his product at some exorbitant cost. Scientists have been experimenting in transplanting individual hair follicles, but this has not been widely practiced due to safety factors and cost. Dandruff does not cause baldness. Every day it is normal to lose a certain number of hairs, but these are eventually replaced with new ones.

## Bust Developers

Because of the increased emphasis placed upon a woman maintaining her sexual image, advertisers and quacks have made a voluptuous figure the desire of every female. Since many young ladies have not been amply endowed by nature, they will seek remedies, based upon hope and desire, to increase their bust size.

An advertisement may read:: "Yes, it is possible to add three full inches to your bustline in just eight short weeks through use of the bust exercise." Usually a before and after layout of photographs accompanies the advertisement.

Recently while discussing quackery in a health class, a coed admitted that she had enclosed a dollar in answer to an advertisement in a maga-

7. "Facts About Quacks," *Today's Health,* February, 1968, p. 72.
8. *The Medicine Show,* p. 169.

zine selling bust developers. Her plain-wrapped package arrived in the mail. Eagerly she opened the package only to find an enlarged photograph of a man's hand. Needless to say, the coed was disappointed. Here again, the element of hope and the small amount of money spent prevented a legal investigation of such quackery and false advertising.

## Cancer Treatments

Cancer is only arrested or cured by means of surgery, use of radium and x-ray, laser beam, and in some instances chemotherapy. The Food and Drug Administration estimates that Americans spend more than ten million dollars each year on phony cancer cures.[9]

The cancer patient who risks his life in the hands of a quack is wasting *precious time* of his life. Cancer can be cured if diagnosed early enough. If the patient seeks phony remedies, the disease may advance into secondary stages which are difficult for a physician to treat.

Fear often motivates the patient to self-medication of pills, or machines. Some individuals fear surgery or chemotherapy. Unfortunately, cancer cures are not obtained by taking daily tablets of some kind. Others fear social discrimination, death, cost for treatment. Others may give up hope and hide their ailment until it is too late.

Cancer quacks often promote escharotic salves, plant roots, red clover tea, and apricot kernels as "cancer drugs." Some imposters advocate that cancer is caused by a chemical imbalance of alkaloids and acids. There is no medical scientific proof of such a statement. Other quacks suggest special diets for the cancer victim. Krebiozen was once a very popular serum promoted as a cancer cure. The American Medical Association states, ". . . there is no scientific evidence, that any vaccine or serum, including Anticancergen Z-50 and Krebiozen, is useful in the treatment of cancer on human beings."[10]

## Cold Remedies

The leading respiratory ailment in the United States is the common cold. It costs Americans five billion dollars in lost wages and medical expenses. Statistics show Americans suffer 230–500 million colds each

9. "Facts You Should Know About Health Quackery," p. 8.
10. "Facts About Quacks," p. 72.

year. Currently over one billion is spent on over-the-counter cough and cold remedies.

Yet our advertisers continue to promote cold cures and remedies, when scientists cannot discover the prevention or cure of this viral nuisance. We learn of vitamins, alkalizers, antihistamine drugs, inhalers, salves, vaccines, and liniments that will treat this common ailment. Some may give you temporary relief, although psychological in nature; none can cure a cold.

Some may dry your dripping nose, others do nothing and are harmless, while some may aggravate already annoying conditions.

Dr. Sol Katz, an authority on respiratory diseases says most remedies are safe if directions are followed. Most contain analgesic of aspirin. Some, however, are potentially dangerous. Antihistamines may cause drowsiness and dizziness and when taken with alcohol can be very dangerous. For instance *Nyquil* is 25 percent or more alcohol. Since it is logistically impossible, as well as unnecessary, for all patients who have common cold to be seen by a physician, much temporary relief can be felt by proper use of simple aspirin.[11]

Every consumer should read a remedy's label for warnings and use of the medication. Although some consumers may buy their cold remedies, still others will concoct their own home remedies. Some of these home remedies have been passed down through generations of families. For example:

1. Drinking whiskey and tea.
2. Sipping tablespoons of cod liver oil.
3. Drinking citrus fruit juices.
4. Wearing herbs about the neck.
5. Applying ointments and salves about the chest.

The average American experiences three colds a year and the viral infection lasts about a week *regardless* of diet, drugs, inhalers or salves used to head them off.[12]

## Cough Remedies

There are about 600 different types of cough remedies that may be purchased at a drug store without a prescription. When an individual coughs, it is due to an irritation somewhere in the respiratory system

11. Sol Katz, M.D. "Evaluating Cold Remedies," *Todays Health,* February, 1974, p. 18.
12. *The Medicine Show,* p. 15.

and is a reflex action controlled by the brain. Coughing is frequently a symptom accompanying the common cold.

Many cough remedies are simply placebos—a formula causing no harm or doing any good, but contributing to the psychological satisfaction of the consumer that they will cure his ailment.

Codeine, dextromethorphan, and antihistamines are popular ingredients used in cough syrups. Some states are now requiring by law prescriptions for cough remedies, particularly those with codeine. In California, for example, one may not purchase a cough syrup over the counter that contains codeine. With the current unrest regarding abuse of various drugs, it is wise for enforcement of this kind to be considered in all states as a precautionary measure. The psychological value of these products is of significance. If a person believes in a remedy, he will probably achieve relief—regardless of cost, or the amount of advertising.

Actually candy drops, hot drinks, and rest will help the simple cough as much as anything on the market. However, *if a cough persists several days, consult your physician* for an accurate diagnosis to confirm that it is not a more serious ailment.

## Cosmetic Quackery

Cosmetics may truly enhance our appearance or hide undesirable marks, but they do not perform miracles. Women, in particular, strive to stay young and look beautiful. Why? Because advertising has emphasized youthful, beautiful women to the point where we now find grandmothers with padded bras, false eyelashes, miniskirts, and long stringy hair. Many women will waste money to rejuvenate their skin or erase their wrinkles.

There are no creams, jellies, lotions, or masks that will remove wrinkles. Purchasing a $1.00 bottle of lotion or a $20.00 bottle will produce the same effect—hope and/or psychological contentment.

Many quacks lurk in the cosmetic industry often leaving individuals with skin problems, not only a more serious physical problem but an emotional problem as well. Consider the case of Mrs. Ceil Hatfield, a former model who read an ad in a newspaper, "Be a Beautiful New You in 10 Days." The ad promised Mrs. Hatfield she could peel years away at a Miami Beach health spa and she would look younger and be wrinkle-free. She was admitted to the spa, where they used a process called "face peeling" or chemosurgery, with no medical authority. (Plastic surgeons are only experimenting themselves with this risky process.) When the tape was finally removed, her face was marred with ugly lines where they had used chemicals to burn layers of the epidermis. Anguish and pain followed and Mrs. Hatfield discovered from a dermatologist that the cells were destroyed so severely that she was incapable of growing new healthy skin. Since her experience, her medical and drug bills have totaled close to $10,000. With the aid of her attorney she was able to collect $75,000—40 per cent of which went for attorney fees. But the emotional scars were also severe and are permanent.[13]

Quick-tanning products and various shampoos for the hair are other items to be studied carefully to see if they perform as advertised.

## Dental Plates and Dentifrices

False teeth are even advertised by means of mail order, obviously an impractical and unsafe method. Often the aged fall victims to this gimmick because of the rising cost of dentistry.

Dentifrices are simply an aid in brushing and cleaning of the teeth. No toothpaste alone can prevent caries or cavities, regardless of "Look mom . . . no cavities; I brush my teeth with ——." The American Dental Association has given its sanction and approval of only two dentifrices. *Crest* was the first, with the presence of stannous fluoride. More recently the ADA in late 1969 approved *Colgate-Palmolive* with the presence of MFP fluoride. Both brands may use the ADA seal in advertising. The toothpaste must be used with regular brushings, however, and the user must have a good diet. (Even better prevention of caries would be topical fluoride treatment by a competent dentist.) Proctor and Gamble manufactures both *Crest* and *Gleem*, and since the ADA approval *Crest* sales have soared above those of *Gleem*. What does P & G do? It merely steps up the advertising and promotion of *both* of their products. The question arises: Why, since *Crest* is so superior to other toothpastes (witness P & G's own ads), does P & G manufacture and sell *Gleem* as well?

## Health Foods

Food faddists or quacks generally pose as qualified scientists or as health lecturers, and promote food products that will prevent disease. Nutrition

---

13. Barbara Lindeman, "You're Not Mrs. Hatfield," *Today's Health,* Feb., 1971, pp. 25–27.

quacks are gifted orators and may give free speeches or "helpful" talks over the radio. The basic reasoning they give for considering their product follows these lines:

1. Diseases are due to diet
2. Soil depletion causes malnutrition
3. Food supply is overprocessed
4. People suffer from subclinical deficiencies[14]

All of these reasons are false statements, but to the uninformed, they may sound logical. Actually, if an individual eats three balanced meals from each of the four food groups, it is completely unnecessary to buy pills or capsules to supplement a diet. Most food items are vitamin or protein enriched today. Although taking a vitamin pill a day will not likely harm you, it is truly an unnecessary practice.

To rely on health foods to keep you well can be dangerous as well as expensive. Yoghurt has only the same basic nutritional value as milk, and sea salt containing iodine is adequately supplied in a diet containing seafoods and iodized salt.[15] Nor is honey a cure for a cough, root beer a tonic for nerves, or blueberry juice a cure for diabetes.

With the current interest in ecology, our diets and food habits are being explored, investigated, and experimented with not only by government officials but by many young people. While the government is rating the safety of our foods, many concerned ecologists are returning to the naturalist movement in nutritional planning.

These followers feel that our food comes to us "not as nature intended but altered by man during both growth and processing." The truly devoted may even grow their own food without chemical fertilizer or pesticides, and will eat no meat from animals which have used antibiotics. Because of this new nutritional health interest, country-style stores are springing up on both coasts selling only organic foods, often at exorbitant prices. One mail order store is the Walnut Acres store in Pennsylvania, which ships organic foods to a group in Phoenix, Arizona, usually 700–800 pounds a month. In Berkeley, California, food co-ops have been formed. One store there, called Wholly Foods, in operation only seven months, has already reported a booming capitalist entrepenurial success. To meet the demands of the under-30 age group, a nationwide subindustry is growing at a rapid pace. At the University of

14. "Your Money and Your Life," p. 12.
15. *Ibid.*

California at Santa Cruz, students may choose an organic vegetarian menu and even have in their cafeteria a "natural" food line.[16]

Because organic and natural foods are expensive (and only research and long-term experimentation will test the validity of our returning to primitive ways of marketing our foods), health food quacks are capitalizing in the new area. Organic foods may not harm an individual nutritionally, but many are often misrepresented. Most nutritionists and physicians still advocate eating balanced diets from the basic four food groups. Any change in diets or nutritional intake should be made upon the advice of a physician.

## Health Books

There is no book that can adequately diagnose or substitute for a physician's consultation. Yet diet plans and books have made best-seller lists. Since these books sound authoritative, and since many readers will take the written word as the truth, many are misinformed. Many hardbound and paperback books have appeared on the market promoting the natural food movements and advocating a return to organic diets. Many may be written by qualified nutritionists, but others are not and readers should be aware of the backgrounds of the authors. For example, Herman Taller in 1961 published a book *Calories Don't Count*. A review of it by Philip White, Executive Secretary, Council on Foods and Nutrition of the American Medical Association, pointed out that Dr. Taller's book failed to publish supporting clinical evidence or to note well-documented criticisms. Dr. Taller was eventually found guilty on six counts of mail fraud and a Food and Drug Administration violation in which he was fined $7,000 and placed on probation.[17]

## Health Clubs and Massage Parlors

The seventies have brought about an awareness, particularly through the media, on looking and feeling young, regardless of your age. Since this is a current trend many new health clubs, spas, and massage parlors have sprung up overnight to capitalize on the consumer's interest and desire to look and feel physically in shape. Most authorities in

16. "The Move to Eat Natural," *Life*, Nov. 11, 1970, pp. 45–50.
17. Marjorie Burns, *Nutrition Books: A Guide To Their Reliability* (Ithaca, New York: Cornell Extension Bulletin 1158, May, 1966).

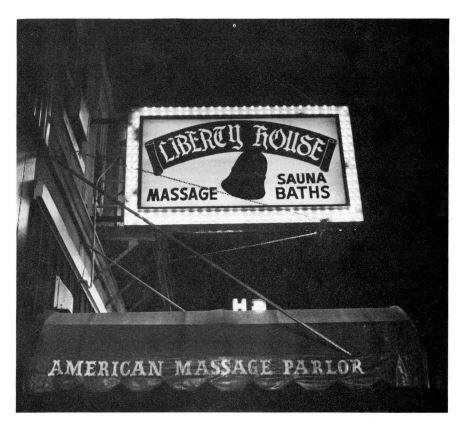

The desire to be physically attractive has resulted in the establishment of a wave of massage parlors across the country.

physical fitness concur that regular, proper exercise such as walking, swimming, running, and cycling are excellent and inexpensive methods toward this goal as well as for the circulatory and cardiac benefits that may result.

Frequently the beautiful facilities of the health spa or club are staffed by unqualified instructors, and although all the equipment and saunas are not likely to harm one, it is an expensive way to achieve physical fitness.

In Los Angeles there are more than 150 massage parlors doing a fifty million dollar a year business.[18] Americans spend money on massages thinking they have sound healthful results. True a massage will momentarily make one feel better as one relaxes, but it will not cure health ailments. Any such claims are phony. Most parlors and spas do not hire specialists in physical therapy. Many are actually attractive, physically fit looking people who know very little about physical fitness or massage. In the hands of trained personnel, however, there can be psychological and physiological benefits.

There are generally two kinds of commercial massage parlors—the straight and the sexy. The straight usually use the "look, but do not touch" approach; the sexy parlors may be disguised houses of prostitution. Most parlors charge about ten dollars per hour and provide steam baths, swimming pools, and even a snack bar. In most massage parlors known homosexuals and alcoholics are barred from services as they are a detriment to the business. [19]

Physicians agree that although massage parlors are not that harmful to most people, their activities can be detrimental to patients who have varicose veins, diabetes, or diabetic neuritis. Anyone with a cardiac or respiratory problem should also stay away from sauna rooms.

## Hemorrhoid Treatments

Hemorrhoids or piles are clusters of varicose veins located in the lower rectum or anus. Usually they occur in adults between the ages of thirty to fifty. Because people are afraid of their anus area, they will not seek a physician's advice when anal bleeding begins. Since there are several varieties of hemorrhoids (internal and external), self-medication of suppositories and other drugs may be dangerous. True, they may temporarily relieve pain, but they are not curing the situation. A warm bath three or four times a day can provide temporary relief just as well. In severe cases, physicians generally perform surgery to remove these rectal vessels. Mild external hemorrhoids may heal gradually if hard stools cease to occur.

## Impotency Cures

There is no self-medication that will insure sexual vitality. Since sexual activity is emphasized by society for the masculine male, hucksters are quick to find phony products for sexual rejuvenation. Their advertise-

19. *Ibid.*, p. 41.

ments are generally sent in a plain envelope to the head of a household. One company is still promoting the male rigiditor for those who no longer are able to have an erection. The flyer reads: "The Male Rigiditor —it solves one of man's most serious problems—no drugs—no hormones." This handy item costs $10.00 and a lot of nerve. Another advertised item has been the electro-magnetic massager that is supposed to increase sexual activity and stimulate one's organs. Those items are among the oldest of all health hoaxes.

## Tobacco Cures

Since the Surgeon General's (Dr. Luther Terry) Report of 1964 concerning the smoking controversy, Americans have been trying to quit smoking or reduce the number of cigarettes that they smoke. Smoking is now linked with chronic diseases and so gimmicks are manufactured to help the individual stop smoking. There is no known drug or combination of drugs that can cure the tobacco habit by themselves. It takes the desire and will power of the smoker to stop, though psychologically for a person to invest in a product to stop smoking may help him to abstain.

## Weight Reducers

For most Americans the cause of obesity is simply overeating. In some cases the tendency to be overweight may run in families, or there may be glandular difficulties. Therefore, proper dieting is essential in maintaining your weight, and should be supervised by your family physician. Vitamin-mineral preparations have no reducing elements. Avoid products that have you give up meals for their product. Certain low-calorie diets given by a physician will alleviate hunger and discomfort, as well as provide a sensible method of reducing.

Sweating, massage, sauna baths, laxatives, girdles are advertised, and time and money are often wasted in an effort to lose weight with them, but often no weight is lost even after experiencing the discomfort.

Weight conscious Americans continue to spend millions of dollars hoping to peel off fat through some slim-quick gimmick. Dr. Morton Glenn of New York Medical School states "I know of no mechanical device that will cause a person to lose or redistribute his weight." One takes off pounds by means of fewer calories and regular exercise, but not with gadgets. Glenn also comments, "There is no proof you can vibrate fat, all these machines do is jiggle fat."[20]

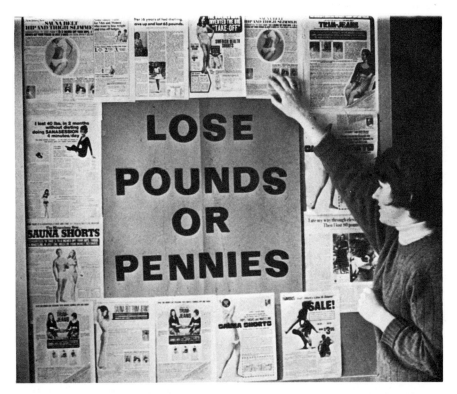

Caution is needed in analyzing advertisements that suggest crash diets or weight reducing gadgets. One should only diet under the supervision of a physician.

Aware of these misleading claims, the legal department of the U.S. Postal Service and the Food and Drug Administration are trying to zero in on the problem. Mail order weight reducing methods and devices have been a major fraudulent scheme to swindle consumers. Because no government agency is authorized to demand proof that a device is effective and safe prior to sale, anyone can go into the business. Then the

20. "Gadgets That Promise to Slim You Quickly," *Changing Times,* January 1974, p. 19.

government must investigate any false claims, which takes time and money. Future legislation which would require all manufacturers of medical devices to furnish effectiveness and safety data could reduce many phony items from the market. Meanwhile, one's best defense for weight control would be to eat sensibly with low calorie diets, exercise regularly, or perhaps enroll in an exercise program at the local YWCA or YMCA under a qualified instructor and program.

## Identifying Quacks and Nostrums

How does one identify a phony or a fake product? There are some general questions and points to remember when learning to become a wise consumer. The American Medical Association offers the following:

### HOW TO RECOGNIZE A QUACK
1. The quack often uses a special or "secret" formula or machine that he claims can cure disease.
2. He may promise or imply a quick or easy cure, or he may talk about "pepping up" your health.
3. He advertises, using his "case histories" and testimonials from his "patients" to impress people.
4. He refuses to accept the tried and proved methods of medical research and proof. He clamors constantly for "medical investigation" and recognition, but he avoids a test or stops short of giving the data needed for a scientific evaluation.
5. He claims medical men are persecuting him or that they are afraid of his competition.
6. He claims that his method of treatment is better than surgery, x-rays, and drugs prescribed by a physician.[21]

With so many products on the market, a mobile complex society, and flexible laws, there are basically only two deterrents able to counteract quackery: (1) a wise and intelligent, informed consumer, and (2) sound enforcement of our laws. Instead of complaining to yourself or to your friend, it is your responsibility to report suspicious persons and products. The consumer must and can protect himself.

21. "Facts on Quacks—What You Should Know About Health Quackery" (Chicago, Ill.: American Medical Association, Dept. of Investigation.)

## A Turkey With the Mumps?

On May 24, 1963 Mrs. Jackie Metcalf, a 22-year-old Torrance housewife, submitted blood samples from a turkey, a sheep and a pig to Dr. Cynthia Chatfield, a chiropractor and co-operator with her mother, Dr. Ruth Drown, of one of America's largest radionic device swindles.

Labeling the bogus blood samples as specimens from her three children, Mrs. Metcalf secured diagnoses from Dr. Chatfield, at $50 each, that her children were suffering from chicken pox and mumps, and was told how to set the dials on her own (Drown-supplied) treatment device for these conditions.

But Mrs. Metcalf wasn't exactly a typical patient. As an undercover agent for the Bureau of Food and Drug Inspections of the State Department of Public Health, her job was to obtain evidence with which to determine whether or not the operation was fraudulent. Over a period of 37 years, Drown Laboratories had treated 35,000 patients, boasted Dr. Drown.

The Drown Theory is described in one of the firm's booklets:

"We *diagnose* by placing the patient (or his blood crystal) in a lateral 'hook-up' to the instrument. When we *treat* we hook up the patient (or blood crystal) in series with the instrument, using an electrode on the solar plexus of the patient (or with the blood crystal hooked up to the electrode) which causes the patient to take the place of a dry-cell battery. We turn the dials to the disease rates and areas of the body affected, and the instrument is grounded. The patient is treated by his *own energy*. . . ."

Christine Weber, "Health Quackery May Kill More People Than All Crimes of Violence," *California's Health*, vol. 24, no. 5, January 1967. Reprinted by permission of the State Department of Public Health, Berkeley, California.

## The Food Dollar

The "hows" of purchasing nutritious foods on a budget is a subject that has a familiar ring to all of us. Wise buying of groceries calls for budgeting and planning.

The average American family divides its food dollar according to this pattern.

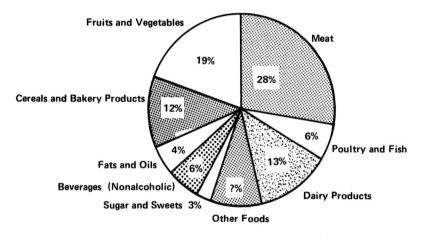

Regardless of income level, the average American family divides its food dollar according to this pattern (weight of food on fresh market basis). (From *Grocery Industry Barometer.* Washington D.C., Grocery Manufacturer's of America, Inc., 1970. Based on "Food Consumption of Household in the U.S.," Spring 1965, Agric. Res. Serv., U.S.D.A.

**What proportion of the income should be spent for food?** In general, the less the income, the greater the proportion of it that must be spent for food in order to secure a nutritionally adequate diet. While the "average" American spends 16 percent of his disposable income on food, an American family at a low income level may have to spend over half, in some cases, of their total income for food in order to obtain a "minimum-cost adequate diet."

The three main ways of reducing the cost of an adequate diet are:

1. *Use a larger proportion of the less expensive food groups.*

Most of us do not need to subsist on a minimum-cost diet, but for those who do the problem is how to make such a diet adequate for body needs. One of the main problems is to get enough calories to satisfy hunger, to provide energy for work, and to keep warm.

Cereal products and starchy vegetables may be used more safely in large quantities than sugar or fats, because sugar and fats are mainly energy foods and they provide a one-sided diet. When a large percentage of cereal products are used in the diet, it is important that whole-grain or enriched products be used, since these carry a valuable bonus in minerals and vitamins, which the highly milled products do not provide.

Obviously, adequate amounts of energy sources alone do not suffice to maintain health. The necessary quota of all essential nutrients must also be met.

2. *Substitute cheaper for more expensive foods within the same food group.*

Substitution of cheaper for more expensive foods within the same group is another way to reduce food costs and is the best program to follow when only moderate reduction of food expense is required, because none of the nutritive advantages of the higher cost diet are sacrificed. For example, one can have the advantages of using fruits and vegetables liberally but keep down cost by selecting only the least expensive kinds of fruits and vegetables. Considerable reductions in costs may be made, by using cheaper substitutes for the more expensive foods in the same group.

There are wide differences in costs within the different food groups. The cost difference depends considerably on whether one buys fat in the form of cottonseed oil or olive oil, and protein in the form of dried skim milk, dried legumes and whole grain cereals, or eggs and beef steak.

Because meat is usually the most expensive item of the diet, low-income families are advised to serve cheaped cuts (such as chuck, breast of veal, shoulder of lamb, and ground, organ, and stew meats) only three or four times a week, and to use fish, legumes, and an egg or cheese dish on the other three or four days.

3. *Eliminate waste in buying, storing, cooking or serving foods.*

Efficient buying and preparation of food are the most satisfactory means of all to reduce food costs, because they involve no diminution in the variety, attractiveness, or nutritive value of the menu. By merely "stopping the leaks," enough saving may be effected to provide a better diet at less cost. Such waste can occur in the course of buying, storing, preparing, or serving foods.

Considerable money savings can be effected by thrifty marketing. In general, buying in larger quantities, watching for special bargains on certain foods, going to the market to select perishable foods that are of good quality, and selecting less expensive types or brands of food when these are suitable, all result in lowering the food bill.

Read package labels to know what you are paying for. Ingredients are listed in descending order of amount present.

## Inexpensive Sources of Various Nutrients

| Nutrients | Food Sources |
|---|---|
| Energy | Fats, oils, flour, cereals, breads, potatoes, sugar, dried beans or peas, and peanut butter. |
| Protein | Dried beans or peas, peanut butter, whole-grain cereals or breads, milk (especially dried skim milk), cheaper cheeses, eggs, poultry, and less expensive meats and fish. |
| Calcium | Milk (especially dried skim milk), ice milk (dessert), cheese, dark green leafy vegetables, whole-grain products, and legumes. |
| Iron | Dried beans or peas, liver, whole-grain or enriched breads or cereals, dark green leafy vegetables, eggs, less expensive meats, potatoes and sweet potatoes, and prunes. |
| Vitamin A | Dark green and deep yellow vegetables, liver, fortified margarine, canned tomatoes, prunes, and less expensive cheeses. |
| Vitamin C | Canned or frozen citrus fruit juices, canned tomatoes, raw cabbage, some dark green and leafy vegetables, and potatoes. |
| Thiamin | Dried legumes, whole-grain or enriched bread and cereals, liver, inexpensive cuts of pork, and potatoes. |
| Riboflavin | Milk, ice milk (dessert), cheese, whole-grain or enriched breads, eggs, dried legumes, and dark green and leafy vegetables. |
| Niacin | Dried beans or peas, peanuts or peanut butter, whole-grain and enriched cereal products, meat, poultry, fish, some dark green, leafy vegetables. |

L. Bogert, G. Briggs, and D. Calloway, *Nutrition and Physical Fitness*, (Philadelphia, W. B. Saunders Company, 1973), p. 407.

## Some Guidelines in Menu Planning

*General Rules*

1. Use the whole day as a unit rather than the individual meal. Make breakfast relatively simple and standardized, then plan dinner, and lastly plan luncheon (or supper) so as to supplement the other two meals.
2. Use some foods from each of the food groups (carbohydrate foods, protein-rich foods, fatty foods, fruits, and vegetables) daily and usually in each meal.
3. Use some raw food at least once a day.
4. Plan to have in every meal at least one food which has staying quality or high satiety value, at least one food which requires chewing, one which contains roughage, and generally some hot food or drink.
5. Combine (or alternate) bland foods with those of more pronounced flavor.
6. Combine (or alternate) soft foods with those crisp in texture.
7. Have variety in color, form, and arrangement of foods.
8. Alternate simple and less nutritious dishes with those which are of higher protein and/or fat content, and hence slow down digestion in, and emptying of, the stomach.
9. When more foods are served at one meal, decrease the size of the portions and use fewer rich foods. When a more simple meal is desired, use a few nutritious, easily digested foods, and serve larger portions.

*Don'ts*

1. Avoid using the same food twice in one day without varying the form in which it is served, except staples such as bread, butter, and milk.
2. Do not use the same food twice in the same meal, even in different forms.
3. Do not use the same foods too constantly, even from day to day.
4. Avoid monotony of color, texture, etc., in any one meal or in the daily dietary.

Waste in the kitchen may occur in many ways, some of the chief ones being: (1) discarding portions of food which have nutritive value (vegetable trimmings, meat trimmings, cooking water, liquid from canned vegetables) which are suitable for cooking, (2) burning foods or careless scraping of them from cooking utensils in serving, or (3) failure to utilize leftover foods properly, (4) food wasted at the table by taking too large individual portions or, in one way or another, rendering what is not eaten unfit to serve again, and (5) spoilage of food through improper care in storage.

## Sources of Protection

### The Food and Drug Administration (FDA)

The FDA's responsibility is to protect the consumer by insuring (1) that there is enforcement of the Food, Drug and Cosmetic Act; (2) that periodic inspections of food, drug, device and cosmetic establishments are maintained; (3) that industry is assisted in setting up controls to prevent violation; (4) that all of the aforementioned are legitimately labeled and packaged; and (5) that certain household products that may be hazardous carry adequate warning labels.[22] The FDA also tests drugs and investigates the safety of colors and ingredients in various products. (Besides investigating the safety of cyclamates, it also issued the ban on thalidomide in 1962, which has been proven to be a birth-deforming substance.) No new additives may be used until the company presents satisfactory evidence to the FDA that the properties are safe when given to animals. The FDA *does not control the supervision of advertising techniques,* however. Over 900 inspectors are employed in over 18 district offices throughout the United States. The FDA also employs its own legal staff to prepare for court cases.

### The Federal Trade Commission (FTC)

The FTC's responsibility is to supervise the advertising of all foods, drugs, cosmetics and devices aired via mass media. Since there are more than 4,000 radio and television stations, and since the FTC has a limited budget and few staff employees, its effectiveness is limited to date. To make its work even more difficult, advertisements are not reviewed before they appear, so the commission must find the advertisements and prove them false or misleading. *After* finding them, it conducts tests, investigations, and finally notifies the advertiser. The advertiser may

22. "FDA—What It Is and Does" (Washington, D.C.: U.S. Department of Health, Education and Welfare, Food and Drug Administration), no. 1.

change the advertisement or may contest in court—another period of delay. It took the FTC 16 years to prove that "Carters Little Liver Pills" did nothing to aid the liver.[23]

## The Post Office

Many quacks hide by using the mail order techniques. No one can use the U.S. mail for purposes of fraud. The Fraud Statute of 1872 prohibits sending materials through the mail with intent to defraud. Any consumer who believes an item or material sent to him through the mail to be fraudulous should report it to his local post office.

## Other Sources

The American Medical Association, the Better Business Bureau, the U.S. Chamber of Commerce, and the American Dental Association—these organizations stand as reliable organizations to educate and assist the public through their findings. They also are concerned about fraudulent practices and products. But it is still up to the individual consumer to register his complaint with a reliable source before proper action can be taken.

## Consumer Responsibility

Every consumer should analyze his purchases carefully. Here are some points to consider when ready to make purchases:

1. Rely on the advice of your physician when considering the purchase of specific products that claim health benefits.

2. Avoid purchasing special health foods and vitamin supplements unless prescribed by a physician.

3. Recognize the modern quack and his sales pitch.

4. Be cautious of health products promoted by a door-to-door salesman.

5. Be alert when reading advertisements for health products.

6. Look for proprietary drug products (nonprescription drugs) that

23. Ralph L. Smith, *The Health Hucksters* (New York: Hillman–McFadden, 1961), p. 187.

bear the letters U.S.P. or N.F., meaning they meet the criteria established by the United States Pharmacopeia or National Formulary.

7. If suspicious of a fraud or a quack, seek the assistance of reliable organizations, and don't hesitate to report your suspicion, regardless of cost.[24]

## Health Services

Some decades are remembered for scientific discoveries or progress in technology. The 70s may well become the years remembered for medical costs soaring out of control and political red tape preventing controls to aid the consumer. So Senator Abraham Ribicoff claims.

"For millions of Americans the symbol of medical care in the 70s is not Red Cross, Blue Cross or the physician's insignia, it is the dollar sign. It is also the doctor shortage, the crowded facilities, and the devasstating needs of the poor."[25] Ribicoff also predicts hospital care will cost $950 a day by 1980. Currently some hospitals will not admit a patient without a $350 deposit. In Illinois, reports reveal that over 150 communities are without a doctor. In Los Angeles, one nurse may care for seventy patients. In Tulsa, Oklahoma, authorities reveal that medical bills account for 60 percent of all bankruptcies.

Good health care for the entire citizenry is one of this country's most serious unresolved problems. The government has been studying health services and the delivery of medical care for years, but progress has been painfully slow.

In some parts of the country health services are excellent but costly. In other metropolitan areas the per capita ratio of doctors to patients is adequate, but it is the poor who can't afford services; furthermore, many people who live in rural areas are currently deprived of medical care. Some political leaders foresee legislation requiring all new physicians to spend two years service by practicing in a needy area. One of the government's immediate solutions has been allocations of federal grants combined with state and local funds to establish clinics and primary health care centers, staffed by qualified medical personnel. New centers are beginning to spring up in remote rural areas, but time will only prove if

24. W. Cushman, M. Beyrer, M. Solleder, and R. Kaplan, *Positive Health, Designs for Action* (Columbus, Ohio: Charles Merrill 1965), pp. 132–33.
25. Abraham Ribicoff. *The American Medicine Machine,* (New York: Saturday Review Press, 1972), p. 12.

these new clinics can be self-supporting due to overall increase in expenditures of medical facilities, staff, and supplies.

More recently has been the new legislation to create Health Maintenance Organizations (HMO). Between now and July 1, 1978 the government will contribute 325 million dollars for establishing more HMOs. The HMO is a plan of prepaid group health programs. It guarantees most basic medical services to a group of subscribers for a fixed fee which is paid in advance. HMO physicians usually work in group practices. In California, The Kaiser plan proved successful and probably pioneered the future for the HMOs now being established. Officials predict the establishment of 400 new HMOs will bring membership to 20 million. In 1963 there were only 3 million members, but because the HMO stresses preventive care and paramedical assistance in a group practice situation it has proved to keep medical costs down for the consumer.

In order to receive federal monies every HMO must now provide:
- physician services.
- in patient/out patient services including lab fees.
- emergency care.
- health care at home.
- medical treatment for drugs and alcohol.
- short term psychiatric care.
- complete physical checkups.
- dental exams for children under 12.[26]

Costs for a family will generally be between $49–$65 a month. Supporters say it is still cheaper than the traditional fee for service because of its emphasis on preventive care and health education. Medical personnel are now in heated debate over advantages and disadvantages.[27]

Although hospital costs have risen 170 percent from 1960 to 1970, and doctor's fees have increased by 60 percent, the challenge of building a modern system of health care and delivering health services to everyone in a just and economical way will not occur overnight. Yet it is also true that it will not be accomplished if pilot programs aren't begun, if procrastination continues and lengthy political debate hinders activity. Whether the HMO is going to be the new, effective means of delivery remains to be seen. Many doctors will fight for fee-for-service and solo practice.

26. "One Stop Health Care: How It Works." *U.S. News and World Report,* Jan. 21, 1974.
27. *Ibid.*

## Health Maintenance Organizations

| *Advantages* | *Disadvantages* |
|---|---|
| 1. Relieves doctors from billing, collecting | 1. No follow-up on certain cases |
| 2. Regular income, days off for physician | 2. Too routine |
| 3. Opportunity to talk to colleagues daily | 3. Fees too low, salary not as high |
| 4. Access to latest equipment | 4. Human values are lost as medicine becomes more socialized |

The medical profession, which was the most honored of all, is under attack with what many label as an overmanaged condition. The profession, peculiarly isolated from political process, failed to comprehend what was going on around it. Now the consumer of medical services demands his rights to know more. Peer review and a professional standards review organization have had to come into being through government legislation.

If people are to be well served, physicians must not be shackled, and dispassionate discussion must prevail in the promulgation of public policy for medicine.[28]

Physicians are scarce and not available in all parts of this prosperous land. Because demand is high and supply is low, the medical imposter intrudes. Our society is so mobile that many families fail to establish the services of a family physician or the general practitioner until an emergency arises. Often they are then angered or dismayed to learn of the shortage of doctors, and the high cost of health services.

In selecting a reliable physician in a community, you can check the AMA listing in the local library to evaluate the medical qualifications of a physician. To become a licensed medical doctor in all states requires four years of college and an additional three or four years of medical school, which is generally followed by some type of internship for several years. The individual must pass National Board examinations, which may

28. Clark Wescoe. "Overmanagement of Medicine," *Science*, Jan. 18, 1974, vol. 183, no. 4121, p. 155.

permit him to practice in reciprocating states where the examinations are the same. Some states require additional state medical examinations Having passed the required examinations, the doctor is licensed to become a general practitioner or family physician. Anything of a serious, specialized nature affecting a patient should be referred to a medical specialist. Medical specialists must take advanced training plus practice in the special area for several years and pass a special examintion by an American Examining Board.

## Medical Specialists

The definitions of medical specialists listed below have been adapted or quoted from John Sinacore's *Health, A Quality of Life.*[29]

**Allergist.** One who treats and diagnoses body reactions which show hypersensitivity to drugs, pollens, foods, animals, or other things (a subspecialty of internal medicine).

**Anesthetist or Anesthesiologist.** One who administers an anesthetic to effect a loss of consciousness (general anesthesia) or a loss of sensation in a specific location (local anesthesia).

**Cardiologist.** One having special knowledge and experience in the diagnosis and treatment of heart disease (a subspecialty of internal medicine).

**Dermatologist.** A practitioner who specializes in the diagnosis and treatment of curaneous lesions and the related systemic diseases; a "skin" specialist.

**Endocrinologist.** One who deals with the internal secretions of the ductless glands and their physiologic and pathologic relations.

**Epidemiologist.** One who specializes in the study of the determinants and distributions of disease prevalence.

**Gastroenterologist.** A specialist in the diseases of the digestive system.

**Gerontologist or Geriatrician.** One who specializes in the science of the physiologic and pathologic changes incident to old age.

**Gynecologist.** The physician who specializes in the branch of medicine which has to do with the diseases peculiar to women, primarily those of the genital tract, as well as female endocrinology and reproductive physiology.

**Internist.** A physician trained in internal medicine, which is the medical specialty concerned with illnesses of a nonsurgical nature, mainly in adults.

**Neurologist.** A specialist in the nonsurgical treatment of diseases of the nervous system.

**Neurosurgeon.** A specialist in the diagnosis and surgical treatment of the nervous system.

**Obstetrician.** One who is skilled in the medical care of a woman during pregnancy and in childbirth and the interval immediately following.

**Ophthalmologist or Oculist.** A specialist in diseases and refractive errors of the eye.

**Orthopedist or Orthopedic Surgeon.** One who specializes in the branch of surgery that has to do with the treatment of chronic diseases of the joints and spine and the correction of deformities.

**Otolaryngologist.** A specialist in the diseases of the ear and larynx.

**Otologist.** A specialist in the diseases of the ear.

**Otorhinolaryngologist.** A specialist in the diseases of the ear, nose, and larynx.

**Pathologist.** A specialist in the identification of disease through the analysis of body tissues, fluids, and other body specimens.

**Pediatrician.** A medical practitioner who specializes in the prevention, diagnosis, and treatment of diseases in children.

**Plastic Surgeon.** The physician who specializes in the branch of operative surgery that corrects or repairs deformed or mutilated parts of the body.

**Proctologist.** A specialist in the science that deals with diagnosis and treatment of the colon, rectum, and anus.

**Psychiatrist.** A specialist who deals in the interpretation and treatment of mental and personality disorders.

**Radiologist.** A physician who is skilled in the diagnostic and therapeutic use of x-rays and other forms of radiant energy.

**Rhinologist.** A specialist who deals with the disorders of the nose.

**Surgeon.** A specialist who treats diseases through operative measures.

**Urologist.** The physician who specializes in the study, diagnosis, and treatment of diseases of the genitourinary tract.

29. John Sinacore, *Health, A Quality of Life* (New York: Macmillan, 1968), p. 273.

Receiving increased attention when a family chooses a doctor has been the osteopathic physician, the holder of a D.O. degree, or doctor of osteopathy. Some feel that osteopaths have equal training to general practitioners. An osteopath is licensed to practice osteopathic medicine and surgery in every state. The theory and practice of the American Osteopathic Association is closely aligned to the medical profession. Osteopaths must go to one of the 5 osteopathic colleges which require 4 years of training and an additional year of internship in one of 90 osteopathic hospitals.

Choosing a family doctor or specialist is an important decision. Before making such a decision the following questions should be asked:

1. Is he a graduate of a recognized school of medicine?
2. Is he licensed to practice medicine?
3. Is he a member of available medical societies?
4. Is he on the staff of a reputable hospital?
5. Has he had experience in the desired area?
6. If a specialist, has he had advanced training in his field?
7. Is he respected in the community and by his associates?
8. Does he inspire confidence in you as a patient?

It may involve some effort to find answers to these questions, but the information *is* available in all communities. It can be found in the following manner:

1. Referral by a former medical advisor
2. Referral from a local, county or state medical association list of licensed physicians and their educational background
3. Referral from local hospital lists of doctors in the area
4. Referral from the local health department
5. Referral from neighbors and health personnel who can assist in establishing a physician's reputation
6. Finally, by making an appointment with the physician and evaluating him from a personal point of view

## Dentists

Did you know that the leading disease among school age children is caries (dental cavities)? Because of poor nutritional habits, Americans and their families are demanding more services from the dental professions for all types of oral problems than ever before. Dentists are licensed to prescribe drugs as well. All states demand passage of strict state board examination requirements, but the dental field also has its areas of specialization. Sinacore describes them as:

**Endodontist.** One who specializes in the diagnosis and treatment of diseases of the pulp (or nerve) of a tooth. This speciality embraces methods of pulp conservation as well as tooth retention once infection at the root has developed.

**Orthodontist.** The dental specialist who is concerned with the correction and prevention of irregularities of the teeth and malocclusion of the jaw.

**Pedodontist.** One who specializes in the treatment of dental ills of children.

**Periodontist.** A dentist who specializes in the treatment of the supporting tissues of the teeth.

**Prosthodontist** is concerned with the construction of special appliances (dentures, bridges, crowns) to compensate mechanically for oral deficiencies such as tooth loss and cleft palate.

**Oral surgeon.** One who specializes in extraction of teeth and surgical procedures involving the soft tissues of the oral cavity.

## Health Insurance

U.S. doctors' fees are rising twice as fast as consumer prices, hospital costs are soaring, and present health insurance programs, public or private, are currently inadequate to meet health requirements for this country. Since 1912 dozens of national health programs have been discussed and studied. In 1968 after the government finally initiated Medicare for the elderly and Medicaid for the needy, 20 percent of all Americans under 65 had no hospital insurance, 22 percent had no surgical insurance, and 97 percent had no dental insurance. Although the U.S. has been reluctant to establish a national health insurance program, Britain, Canada and Japan have had successful programs for some time.

The U.S. Department of Health, Education and Welfare reported that individual health care costs will continue to rise due to higher salaries for health personnel, and increased hospital service and administrative costs. As health costs rise, and health services become less and less accessible, interest has grown in extending the health insurance principle to all citizens by means of legislation.

Representative Griffith, who has been a pioneer for national health insurance, pointed out that:

1. The United States is not a leader in longevity even with current funds being spent for health care.

2. Other countries with better longevity rates and with national health insurance programs provide services at a lower cost than in the United States.

3. More than 412,000 persons in 115 counties in 23 states do not have access to physicians.

---

For the family of Norman Quynn, sixty-four, a retired grocer from Waynesboro, Pennsylvania, the future came early —ten years and two months early. They had their $1,000 a day hospital bill on February 16, 1970 when they received a $4,599.90 bill for the four and a half days Mr. Quynn was a patient at the University of Pennsylvania Hospital in Philadelphia. He was admitted at 6:00 p.m. on Sunday and died at 6:30 a.m. the following Friday. Mr. Quynn underwent complex and extensive surgery for a bleeding ulcer that had hemmorrhaged and for other stomach problems. His bill included the following items:

| | | | |
|---|---|---|---|
| Room | $462 | Intensive care | $180 |
| Laboratory | $743 | Intravenous | $139 |
| Pharmacy | $114 | Albumin | $320 |
| Operating room | $395 | Breathing | |
| Tranfusions | $1,430 | press machine | $20 |
| Surgical supplies | $321 | Pulmonary function | |
| Radiology | $145 | study | $60 |
| Cardiology | $40 | Other charges | $134 |
| Oxygen | $96 | | |

The family was stunned by the size of the bill, especially since Mr. Quynn had previously spent the same amount of time in a hospital in rural Chambersburg, Pennsylvania, where he had a kidney removed for $899, or $200 a day.

Source: Abraham Ribicoff, *The American Medical Machine*. (New York: Saturday Review Press, 1970), p. 11–12.

4. One out of 50 Americans cannot obtain a doctor under any circumstances.[30]

Former President Nixon expressed his concern for the health status of Americans by emphasizing what was right with medical care—higher quality, profusion of new techniques, powerful new drugs and splendid new facilities.

On the other hand, he mentioned faults in our present medical care system, one of the biggest being that 60 percent of increased medical expenditures in the decade were due to inflation. Medical costs have soared twice as fast as the cost of living, with hospital costs rising five times faster than other prices. Primary-care physicians and out-patient facilities are short of supply in some areas and emergency care services are limited.

Every year millions of Americans incur large medical expenses, often far surpassing their financial capabilities. Most families plan for a "doctor bill" now and then, but a major medical expenditure is rarely incurred on a planned basis. Related medical expenses frequently overlooked are: help in the home when a housewife is seriously incapacitated; loss of income when the family wage earner has a long illness; custodial care associated with old age; and appliances, special foods, medications, and related medical services.

There will always be families who are temporarily or permanently unable to meet the costs of prolonged or serious illness. Services now available are the following:

1. Public hospitals operated by city or county

2. Some beds available free of charge for the indigent in private hospitals

3. Hospitals sponsored by private groups such as fraternal organizations and religious sects

Most Americans need some type of health insurance in order to be able to afford health care services. Health insurance could be defined as an enterprise of collective security in which the individual makes regular payments, called "premiums," to guarantee and protect himself against an unplanned financial crisis due to a health problem or an accident such as illness, injury, old age, or death. There are basically two types of insur-

---

30. John Sinacore, "National Health Insurance Gains Support In Congress," *Congressional Quarterly Weekly Report,* vol. 28, no. 38, p. 2269 (Sept. 1970).

ance: the tax-supported programs, and the individual insurance programs. Among the government or tax-supported programs offering help to the medically indigent are: Veterans Administration hospitals and medical care; medical care for military personnel and their dependents; medical care for those with special diseases, such as mental disease, communicable diseases such as tuberculosis and venereal diseases, and rare diseases, such as leprosy, treated at the Public Hospital, in Louisiana.

The most broad-based tax-supported program of medical insurance is the Medicare program. This protection was instituted in 1965 to cover all persons over 65 years of age, regardless of need. It is not a voluntary program but is compulsory, with all persons contributing through Social Security.

Part one of Medicare deals with payment of hospital bills. The major benefits of this part include: 90 days hospitalization, with the patient paying $40.00 for the first 60 days and $10.00 a day after that; 100 days of post-hospital care in a Medicare-approved nursing home at $5.00 a day after the first 20 days; 100 home visits by a nurse, therapist, or related health worker after a hospital stay of at least 3 days; 190 days psychiatric hospital care during a lifetime; and outpatient services with the patient paying the first $20.00 and 20 percent of the cost above that for all services rendered during the 20-day period.

Part two of Medicare is a voluntary program designed to defray other medical expenses incurred. Persons 65 years and older desiring to participate in this program pay $4.00 per month as a premium, the first $50.00 accumulated per year, and 20 percent of the expenses above that. The major benefits of this program include: physician and surgeon services including necessary specialists; 100 home health visits a year, regardless of hospital stay; diagnostic x-ray and laboratory tests; x-ray, radium, and isotope therapy; ambulance services; medical appliances; and outpatient psychiatric treatment, limited to $250.00 per year.

The Medicare program is a great help to many people, but it does not provide for out-of-hospital medications, long illnesses requiring long hospitalization and doctor bills, nor custodial care in nursing homes. Therefore, many people find it advisable to carry some type of individual insurance in addition to Medicare.

There are basically five types of individual insurance programs available, regardless of the issuing company. They are all a contract between the policy holder and the issuing company, whether issued on a group basis or individually.

Loss of income protection is designed to protect a family if the breadwinner is incapacitated for a prolonged period. It guarantees a given percentage of income for a limited amount of time, usually 50 percent of the income for one year or more.

Hospitalization coverage provides for room and board and related hospitalization expenses for a given number of days.

Surgical expense insurance provides for a set amount of coverage for each specific type of operation to be used to cover operating room costs and surgeon fees.

Protection against regular medical expenditures is a type of insurance becoming more popular in recent years. It allows for routine visits to a doctor's office and his home visits. Some policies will cover medication and related expenses.

Major medical insurance protects against the "catastrophic" illness. It covers medical and hospital bills incurred during major or long-term illnesses and can be written with a deductible amount, as with automobile insurance.

No matter what type of insurance is purchased, or whether or not it is purchased on an individual basis or on a group plan at the place of employment, it is wise to deal with a reputable insurance company and to keep in mind three things:

1. How much medical expense can an individual afford to pay himself?
2. For what type eventuality does one desire protection?
3. Does the policy actually allow for the above?

Two of the most serious risks are loss of income due to injury or illness and the catastrophic medical costs. No major medical insurance is inexpensive and odds are the cost will increase. No present rates can be guaranteed for the future, so one should obtain all the health insurance one can afford even if sacrifice may be involved. Disability insurance is the most practical and effective way of offsetting risks. Such insurance replaces a large portion of an individual's paycheck for whatever one pays for the benefits, provided one is disabled. Total disability refers to complete inability to carry out duties of a present job for a period stated in one's policy. The noncancellable policy is usually the safest and best form of protection one can buy.[31]

31. Gayle Richardson, *Am I Covered,* (Indianapolis: Unified College Press, Inc., 1973).

Many legislators feel that the Medicare and Medicaid programs must be replaced because their services are limited to the poor and to the elderly. Private health plans often fail to meet needs because of no comprehensive coverage, and they are also generally unavailable to individuals of limited incomes.

In December of 1970 Congress passed a bill authorizing 225 million dollars to be spent over the fiscal years 1971–73 to assist hospitals and medical schools in relieving the shortage of doctors in general practice. It also provided aid for medical students and hospitals concentrating in the area of family medicine.

Health, Education and Welfare Secretary Elliot L. Richardson commented, "Impressive growth in the number of people covered by health insurance conceals the fact that only 29 percent of all personal health expenditures were paid by insurance in 1968."

Health insurance coverages many times are riddled with loopholes and fine print. They may promise complete coverage but in a crisis there may be less protection than one thought and more expenses than one can afford.

The American Medical Association opposed national health insurance. They favored a free health insurance plan for the poor financed by the federal government. Persons with an income would receive a tax credit for their premiums based upon a sliding scale. They called their proposal, which encouraged everyone to purchase comprehensive health insurance, "Medicredit." Legislators didn't feel this plan was in the best interest of the consumer.

Representative Griffith of Iowa introduced a plan in June, 1970, as did Senator Kennedy in August. Later they combined their efforts and called their proposal the "Human Security Program." Senator Edward Kennedy, chairman of the Health Subcommittee of the Labor and Public Welfare Committee, desired a working partnership between public and private sectors, with the estimated program to cost about 40 billion dollars. His basic program stemmed from the efforts of a task force of 100 members originally formed by Walter Reuther.

Kennedy's "cradle-to-the grave" concept benefits health care for everyone with complete federal control and abolishment of private insurance companies, but it is a costly program to taxpayers. Kennedy justified his plan after listening to personal accounts of medical inadequacies when serving on the Senate Investigation Committee hearings in this area.

As a believer and crusader for health care for every American, he states, "Just as Franklin Roosevelt's Social Security Program of the 30s brought hope to a nation mired in a great depression, so I believe the Health Security Program in the 70's can guarantee good health care to our people and lead us out of the crisis we now face in our health system."[32] Private health insurance companies served a good purpose at one

> "I am shocked to find that we in America have created a health care system that can be so callous to human suffering, so intent on high salaries and profits, and so unconcerned for the needs of our people.
> I believe good health care should be a right for all Americans. Health is so basic to a man's ability to bring to fruition his opportunities as an American that each of us should guarantee the best possible health care to every American at a cost he can afford."
>
> Source: Edward Kennedy, *In Critical Condition, The Crisis in America's Health Care,* (New York: Simon and Shuster, 1972), p. 252.

time, but it does appear America has outgrown the system. Private companies appear to be burdened with high medical costs, more technicalities in policies and lower profits to themselves. Kennedy would like to utilize these private sectors under a nationalized health insurance program with the government picking up the tab.

Former President Nixon's plan costs would have approximated 4–6 billion in contrast to Kennedy's 40 billion estimate. The businessmen in the country would have felt the crunch of Nixon's plan since the employer would have payed for 25 percent of coverage. The plan would have averaged $445 a year per family. Critics of Nixon on this issue felt that it overburdened employers and employees in its zest for government economy. Any plan that can help curtail present medical costs should help a citizen achieve his basic right to good health. Judging from past evidence, we may not have progressed very far in actualizing human concern for the well-being of others, for it was Aristotle who said, ". . . If we believe men

32. Edward Kennedy. *Viewpoint,* vol. 3, no. 3, 1973, Ind. Union Dept. AFL-CIO.

have any personal rights at all as human beings, they have an absolute right to such a measure of good health as society, and society alone, is able to give them."

After continued pressure led by Democrats, President Nixon was forced to draft his administration's own proposal for a national insurance plan, although he had campaigned against national health insurance in 1968. In February, 1971 President Nixon offered a plan which may be in effect by 1977. His plan calls for increased health care programs, and requiring health insurance for 80 percent of the population through employer-employee contributions. (Senator Kennedy's plan would cover the nation's entire population.) Under the Nixon plan, the employer would pay 75 percent of the cost for families with children having an annual income of more than $3,500. The government would pay the entire amount for families with less than $3,500 income.

Nixon's proposal for compulsory coverage has been criticized by some as a prospective boon to the insurance industry. The Nixon package appears to involve minimum cost for a program that would attempt to resolve the nation's health crisis and increasing costs. His plan would include all maternity care with no deductibles and well-child clinics to include vaccinations. Senator Kennedy is opposed, since he disagrees with the principle of involving private insurance industries. Many speculate that Blue Cross and Blue Shield could be used to underwrite the employer insurance and family health insurance plans.

## Questions for Study and Discussion

1. Do you think self-medication is dangerous?
2. When do you feel you last fell prey to a quack or a nostrum?
3. What health products are currently on the market that you feel should be more carefully investigated?
4. Why has the FTC been so lenient with the advertising of health products?
5. What health advertisements today do you feel are misleading?
6. Why are people afraid of hospitals?
7. Why is the American public ignorant about health and life insurance?
8. Is there presently a shortage of physicians? If so, what effect does this have on our nation's health?
9. Is there a need for a change in the existing types of health insurance? What would you suggest?

10. What is the role of voluntary health organizations such as the American Cancer Society and the American Heart Association?

## References

American Assembly. *Health of Americans,* Englewood Cliffs, N.J.: Prentice Hall, Inc., 1970, p. 209.

Cushman, Wesley P.; Beyrer, Mary K.; Solleder, Marian K.; Kaplan, Robert. *Positive Health Designs for Action.* Columbus, Ohio: Charles E. Merrill, 1965, pp. 123–46.

"Facts About Quacks." *Today's Health.* February, 1968, p. 58.

"Facts You Should Know About Health Quackery." Educational Division, Better Business Bureau, 1957.

"FDA—What It Is and Does." Washington, D.C.: U.S. Department of Health, Education and Welfare, Food and Drug Administration, No. 1.

Furlong, William. "Getting a Massage That Won't Rub You The Wrong Way." *Today's Health,* May, 1972, p. 41.

Furlong, William. "You and Your Dangerous Health Practices," *Today's Health,* October, 1972, pp. 54–60.

"Gadgets That Promise To Slim You Quickly." *Changing Times,* January, 1974, pp. 19–21.

Katz, Sol. M.D. "Evaluating Cold Remedies." *Today's Health,* February, 1974, pp. 18–21.

Kennedy, Edward. *In Critical Condition, The Crisis in America's Health Care,* New York: Simon and Schuster, 1972, p. 252.

"National Health Insurance Is On The Way." *Business Week,* January 26, 1974, pp. 70–71.

"One Stop Health Care: How It Works." *U.S. News and World Report,* January 21, 1974.

"Pills and Potions for Indigestion." *Changing Times,* 21 (February, 1974): p. 39.

Ribicoff, Abraham, Sen. *The American Medical Machine,* Saturday Review Press, New York, 1972, p. 212.

Richardson, Gayle. *Am I Covered?* Indianapolis: Unified College Press, Inc., 1973, p. 309.

Sinacore, John. *Health, A Quality of Life.* New York: Macmillan, 1968, pp. 251–86.

Singer, Steve. "When They Start Telling You To Lose Weight." *Today's Health,* November, 1972, pp. 47–49.

*The Medicine Show.* Editors of Consumer Reports, Consumer Union Publication. New York: Simon and Schuster, 1961.

*Viewpoint,* vol. 3, no. 3, Third Quarterly 1973, Industrial Union Dept. AFL-CIO.

Weaver, Peter. "Toward More Effective Labeling," *Today's Health,* February, 1974.

Wescoe, W. Clarke. "Overmanagement of Medicine," *Science*, 183 (January 18, 1974): 155.

"Your Money and Your Life." Food and Drug Administration Catalog of Fakes and Swindles in the Health Field, U.S. Department of Health, Education and Welfare, No. 19, October, 1968.

# 9

# Nutrition

## General Concept

Nutrition is an important factor in the promotion of health and the prevention of disease. Evidence mounts that Americans who fail to attain a diet optimal for health can be found at every socioeconomic level.

## Outcomes

The student should be able to:
1. Identify the major nutrients required by the body to maintain health.
2. Demonstrate ways in which nutrients are used by the body.
3. Select the basic elements of a balanced diet for himself and his family.
4. Demonstrate that a variety of cultural food patterns can maintain good nutrition.
5. Explain the different nutritional needs of people throughout the life span.
6. Identify the major nutritional problems in contemporary society and be aware of the preventive aspects of these diseases.
7. Distinguish truths from myths about food and nutrition.

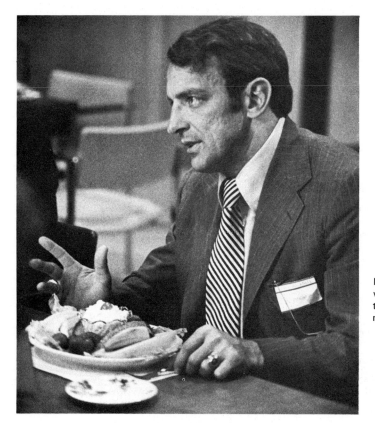

Meals should be socially gratifying with a time for pleasant conversation as well as meeting functional nutritional needs.

8. Identify inexpensive sources of various nutrients for wise food purchasing.

## Nutrition—What's It All About?

The present interest in saving the environment has united many diverse groups towards a common goal. From all levels of society people have climbed on the ecology bandwagon to promote balance with nature and the preservation of our country's resources. While the average American was becoming concerned about the environmental problems the youth subculture was adopting dietary patterns based on the concept of nature. Some of these concepts are healthful; others are questionable.

One ray of sunshine in this rather confused scene has been a greater public awareness of the importance of nutrition. The modern day consumer is bombarded with the need to discriminate between fact and fiction. Along with the awareness of nutrition has come a great deal of misleading information about food. To have the consumer become more knowledgeable about his nutritional needs will require a monumental effort from nutritionists, sociologists, anthropologists, economists, psychologists, agriculturalists, politicians, teachers, and public health workers. This diverse group of experts is required because nutrition is the study of the food man eats and the use of this food in the body.[1] Nutrition for each individual doesn't just happen. It is an accumulation of lifetime habits beginning at birth. Food patterns vary from individual to individual and culture to culture. These food patterns become more rigid as an individual ages and it is difficult at best to alter dietary patterns.

## Nutrition—What Combo Makes You Swing?

In learning to play a guitar there are some basic chords to learn, and with these chords you can compose a variety of tunes. With nutrition after you learn the basic elements you can develop your own individual

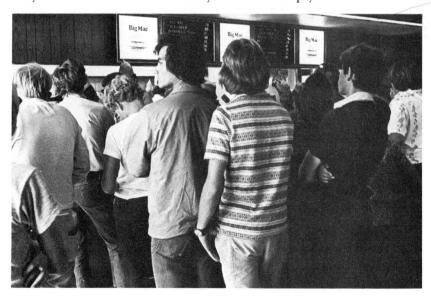

Dependence on fast foods and snacks threaten nutritional balance and weight control.

1. Stare, F. J. and M. McWilliams, *Living Nutrition*. (New York: John Wiley & Sons, 1973), p. 29.

dietary pattern using a combination of foods, depending on your preference, whether it be a typical American diet or a good vegetarian diet. Many combinations can work, as long as the basic nutrients are included in order to maintain good health.

These needs are satisfied by substances called nutrients which are found in the food man eats. These nutrients are further defined as carbohydrates, fats, proteins, minerals, vitamins, and water. The body depends on food for about 52 different nutrients. The physiological function of food may be divided into three general categories: the need for food materials to supply energy, the need for food materials to build and maintain the cells and tissues, and the need for food materials to regulate body processes.

## Food Nutrients to Supply Energy

The nutrients in foods which supply energy include carbohydrates, fats (lipids), and proteins. Under normal conditions of health and good eating habits the body will derive most of the energy needed from the carbohydrates and fats in food. Even though protein is generally classified as a tissue-building or repairing nutrient, it can be used as a source of energy. Protein is used for energy when there is insufficient carbohydrate and fat in the food intake to meet the energy demands. Protein foods are more expensive and less plentiful than either carbohydrate or fat foods. Using protein for energy has been compared to burning costly cherry wood when a cheaper wood, such as pine, would give the same amount of heat. Inasmuch as the primary function of food is to supply the body with energy-producing materials, the energy demand must be satisfied before the body uses food for building and maintenance, or regulation.

## The Need for Food Nutrients to Build and Maintain Body Tissue

Nutrients used in the building and maintenance of the body are proteins, minerals, and water. Each cell and tissue contain some of each of the body building nutrients.

## The Need for Food Nutrients to Regulate Body Process

All of the nutrients with the exception of carbohydrates and fats play a role in the regulation of the body processes. The proteins, the minerals, the vitamins, and water each perform regulatory functions essential to the normal functioning of the body.

## Carbohydrates

In typical American diets, carbohydrates provide between 45–55 percent of the day's calories. All carbohydrates contain carbon, hydrogen, and oxygen. A single classification of carbohydrates important in nutrition is:

1. Compounds with one carbohydrate unit are called monosaccharides. Glucose, fructose, and galactose are monosaccharides.
   a. Glucose, sometimes called dextrose, is found in sweet fruits such as grapes and in vegetables such as sweet corn. Glucose is the most important sugar in this class. It is the form of carbohydrate circulating in the blood and is utilized by the tissues for energy.
   b. Fructose, or fruit sugar, is the sweetest of all sugars. It occurs in honey, ripe fruits, and many vegetables.
   c. Galactose results from the breakdown of lactose, or milk sugar. It does not occur in the free state in nature.
2. Compounds with two carbohydrate units are called disaccharides. Sucrose, maltose, and lactose are the three disaccharides contained in the foods of the diet.
   a. Sucrose, the table sugar with which we are familiar, is found in sugar cane, sugar beets, and in many fruits and vegetables.
   b. Maltose, or malt sugar is found in malted products such as cereals and beer.
   c. Lactose, or milk sugar is produced by mammals. It is not very soluble, and is much less sweet than the other single or double sugars.
3. Compounds with more than two carbohydrate units are called polysaccharides. Polysaccharides include starch, glycogen, and cellulose.
   a. Starch is the form in which plants store carbohydrate, and thus is the primary source of energy in the diet. Cereal grains, seeds, roots, potatoes, green bananas, and other plants contain considerable starch.

b. Glycogen, the so-called animal starch, is the form in which the animal body stores carbohydrate. Oysters and liver are good sources of glycogen.

c. Cellulose is the most abundant organic compound in the world, comprising at least 50 percent of the carbon in vegetation. Wood and cotton are chiefly cellulose, but the skins of fruits, the coverings of seeds, and the structural parts of edible plants are the only forms of cellulose and hemicellulose with which we are concerned in the study of nutrition. We need a certain amount of cellulose to aid digestion and eliminate waste products in the feces.

How much carbohydrate in foods? The carbohydrate content of some typical foods—shown as percentages of total weight

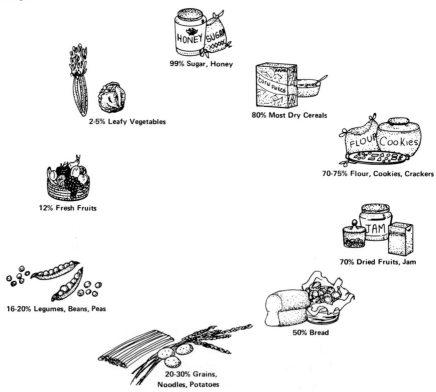

99% Sugar, Honey

2-5% Leafy Vegetables

80% Most Dry Cereals

70-75% Flour, Cookies, Crackers

12% Fresh Fruits

70% Dried Fruits, Jam

16-20% Legumes, Beans, Peas

50% Bread

20-30% Grains,
Noodles, Potatoes

Ronald Deutsch, *The Family Guide to Better Food and Better Health* (Des Moines, Iowa: Meredith Corp., 1971), page 65. Illustration by Diana Dennington Deutsch.

## What Do Carbohydrates Do for Us?

Carbohydrates are essential to the body as a source of energy. They provide a sparing action for protein in the body, because protein is not needed for energy if sufficient carbohydrate is available to supply the body's needs.

> There is often a high consumption of "empty" carbohydrates —as refined sweets and sugars, omitting valuable carbohydrate foods as fruits and vegetables which contain other nutrients. The high incidence of dental caries and disease is also related to frequent consumption of refined sweets.

## Fats

The second great source of food energy is fats. Although the typical American diet provides between 40–50 percent of the total calories from fat, many nutritionists suggest this be reduced to between 30–35 percent.

Fats are made by both plants and animals for extra compact fuel shortage. The form of a fat, whether it is liquid or solid, depends on the kind of fatty acids found in its structure. Generally speaking, fats from animals tend to be hard. Fats from vegetable sources are likely to be in liquid form, and known as oils.

Hard fats tend to be saturated. All the bonds, the atomic linkages, are satisfied, by having hydrogen atoms hooked onto them. Thus the term saturated fat.

Oils do not have all their atomic linkages filled. Thus the oil looks like an incomplete fat. It has vacancies where hydrogen atoms ought to be. So it is called an unsaturated or polyunsaturated fat.

Modern food technology does many complex things with fats and oils to provide such processes, missing hydrogen atoms are added to unsaturated fats. And this is where the familiar label term "hydrogenated" comes from.

Some sources of fat are obvious, or visible. These include butter, margarine, salad oil and fat around meat. Others are less obvious or hidden, such as streaks of fat in meat, (e.g., porterhouse steak), cream, cheeses (except those made from skim milk), avocadoes, nuts, and chocolate.

Animal foods are usually good sources of fat in the diet—butter, beef, or pork. Other meats, however, are fairly low in fat, such as chicken or fish.

Several plants are significant sources of oils. Examples include oil from soybeans, cottonseed, olives, corn, coconut, peanuts, palm, (sunflower and safflower). Margarine may be considered as the vegetable oil counterpart to butter.

## What Does It Do For Us?

Fats are:

(1) an important source of concentrated energy.

(2) the sole source of the essential fatty acid (linoleic acid).

(3) carriers of vitamins A, D, E, and K, the fat soluble vitamins.

(4) helpful in preventing the early recurrence of hunger pangs, after a meal.

(5) significant in their ability to improve the flavor of many foods.

How much fat in foods? The fat content of some typical foods—shown as percentages of total weight

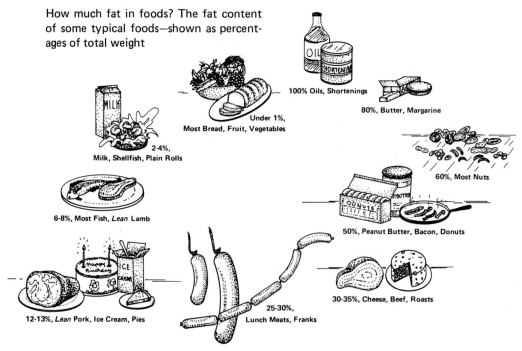

100% Oils, Shortenings

80%, Butter, Margarine

Under 1%, Most Bread, Fruit, Vegetables

2-4%, Milk, Shellfish, Plain Rolls

60%, Most Nuts

6-8%, Most Fish, *Lean* Lamb

50%, Peanut Butter, Bacon, Donuts

30-35%, Cheese, Beef, Roasts

25-30%, Lunch Meats, Franks

12-13%, *Lean* Pork, Ice Cream, Pies

Ronald Deutsch, *The Family Guide to Better Food and Better Health* (Des Moines, Iowa: Meredith Corp., 1971), page 67. Illustration by Diana Dennington Deutsch.

> Some food faddists attach special significance to lecithins as substances with unusual health-promoting properties, particularly in helping to regulate (lower) the level of cholesterol in the blood. They have no such properties.
>
> Lecithins are prepared commercially from soybeans, and also from egg yolks, and are used in many food products as a smoothing or emulsifying agent. They are completely metabolized by the body and, because of the fatty acids they contain, they are generous sources of calories.

## Protein

Protein containing foods are required in the diet to provide the essential amino acids and nitrogen required for growth and maintenance of body tissues. Nitrogen is the distinguishing element in protein. From 12 to 15 percent of the day's calories should be available from protein in the diet.

All proteins are formed from amino acids, which are simple units. Most food proteins are comprised of 12 to 20 amino acids linked together in one large molecule. Food protein is broken down in the body to its component amino acids and these amino acids are used by the cells to create the individual's custom-made protein, according to the specifications of his own genetic coding.

There are two kinds of amino acids: Essential and nonessential. Essential amino acids the body cannot synthesize, and therefore these substances must be obtained from the diet. Eight amino acids are essential and one more is required by human infants.

The essential amino acids are histidine, isoleucine, leucine, lysine, methionine, phenylalanine, threonine, tryptophan, and valine.

Nonessential amino acids can be synthesized from other food sources, as carbohydrate or fat, and are necessary to meet the body's total needs for protein.

If a food protein contains all the essential amino acids it is called "complete". If one or more of the essential amino acids is missing the protein is termed "incomplete".

The protein from animals with the exception of gelatin is complete protein. This includes meat, fish, eggs, milk, and cheese.

Proteins from plant sources include legumes, which are particularly good sources of protein, wheat, corn, rice, and other cereals. Plant proteins tend to be incomplete protein sources.

If we know how to do it, though, we can combine vegetable proteins so that we get all eight amino acids at the same meal. If we eat one food that is missing four amino acids with another that has those four or eat a food that is short on one amino acid with a food that has an extra supply of that particular amino acid, we'll get complete protein. For example, soybeans have a good supply of seven of the amino acids, but they are low in one amino acid called methionine. Corn meal, on the other hand, doesn't have a good supply of many of the amino acids, but it does have a large amount of methionine, enough to make up for the deficit in soybeans. So if we eat corn and soybean products together, it's as good as eating meat. Remember that if we don't eat enough of all eight amino acids together, our bodies won't be able to use any of these amino acids very well. It's like a typesetter running out of the letter "e" —he or she isn't able to type half the words on a page.

Other combinations of complete protein besides cornmeal and soybeans are:

Grains + Dried Beans

Grains + Brewer's Yeast

Grains + Nuts *or* Seeds + Dried Beans or Milk Products

Grains + Small Amounts of Complete Protein Foods, Such as Eggs, Milk, *or* Meats

Dried Beans + Grains

Dried Beans + Nuts *or* Seeds

Nuts *or* Seeds + Dried Beans

Nuts *or* Seeds + Grains + Dried Beans *or* Milk Products

Nuts *or* Seeds + Small Amounts of Complete Protein Foods, Such as Eggs, Milk, *or* Meat

## What Does It Do For Us?

Protein is present in every cell in the body. It is necessary for the building of new tissue and the maintenance of tissue already formed. In addition it provides the raw materials for the production of antibodies, enzymes, and hormones. Protein helps to regulate the body's fluid balance and acid-base proportions. It can be used for energy, although if used for energy it is not available for use in the other important functions.

The greatest need for protein in proportion to body size is for infants and young children. As people mature, the requirement in relation to body size decreases gradually until the fairly stable requirement of adulthood is reached.

## Minerals

Although minerals account for less than 5 percent of the body weight, the mineral elements are indispensible. Those required in the diet in the largest quantities include calcium, iron, phosphates, potassium, sulfur, sodium chloride, and magnesium. The trace elements essential for humans include zinc, selenium, magnesium, copper, iodine, molybdenum, cobalt, and fluorine.

In general, minerals help to regulate the body or are important substances in the muscle tissues, body fluids or other body structures. In addition, they help maintain the correct acid-base ratio in the body, regulate fluid (osmotic) pressure, help the blood to clot and promote nerve impulse transfer.

The body needs a number of minerals. While we know it needs specific quantities of some, we are not sure about the need for others. Some, needed in minute quantities, we call "trace" minerals.

## Calcium and Phosphorus

Both are important in maintaining a proper acid-base ratio, in keeping up the bones and teeth and in promoting many body functions. Calcium helps maintain good muscle tone, helps the blood to clot, the heart to beat rhythmically and the nervous system to function.

Phosphorus, among its many functions, maintains normal muscle functioning. It is vital to the metabolism of carbohydrate, fat, and protein. To assure an adequate amount of these two minerals, a pint of mi. or its equivalent should be consumed daily.

Meat and other protein-rich foods are good sources of phosphorus. Cereals and legumes are also. Leafy vegetables contain calcium but, because of their fiber, may hamper its absorption. Some foods, such as

spinach, beets, chard, and rhubarb contain oxalic acid which also interferes with the absorption of calcium.

| Milk Equivalents | | |
|---|---|---|
| Food Item | Percent Of a Pt. Of Milk | Fat Adjustment In Diet Use |
| 1 oz. cheddar, Swiss or similar cheese | .40 | 1 t less |
| 1 oz. cream cheese type: | | |
|     Neufchatel, 25% fat | .03 | 1 t less |
|     Philadelphia, 35% fat | .03 | 1½ t less |
| 5 oz. cottage cheese | .20 | none |
| 5 oz. non-fat cottage cheese | .20 | add ¼ t |
| ½ c. ice cream, 10% fat | .15 | 1 t less |
| ½ c. sherbert, 4% fat | .06 | none |

## Iron and Copper

Anemia may occur because of poor iron absorption or low dietary intake.
Other causes might be a lack of vitamins, a chronic blood loss or a failure
to manufacture enough blood cells in the bone marrow. About 1/10th of
the iron consumed by young, active adults is absorbed.

Green, leafy vegetables; meat; egg yolk; molasses; prunes and other
dried fruits; whole-grain cereals and legumes are good sources of iron.
Organ meats are high in iron; milk and dairy products are not, but what
they do contain is well absorbed.

The diet should supply about 10 mg of iron a day. This is not a
great amount but it is extremely important. Seeing that some iron-rich
food is served daily usually assures an adequate supply. The following
foods will supply the listed milligrams of iron:

| | | | |
|---|---|---|---|
| 1 pt milk | 1.0 mg | ½ c rolled oats | 1.0 mg |
| 4 oz prune juice | 1.5 mg | 3 oz. ground beef | 2.3 mg |
| 1 egg | 1.5 mg | ¼ c raisins | 1.0 mg |
| ½ c Swiss chard | 3.1 mg | ¾ c bean soup | 3.0 mg |
| 1 oz. 40% Bran Flakes | 1.8 mg | 1½ oz. cooked beef liver | 6.5 mg |
| Slice whole wheat bread | 0.9 mg | 1½ oz. cooked pork liver | 13.0 mg |

Copper is also important for manufacturing good blood. Usually
it is plentiful in the diet. A copper deficiency in elderly individuals can
cause a loss of calcium and phosphorus and increased bone fragility.

## Sodium

The body's reserves of bases (alkalies) are largely made up of sodium. These reserves help maintain a proper acid-base balance. Sodium is necessary also for good muscle tone and contraction. It is associated with tissue and fluid functions of the body.

Many foods contain fairly large quantities of sodium such as beets, carrots, or celery. Baking soda or baking powder contain large quantities. So do catsup, Worcestershire sauce, pickles, dry cereals, gravy, soup bases, bakery mixes, and so forth. Many dried fruits and some dried vegetables, such as potatoes, are bleached with sodium sulfite. Some fish flesh is high in sodium and some frozen or fresh fish may be lightly salted to help preserve it.

Read labels of processed foods for their salt content. Canned vegetables and a number of frozen vegetables usually contain about 1 percent salt. A salt brine is used to test for the maturity of peas, lima beans, and so forth for canning or freezing. The mature ones sink to the bottom. This treatment may add so much salt the vegetables cannot be used in low sodium diets.

## Iodine

Thyroxin from the thyroid gland is an important hormone in controlling the speed or metabolic rate at which the body operates. It contains considerable iodine. If the body lacks iodine, the thyroid gland overworks trying to produce enough thyroxin and it may become enlarged, a condition called simple goiter.

Most soils have enough iodine in them to give adequate quantities in the drinking water but in the north mid-central (Great Lakes basin) and northwestern states the drinking water lacks iodine and this area is called the "goiter belt." By using iodized salt, this lack can be made up. Seafoods and fish from the sea have a high quantity of iodine in them. In a salt-free diet in the goiter belt, iodine may be given under medical orders.

## Potassium

As noted, potassium is one of the minerals important in maintaining the proper electrolyte or acid-base ratio in the body. When potassium is lacking, the individual will have a marked lassitude, accompanied by diarrhea and a decreased food intake. Potassium helps the nerves and muscles to function. Meats, their juices and broths, are high in potassium. Potassium is fairly well distributed in most foods but legumes, cereals, nuts, dried fruits, and molasses will have a higher amount than most foods.

When individuals take diuretics (drugs which eliminate excess body fluids via the urine), the potassium level in the body needs to be watched because a diuretic eliminates minerals other than sodium from the body. Too low a potassium level in the body may cause cardiac problems and even heart arrests.

## Other Minerals

There are a number of minerals that may be required in the body, some only in trace quantities. There are others in foods but we do not know their function, if any, in the body or how much of them we need. Since most of these are liberally supplied in a well-balanced diet, there is usually little need to see that they are included.

Magnesium is important in maintaining important body functions. It aids bone formation and is important in the utilization of amino acids. Sulfur is a significant substance in several of the amino acids and in some other body substances. Zinc can be a poison if taken in too great a quantity but in minute amounts it is important in maintaining metabolic reactions and in the functioning of the pancreas.

Fluorine is important in the formation of teeth and perhaps in their maintenance. It helps to create a larger, stronger, harder dental crystal in the teeth, making them last longer and become more resistant to decay. Molybdenum is required in enzyme systems. Chromium is also essential. Aluminum, silicon, and bromine are probably used by the body in small amounts but just how is not known. Similarly, arsenic, nickel, boron, and selenium are metals that may have a function in the body. Selenium and molybdenum can be toxic if taken in too great a quantity.

## Vitamins

Man cannot live on vitamins alone. Minerals, proteins, fats, and carbohydrates are also components of good nutrition. Yet there is a widespread misconception that vitamins are synonymous with good nutrition. Al-

## Fluoride, The Missing Additive

Many experts agree that our most important nutrient, water, ought to have one additive in most regions of the United States. The additive is fluoride, an element which becomes deposited in teeth to make them harder and more resistant to the attack of bacterial acids which cause tooth decay. The American Dental Assoc., American Association for the Advancement of Science, the American Medical Association and the U.S. Public Health Service are only a few of the supporters of the drive to fluoridate water to prevent needless caries (cavities).

"On the basis of available evidence," reads an AMA statement, "it appears that fluoridation decreases the incidence of caries during childhood. Other evidence indicates as well a reduction of dental caries up to at least 44 years of age."

The scientific recommendation is that the fluoride content of water supplies be tested. If they are not naturally endowed with one part per million of fluoride (about a thousandth of a gram to a quart of water) they should be brought up to that standard.

No health risk has proven to be involved, and doctors do not expect to find any in the future. Fluoride is a nutrient occurring naturally in such foods as fish, cheese, meat and tea, though not in sufficient quantity to protect our teeth.

though they are essential elements, all of the nutrients discussed are necessary.

Vitamins are usually grouped according to their solubility. The fat soluble group includes vitamin A, D, E, and K. Ingestion of large amounts of vitamin A and D may be harmful as these two vitamins are stored in the body.

The water soluble vitamins include ascorbic acid (vitamin C), and the B complex vitamins—thiamin, riboflavin, niacin, vitamin $B_6$ (pyridoxine), pantothenic acid, biotin, folacin (folic acid), and vitamin $B_{12}$. No one food contains all the vitamins, but a varied diet encompassing a wide variety of foods will provide all those necessary for optimum health.

The functions of vitamins in the body are frequently interrelated and, if one is lacking, then others in plentiful supply may not be able to function.

**Vitamin A.**  Vitamin A is needed for good vision; a lack of it may cause night blindness or, if the lack is severe, complete blindness. Vitamin A is involved in protein synthesis, tissue repair, maintenance, and growth. The skin may become quite dry if vitamin A is lacking. Xerophthalmia, a dryness of the eye, also results when vitamin A is lacking.

Vitamin A is fat soluble and found in animal fats such as cod liver oil, liver, egg yolk, and butter. A number of foods contain the vitamin A precursor called carotene. The carotenes are yellow pigmented substances some of which the body changes into vitamin A. They are plentiful in yellow pigmented vegetables, such as carrots, sweet potatoes, squash, or in green vegetables, such as broccoli, string beans, etc.

We can store vitamin A in our bodies; this makes it possible to consume a plentiful supply on one day which will be sufficient to last for several more days. An excess of vitamin A can do harm. If too much is taken, hemorrhages start under the skin, the hair thins, the joints become inflamed and skin lesions form. Vitamin A and the carotenes are fairly stable and are only slowly destroyed in storage or cooking.

**Vitamin D.**  Another stable, fat soluble vitamin is vitamin D. It can be found in fish liver oils, cream, butter, eggs, and so forth. It can also be made in our bodies by the action of the sun's ultra-violet rays. We can manufacture vitamin D by radiating foods containing certain fats with ultra-violet rays. An individual with dark or black skin manufactures less vitamin D than others with fairer skins. (Some now think vitamin D may be a hormone more than a vitamin).

Vitamin D is needed for proper utilization of phosphorus and calcium and, although no requirement of quantity needed has been established for older people, it is quite possible a lack can result in insufficient calcium and phosphorus being deposited in the skeletal system. Children lacking vitamin D develop rickets. Again, too much can be taken and the body can store it.

**Vitamins E and K.**  Vitamin E is essential for smooth muscle functioning. In human beings it seems to be effective as an antioxidant of fats, and other body substances. It may be helpful in circulatory problems and in utilizing amino acids. Vitamin K may be impaired if the gall bladder does not supply enough or good enough bile salts to emulsify fats containing vitamin K. Excess aspirin or sulfa drugs interfere with the blood coagulating properties of vitamin K. Both vitamins E and K are oil soluble and are fairly stable. Usually our foods furnish all we need of them. It is possible that microorganisms can manufacture vitamin K in our intestinal tracts.

A growing interest in vitamin E is developing in nutritional circles although, as yet, there is little evidence that vitamin E plays roles in human nutrition other than those described above. Vitamin E has been found to be essential to the metabolism of unsaturated fatty acids and as the intake of unsaturated fatty acids increases so must the intake of vitamin E. However, foods high in unsaturated fatty acids also carry a liberal supply of the vitamin so there is little danger of a shortage in the body for this metabolic purpose. Claims that vitamin E may be effective in reducing problems in sclerosis, nephritis, diabetes, hypertension or the heart have not been substantiated and administration for these purposes may be harmful to the individual.

**The B-Vitamins.** The B-vitamin group, or B-complex, once was thought to be one vitamin. Because what we thought was one turned out to be a group, we designate them sometimes as $B_1$, thiamine; $B_2$, riboflavin; etc.

**Thiamine.** Vitamin $B_1$, or thiamine, is needed to develop a good appetite, to burn carbohydrates and for good nerve functioning. If we do not have enough, we develop a disease called beriberi, a condition typified in part by constipation and tenderness of the calf muscles. Good sources of thiamine are whole-grain cereals, enriched cereals, yeast, meats—especially pork and liver—legumes and milk. Since the quantity of thiamine one needs is governed by the amount of carbohydrates burned, the quantity needed is less as carbohydrates are reduced. Thiamine cannot be stored in the body so each day we should consume what we need.

**Niacin.** A lack of niacin can cause pellagra, a disease evidenced by skin sores in the same place on the left and right sides of the body, diarrhea, mental deterioration, and even death. Niacin is important in developing energy and combines with thiamine and riboflavin to do this.

Niacin is plentiful in nuts, especially peanuts, brewer's yeast, meats, and enriched cereals. The body can manufacture it from tryptophan, an amino acid. Milk is a good source of niacin.

**Other B-Complex Vitamins.** The remaining B-vitamins, $B_6$, (pyridoxine) $B_{12}$, folic acid, biotin, and pantothenic acid are needed in small quantities by human beings but how much is needed of some of them, we do not as yet know.

Pyridoxine ($B_{12}$) is important in protein metabolism and in converting tryptophan to niacin. It is also involved in the metabolism of some fatty substances. $B_{12}$ is found in most of our foods but is plentiful in fish, poultry, meat, cereals, dairy products, soybeans, nuts, and organ meats. Brewer's yeast is extremely high in it. The body can also manufacture it if given the proper materials.

Folic acid is found in leafy (foliage) vegetables as well as liver, legumes, yeast, asparagus, and broccoli. It is important in cell functioning and in blood formation. A lack of folic acid affects the oxygen-carrying power of the blood. The vitamin is helpful in some anemias.

Pantothentic acid is found in plentiful supply in the same foods in which pyridoxine is high. It is important in body metabolic processes. It supports the nervous system and is involved in the function of the adrenal glands and in body oxidations.

**Vitamin C.** Scurvy, a disease once common in sailors because they were unable to get fresh fruit or vegetables, is caused by a lack of ascorbic acid or vitamin C. This vitamin is plentiful in citrus fruits, tomato juice, cabbage, many fresh berries and will be in good supply in bean sprouts, broccoli, cauliflower, fresh leafy greens, melons, turnips, rutabagas, kohlrabi, okra, onions, parsnips, fresh peas, peppers, persimmons, pimientos, fresh pineapple, potatoes, rhubarb, and spinach.

Vitamin C is one of the most perishable vitamins. It oxidizes easily; a pitcher of orange juice left in a refrigerator overnight will lose very little, however, because it is acid and low in oxidizing enzymes. Mincing vegetables finely quickly results in oxidation. Cooking foods in lots of water encourages leaching of the vitamin. Heating destroys it when exposed to air or copper equipment, especially if the food is cooked in an alkaline medium. (Soda, again, is effective in destroying it if added to the cooking water.) Because the body cannot store large quantities of it, one should receive an adequate amount each day.

Ascorbic acid is important in the formation and maintenance of tissue, bones, teeth, and blood. Cuts and wounds of individuals low in ascorbic acid heal with difficulty. Vitamins A and C seem to work together closely and a lack of one of them in the diet may hamper the functioning of the other.

**Water.** Water makes up approximately 70 percent of the body weight. It is therefore vital to life. Water is used in the body in a variety of ways:

1. As building material for all cells.
2. As a solvent for nutrients and waste materials.
3. As a lubricant for joints, organs and cells.
4. As a regulator of body temperature through evaporation from the lungs of skin.

Sources of water for the body include fluids, foods, particularly fruits and vegetables, and the water produced by the metabolism of the energy nutrients within the tissues. Factors such as climate and physical activity will affect the amount of water needed by the body. The recommendation of 6–8 glasses liquid daily is only a guide.

## Alcohol

Ethyl alcohol is a substance closely related to carbohydrates and fats. It can be burned in the body just as they are burned. Pure alcohol (100% or 200 proof) gives 7 calories of heat or energy per gram; 2 oz. of 80 proof whiskey (40%) will give 168 calories or nearly as much as a baked potato with a pat of butter. Normally, the caloric value of nonsweet alcoholic spirits is equal per ounce to the numerical value of the proof; for instance an ounce of 100 proof spirit yields about 100 calories. This rule does not apply to wines, beers, ales, and so forth that are of lower proof.

### Calories In Some Alcoholic Beverages

| Beverage | Calories | Beverage | Calories |
|---|---|---|---|
| Beer or ale, 8 oz. glass | 115 | Dry dinner wine, 3 oz. | 80 |
| Sweet liqueurs, 1 oz. | 75 | Sherry, 3 oz. | 85 |
| Brandy, 70 proof, 1 oz. | 60 | Sweet wine, 3 oz. | 120 to 150 |
| Eggnog | 338 | Champagne, 3½ oz. | 90 |
| Gin, rum, whiskey, 80 to 86 proof, 1½ oz. or jigger | 120 | Hard cider, 6 oz. | 75 |
| | | Dry martini, 4 oz. | 200 |

## What Your Body Does with the Food You Eat

Have you ever come in from swimming or playing tennis and been so hungry you could hardly wait for the hamburger cooking on the grill? When you swim, play tennis, or exercise a great deal, your cells work extra hard. All food that reaches them is used to provide you with extra energy. Then you start to get hungry as your brain has received a message that your stomach is empty. Before foods reach your cells and become a part of you, they must be changed into a useable form. This change is called digestion.

## Digestion in the Mouth

As you eat your hamburger—perhaps with a bun, an apple, and drink some milk—your teeth chew the solid food into smaller particles and at the same time mix it with saliva. The saliva flows from your salivary glands and the moist saliva aids in swallowing and passage into the stomach. Saliva is a digestive juice containing water, mucus, and a digestive enzyme, amylase. Chemical changes take place in foods as a result of digestive enzymes. Your saliva changes the carbohydrate, or starch, in the bun and apple into surplus carbohydrates, or disaccharides. To aid this process, it is important to eat slowly and chew food well.

What happens to the hamburger and milk in your mouth? Very little, except that your teeth grind up the hamburger and it tastes good.

When food leaves your mouth, it passes into a 10 inch tube called the esophagus. A series of ring-like muscles, called the sphincter muscles, squeeze the food along until it reaches the stomach. This action is much like moving a bead along the length of a soda straw, squeezing the straw behind the bead each time it is moved.

## Digestion in the Stomach

In the stomach, strong muscles churn the food into a thick mass, called chyme. Hydrochloric acid and the enzyme, pepsin, begin to split the proteins in the hamburger, the milk, and the bun to smaller, more soluble parts called polypeptides. The liquid milk is changed into soft curds.

Protein from the meat, milk, and bun are only partially digested as they move into the small intestine. The fat portion of the milk and meat and bun leaves the stomach more slowly. Fats are known to have "satiety value". That is they delay the feeling of being hungry and aren't digested until they reach the small intestine.

## Digestion in the Intestine

Next to the upper part of the small intestine there are two organs: the pancreas and the gall bladder. They are connected to the intestine and supply juices and enzymes to complete the digestion of carbohydrates to simple sugars and glucose. Cellulose and other indigestible carbohydrates are moved along into the large intestine and are finally excreted.

Bile from the gall bladder begins to emulsify the fat so that it becomes soluble in the liquified food materials. Two enzymes, pancreatic

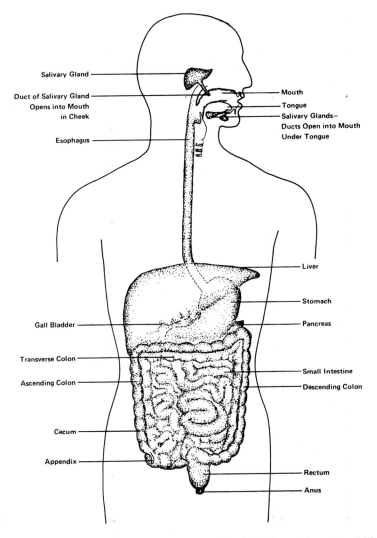

Salivary Gland

Duct of Salivary Gland
Opens into Mouth
in Cheek

Esophagus

Mouth

Tongue

Salivary Glands—
Ducts Open into Mouth
Under Tongue

Liver

Stomach

Gall Bladder

Pancreas

Transverse Colon

Ascending Colon

Small Intestine

Descending Colon

Cecum

Appendix

Rectum

Anus

F. J. Stare, & M. McWilliams, *Living Nutrition*, (New York, John Wiley and Sons, Inc., 1973) p. 251.

lipase and intestinal lipase split the fat molecules into smaller fragments so that they can pass through the intestinal wall.

Pancreatic and intestinal enzymes also complete the breakdown of the protein polypeptides into individual amino acids.

What happens to minerals and vitamins? Very little. The vitamins and mineral compounds dissolve as a part of the break-down process of the other nutrients. They then become part of the digested liquid in the small intestine.

You would never recognize the hamburger, apple, and milk now. You have a liquid that contains all of the dissolved food materials. This liquid passes through the intestinal wall into the blood stream. Any indigestable material or waste passes into the large intestine and leaves the body.

## How Food Reaches Your Cells

The second step in getting food to your cells is that of transporting the nutrients to all parts of the body. The transportation system is your blood stream. The blood, as it passes through organs and tissues, adds or removes materials as a part of its journey in the body. The plasma portion of the blood fulfills two functions: it carries dissolved nutrients to the cells, and picks up waste materials from these same cells. The red blood cell portion of the blood carries oxygen to the cells and also carries away the waste carbon dioxide. The nutrients after being digested enter the blood stream via the vessels in the small intestine.

Proteins from your hamburger, milk, and bun appear in the bloodstream as individual amino acids where each cell takes those it needs for growth and repair. Each cell chooses only those amino acids it needs to build its own unique tissue.

Carbohydrate which has been broken down to glucose is also supplied to the cells, with additional storage sites in nearby muscles and in the liver. If there is more glucose in the blood than your cells need, some is removed and stored in the liver as the animal form of starch known as glycogen. The liver has the ability to reconvert glycogen back to glucose if the glucose level in the bloodstream drops too low. Or fats and proteins may be converted by the liver to glucose.

If fats are not needed for immediate energy, they are stored in the body as reserve energy. This may result in overweight and eventually obesity. They are stored in a number of areas: just under the skin so that body heat does not escape too quickly; around the vital organs as a protective cushion; and even in the bone marrow.

Individual cells make selective use of the vitamins and minerals, dependent on their need and function.

## The Many Ways to Mix and Match for Good Nutrition

Men and women in different parts of the world have developed diets of striking diversity. As much as these diets differ, they all have been capable of sustaining life over a long period of time and have, in addition, given much enjoyment in eating. Let's look at some typical foods in various cultural food patterns represented in American community life to see how nutrients are supplied.

1. *Mexican-American Diet*

   Carbohydrates — Corn and flour tortillas, atole, pinto beans, oranges, pasole, rice.

   Fats — Lard, cheese, beef, chicken, avocado.

   Protein — Cheese, chicken, beef, pinto beans, tortillas, rice.

   Vitamins — Chili pepper, pinto beans, tomatoes, citrus fruit, carrots, tortillas.

   Minerals — Corn tortillas, beans, cheese.

2. *Black (Southern)*

   Carbohydrates — Grits, biscuits, cornmeal, black-eyed peas, beans, rice.

   Fats — Fat-back, lard, ham hocks.

   Protein — Chitlins, pork, chicken, game, fish, beans, rice, organ meats.

   Vitamins — Greens, sweet potatoes, pork, black-eyed peas, beans.

   Minerals — Greens, beans, organ meats, chicken, pork, hominy.

3. *Chinese-American*

   Carbohydrates — Rice, snow peas, melons, celery, mushrooms, bean sprouts, pineapple.

   Fats — Soy, sesame, peanut oils, lard.

   Protein — Pork, chicken, duck, fish, eggs, soybeans.

   Vitamins — Cabbage, chinese greens, carrots, green pepper, pineapple, mandarin oranges, bean sprouts, mushrooms.

   Minerals — Chinese greens, organ meats, fish, pork, chicken, duck.

4. *Anglo*

   Carbohydrates — Bread, corn, potatoes, apples, milk, oranges.

   Fats — Butter, margarine, beef, milk, cheese.

   Protein — Pork, beef, milk, cheese, baked beans, bread, chicken, eggs.

   Vitamins — Bread, green beans, potatoes, tomatoes, beef, milk, butter, oranges, broccoli.

   Minerals — Milk, cheese, beef, organ meats, broccoli.

# Food intake for good nutrition according to food groups and the average size of servings at different age levels*

| Food group | Servings per day | Average size of servings at each age level | | | | | |
|---|---|---|---|---|---|---|---|
| | | 1 year | 2 to 3 years | 4 to 5 years | 6 to 9 years | 10 to 12 years | 13 to 15 years |
| **Milk and cheese** (1.5 oz. cheese = 1 cup milk) | 4 | ½ cup | ½ to ¾ cups | ¾ cup | ¾ to 1 cup | 1 cup | 1 cup |
| **Meat group (protein foods)** | At least 3 | | | | | | |
| Egg | | 1 egg | 1 egg | 1 egg | 1 egg | 1 egg | 1 or more |
| Lean meat, fish, poultry (liver once a week) | | 2 tbsp. | 2 tbsp. | 4 tbsp. | 2-3 oz. (4-6 tbsp.) | 3-4 oz. | 4 oz. or more |
| Peanut butter | | | 1 tbsp. | 2 tbsp. | 2-3 tbsp. | 3 tbsp. | 3 tbsp. |
| **Fruits and vegetables** | At least 4, including: | | | | | | |
| Vitamin C source (citrus fruit, berries, tomato, cabbage, cantaloupe) | 1 or more (twice as much tomato as citrus) | ⅓ cup citrus | ½ cup | ½ cup | 1 med. orange | 1 med. orange | 1 med. orange |
| Vitamin A source (green or yellow fruits and vegetables) | 1 or more | 2 tbsp. | 3 tbsp. | 4 tbsp. (¼ cup) | ¼ cup | ⅓ cup | ¾ cup |
| Other vegetables (potato, legumes) | 2 or more | 2 tbsp. | 3 tbsp. | 4 tbsp. (¼ cup) | ⅓ cup | ½ cup | ¾ cup |
| or | | | | | | | |
| Other fruits (apple, banana) | | ¼ cup | ⅓ cup | ½ cup | 1 medium | 1 medium | 1 medium |
| **Cereals (whole grain or enriched)** | At least 4 | | | | | | |
| Bread | | ½ slice | 1 slice | 1½ slices | 1-2 slices | 2 slices | 2 slices |
| Ready-to-eat cereals | | ½ oz. | ¾ oz. | 1 oz. | 1 oz. | 1 oz. | 1 oz. |
| Cooked cereal (including pastes, rice, etc.) | | ¼ cup | ⅓ cup | ½ cup | ½ cup | ¾ cup | 1 cup or more |
| **Fats and carbohydrates** | To meet caloric needs | | | | | | |
| Butter, margarine, mayonnaise, oils: 1 tbsp. = 100 calories | | 1 tbsp. | 1 tbsp. | 1 tbsp. | 2 tbsp. | 2 tbsp. | 2-4 tbsp. |
| Desserts and sweets 100 calorie portions: ⅓ cup pudding or ice cream 2 3" cookies, 1 oz. cake, 1⅓ oz. pie, 2 tbsp. jelly, jam, honey, sugar | | 1 portion | 1½ portions | 1½ portions | 3 portions | 3 portions | 3 to 6 portions |

* Bennett, M., and Hansen, A., Nutritional requirements. In Nelson, W., editor: Textbook of pediatrics, ed. 8, Philadelphia, 1964, W. B. Saunders Company, p. 123.

## Nutrition and Athletics

The idea that athletes need a diet significantly different from the average person is one that persists in many locker rooms. Feeding athletes an exotic array of health foods or a high protein diet are commonly held ideas. Some schools require that all members of the team eat at a training table so that a rigid diet is faithfully followed. This approach may serve a psychological purpose in raising team morale, but research studies have not substantiated the merits of this nutritional approach.

What recommendations for feeding athletes are sound? Not less than three meals a day are recommended for good nutrition of athletes. For activities such as track or tennis, the pattern of five lighter meals daily may be preferable. These meals should follow the same food patterns that are recommended for the average person, except that portion sizes may be larger. There is some indication that athletes may improve their performance a little by increasing carbohydrate intake.

Contrary to popular beliefs, athletes do not require a higher percentage of protein than other individuals. Serving sizes of protein foods as well as other foods will be increased to provide sufficient calories for the high energy expenditure.

Some coaches have recommended vitamin supplements for their players in the belief that this will provide athletes with more vim and vigor. Research has not shown that performance is improved when levels of vitamin intake are increased.

Salt consumption of athletes should be geared to the replacement of salt lost through perspiration. Except in unusually hot weather, the salt needed to season food is adequate.

## Nutrition for the Adult (20s to 60s)

An individual, upon reaching maturity, bears the imprint of his nutrition during infancy, childhood, and adolescence. Adulthood should be a time of achievement. A person's health, vigor, work capacity, happiness, and contentment reflect, in part, the kind of nutrition that has marked his previous life.

Thus, some people reach adulthood with vigorous, normally functioning bodies and minds. Others permanently carry many nutritional scars as a result of tissue injury. The scars may not be immediately detectable, but animal experiments have shown that faulty nutrition in

Q. My son is on the high school track team. His coach tells the team to eat only tea and toast in the morning and then snack on honey, gelatin powder, and other sweet foods before running a race. Is there real scientific evidence to support these suggestions?

A. The dietary advice of many athletic coaches unfortunately is based more on folklore and custom than on scientific evidence. Since research in this area is limited, even nutritionists must base their suggestions somewhat on logic and theory. The first is, of course, no different for an athlete than for anyone else: a well-balanced diet. It has also been shown that a high carbohydrate diet, the day before a long distance race may be an effective protection against loss of muscle glycogen, the storage form of carbohydrate. But the nature of the diet (as long as it is adequate) does not seem to be a material factor for short-term events.

One study done recently demonstrates the effectiveness of a special diet prior to long distance running. For three days a week before the race, athletes ate a carbohydrate free diet. Then, for the next three days they switched and ate a diet very high in carbohydrate designed to build up body stores of muscle glycogen. They were allowed no heavy exercise. Meanwhile a second group served as controls and ate a regular mixed diet. Three weeks later the two groups switched places and the control group became the study group. Results showed that the best performance for each athlete occurred after eating the special carbohydrate diet. This study constitutes an important beginning in attempting to demonstrate how performance can really be affected by careful dietary control.

As for your son's meager prerace breakfast, I think it is quite safe to suggest that something which is a bit more substantial—such as juice, cereal with milk, toast with butter or margarine—taken well before race time, might be a more sound nutritional practice.

Dr. Jean Mayer, "Food for Thought", Phoenix Republic, Feb. 5, 1973, p. 20.

early life—acting like a time bomb—may induce physical breakdowns in later life. The nutritional needs of the adult must, therefore, be considered both from the standpoint of those who have been well nourished as children and those whose diets were inadequate in the early or teen years.

## Food and Feeding

Dietary needs of adults are the same in quality as those of children. However, the quality of kilocalories in which these nutrients are provided is gradually reduced during the adult years. As declining activity and basal metabolic rate effect this reduction in kilocalories, the selection of foods becomes more critical if one is to provide all the nutrients the body needs for optimum health. An adequate diet for adults can be provided by following the food groups for adults outlined in pages 217–30.

There is a continuing need for calcium and phosphorus for maintenance purposes although growth has ceased. One or two glasses of milk daily are sufficient, particularly if the water consumed has adequate amounts of fluoride (fluoridated water). One of the more recent discoveries in nutrition is that the mineral nutrient fluoride helps the body keep calcium in the hard tissues of the body—the teeth and bones—and prevents it from being deposited in the soft tissues.

The dietary allowances recommended for adults are rather simple to meet if an adult is careful to eat three meals a day and take into consideration the calories in snacks and cocktails. One of the greatest impediments to good nutrition in adults is the attitude that nutrition is not important once growth has ceased. This simply is not so. Every person reflects physically what he eats over a period of time, and adults are the result of dietary patterns over a long period. As in the teen-age period, females are less likely to be well nourished than males during the adult years. Adults need to be aware of shifts in food intake that result from physical alterations such as poor digestion or impaired absorption. If specific foods are eliminated from the diet, other foods containing the needed nutrients or a nutritional supplement will be needed to maintain good nutritional status.

## Nutrition After Age 65

The elderly in our society are required to make many social and psychological adjustments in addition to the physiological changes that accom-

# Food and Nutrition Board, National Academy of Sciences-National Research Council
## Recommended Daily Dietary Allowances,[1] Revised 1973

Designed for the maintenance of good nutrition of practically all healthy people in the U.S.A.

| | Years | | Weight | | Height | | Energy | Protein | FAT-SOLUBLE VITAMINS | | Vitamin D | Vitamin E Activity[5] |
| | | | | | | | | | Vitamin A Activity | | | |
| | from | up to | (kg) | (lbs) | (cm) | (in) | (kcal)[2] | (g) | (RE)[3] | (IU) | (IU) | (IU) |
|---|---|---|---|---|---|---|---|---|---|---|---|---|
| **Infants** | 0.0 | 0.5 | 6 | 14 | 60 | 24 | kgx117 | kgx2.2 | 420[4] | 1400 | 400 | 4 |
| | 0.5 | 1.0 | 9 | 20 | 71 | 28 | kgx108 | kgx2.0 | 400 | 2000 | 400 | 5 |
| **Children** | 1 | 3 | 13 | 28 | 86 | 34 | 1300 | 23 | 400 | 2000 | 400 | 7 |
| | 4 | 6 | 20 | 44 | 110 | 44 | 1800 | 30 | 500 | 2500 | 400 | 9 |
| | 7 | 10 | 30 | 66 | 135 | 54 | 2400 | 36 | 700 | 3300 | 400 | 10 |
| **Males** | 11 | 14 | 44 | 97 | 158 | 63 | 2800 | 44 | 1000 | 5000 | 400 | 12 |
| | 15 | 18 | 61 | 134 | 172 | 69 | 3000 | 54 | 1000 | 5000 | 400 | 15 |
| | 19 | 22 | 67 | 147 | 172 | 69 | 3000 | 52 | 1000 | 5000 | 400 | 15 |
| | 23 | 50 | 70 | 154 | 172 | 69 | 2700 | 56 | 1000 | 5000 | | 15 |
| | 51+ | | 70 | 154 | 172 | 69 | 2400 | 56 | 1000 | 5000 | | 15 |
| **Females** | 11 | 14 | 44 | 97 | 155 | 62 | 2400 | 44 | 800 | 4000 | 400 | 10 |
| | 15 | 18 | 54 | 119 | 162 | 65 | 2100 | 48 | 800 | 4000 | 400 | 11 |
| | 19 | 22 | 58 | 128 | 162 | 65 | 2100 | 46 | 800 | 4000 | 400 | 12 |
| | 23 | 50 | 58 | 128 | 162 | 65 | 2000 | 46 | 800 | 4000 | | 12 |
| | 51+ | | 58 | 128 | 162 | 65 | 1800 | 46 | 800 | 4000 | | 12 |
| **Pregnant** | | | | | | | +300 | +30 | 1000 | 5000 | 400 | 15 |
| **Lactating** | | | | | | | +500 | +20 | 1200 | 6000 | 400 | 15 |

## WATER-SOLUBLE VITAMINS / MINERALS

| | Ascorbic Acid (mg) | Folacin[6] (ug) | Niacin[7] (mg) | Riboflavin (mg) | Thiamin (mg) | Vitamin B6 (mg) | Vitamin B12 (ug) | Calcium (mg) | Phosphorus (mg) | Iodine (ug) | Iron (mg) | Magnesium (mg) | Zinc (mg) |
|---|---|---|---|---|---|---|---|---|---|---|---|---|---|
| **Infants** | 35 | 50 | 5 | 0.4 | 0.3 | 0.3 | 0.3 | 360 | 240 | 35 | 10 | 60 | 3 |
| | 35 | 50 | 8 | 0.6 | 0.5 | 0.4 | 0.3 | 540 | 400 | 45 | 15 | 70 | 5 |
| **Children** | 40 | 100 | 9 | 0.8 | 0.7 | 0.6 | 1.0 | 800 | 800 | 60 | 15 | 150 | 10 |
| | 40 | 200 | 12 | 1.1 | 0.9 | 0.9 | 1.5 | 800 | 800 | 80 | 10 | 200 | 10 |
| | 40 | 300 | 16 | 1.2 | 1.2 | 1.2 | 2.0 | 800 | 800 | 110 | 10 | 250 | 10 |
| **Males** | 45 | 400 | 18 | 1.5 | 1.4 | 1.6 | 3.0 | 1200 | 1200 | 130 | 18 | 350 | 15 |
| | 45 | 400 | 20 | 1.8 | 1.5 | 1.8 | 3.0 | 1200 | 1200 | 150 | 18 | 400 | 15 |
| | 45 | 400 | 20 | 1.8 | 1.5 | 2.0 | 3.0 | 800 | 800 | 140 | 10 | 350 | 15 |
| | 45 | 400 | 18 | 1.6 | 1.4 | 2.0 | 3.0 | 800 | 800 | 130 | 10 | 350 | 15 |
| | 45 | 400 | 16 | 1.5 | 1.2 | 2.0 | 3.0 | 800 | 800 | 110 | 10 | 350 | 15 |
| **Females** | 45 | 400 | 16 | 1.3 | 1.2 | 1.6 | 3.0 | 1200 | 1200 | 115 | 18 | 300 | 15 |
| | 45 | 400 | 14 | 1.4 | 1.1 | 2.0 | 3.0 | 1200 | 1200 | 115 | 18 | 300 | 15 |
| | 45 | 400 | 14 | 1.4 | 1.1 | 2.0 | 3.0 | 800 | 800 | 100 | 18 | 300 | 15 |
| | 45 | 400 | 13 | 1.2 | 1.0 | 2.0 | 3.0 | 800 | 800 | 100 | 18 | 300 | 15 |
| | 45 | 400 | 12 | 1.1 | 1.0 | 2.0 | 3.0 | 800 | 800 | 80 | 10 | 300 | 15 |
| **Pregnant** | 60 | 800 | +2 | +0.3 | +0.3 | 2.5 | 4.0 | 1200 | 1200 | 125 | 18+[8] | 450 | 20 |
| **Lactating** | 60 | 600 | +4 | +0.5 | +0.3 | 2.5 | 4.0 | 1200 | 1200 | 150 | 18 | 450 | 25 |

[1] The allowances are intended to provide for individual variations among most normal persons as they live in the United States under usual environmental stresses. Diets should be based on a variety of common foods in order to provide other nutrients for which human requirements have been less well defined. See text for more-detailed discussion of allowances and of nutrients not tabulated.

[2] Kilojoules (KJ) = 4.2 x kcal

[3] Retinol equivalents

[4] Assumed to be all as retinol in milk during the first six months of life. All subsequent intakes are assumed to be one-half as retinol and one-half as B-carotene when calculated from international units. As retinol equivalents, three-fourths are as retinol and one-fourth as B-carotene.

[5] Total vitamin E activity, estimated to be 80 percent as a-tocopherol and 20 percent other tocopherols. See text for variation in allowances.

[6] The folacin allowances refer to dietary sources as determined by *Lactobacillus casei* assay. Pure forms of folacin may be effective in doses less than one-fourth of the RDA.

[7] Although allowances are expressed as niacin, it is recognized that on the average 1 mg of niacin is derived from each 60 mg of dietary tryptophan.

[8] This increased requirement cannot be met by ordinary diets; therefore, the use of supplemental iron is recommended.

pany the aging process. Modifications in the life-style of the individual and in the functioning of the body result in modified dietary patterns during this phase of life. In particular, the elderly will need to reduce caloric intake while maintaining a highly nourishing diet. Modifications may include a shift toward eating more frequent, smaller meals, a softer diet, and the ingestion of more warm beverages. As a result of growing community awareness of the problems of the elderly, some programs have been implemented to assist its senior residents in overcoming the problems that may cause them to be poorly nourished.

## Current Health Problems Relating to Nutrition

The problems of atherosclerosis and obesity are two common concerns of the American adult population—both those who reached adulthood in a well-nourishd state and those who were overweight in childhood. Improper diet is certainly not likely to be the single causative culprit, but it can play a prominent role in the development of physical problems.

1. Atherosclerosis and Coronary Heart Disease.

   What makes blood vessels close? Today, when researchers look at heart attacks, strokes, senility, and a host of other crippling or life-threatening ills, they see them mainly as symptoms of a single underlying disease—the narrowing and blocking of blood vessels. The ailments appear to differ largely as to where the circulation is closed down. If the block occurs in the vicinity of the heart, for example, we face a coronary; if it is in the brain, or the vessels leading to the brain, we have a stroke.

   In general, the closing off of blood vessels is attributed to atherosclerosis. A condition from which every adult suffers to some extent, this is a kind of corrosion of the inner surfaces of arteries, the vessels carrying red, oxygen-rich blood to every corner of the body.

   How blood vessels are damaged:
   a. A normal vessel in which the blood is free-flowing.
   b. Build-up of deposits on the vessel wall narrows the circulatory passages.
   c. The narrowing reaches a point at which insufficient blood can reach the tissues beyond, causing oxygen starvation.
   d. An embolism (clot) is trapped in a narrowed vessel, closing down circulation.

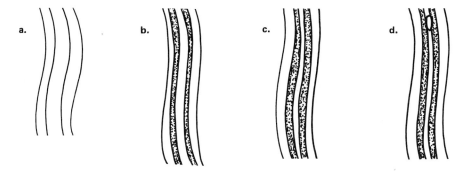

What is the object of all this effort? In general, it is to lower the quantity of certain fat-like substances in the blood by (1) reducing the percentage of fat in the diet to a total of about one-third of the whole diet—a reduction from a typical 45 percent or so: (2) controlling the kind of fat consumed, so that polyunsaturated fats are more plentiful than saturated fats: (3) cutting down the amount of cholesterol eaten in meals to levels quite a bit below those now found in typical American dietaries. All this is mainly accomplished in two ways: by severly trimming the total of animal fats we eat—not easy to do in a nation that gets so much of its protein from animal sources, and by increasing the consumption of certain oils—generally those pressed from specific seeds and beans.

The regime for cardiovascular disease risk factor program includes two alternatives:

a. *Alternative I*

The American Heart Association's General Dietary Recommendation.

1. A caloric intake adjusted to achieve and maintain ideal body weight.

2. A reduction in total fat calories achieved by a substantial reduction in dietary saturated fatty acids. Reduction to 35% is desirable. Less than 10% of the total calories should come from saturated fatty acids and up to 10% from polyunsaturated fatty acids.

3. A reduction in dietary cholesterol—it is recommended that the average daily intake of cholesterol be approximately 300 mg.

4. Dietary Carbohydrate—When the proportion of calories from fat in the diet is reduced the caloric difference will generally be made up with carbohydrate. Dependence on foods containing

complex natural carbohydrates, such as vegetables, fruits, and cereals is preferable to excessive use of refined sugar such as that contained in candy, soft drinks, and other sweets.

5. Salt Intake—The acceleration of coronary heart disease in the presence of hypertension is well recognized, but the casual relationship in man between salt intake and hypertension has not been firmly established. Information available to date from experimental human and animal data suggests that it is prudent to avoid excessive salt in the diet.

6. For patients on a doctor's prescription only:
   a. "Planning Fat-Controlled Meals for 1200–1800 Calories"
   b. "Planning Fat-Controlled Meals for 2000–2600 Calories"
   c. "A Maximal Approach to the Dietary Treatment of the Hyperlipidemias", a handbook for physicians and four diets for patients to be published.

   For the general public, no prescription required:
   a. Two companion booklets—"The Way to a Man's Heart" and "Recipes for Fat-Controlled, Low Cholesterol Meals"

b. *Alternative II—Cardiovascular Disease*

An alternative to the current low fat, low saturated fat, low cholesterol diet emphasizes quantities rather than types of animal foods. This new concept offers variety, decreased waste, economic advantages and lowered saturated fat and cholesterol intakes. The concept was developed by a multi-disciplinary group composed of a private practicing pediatrician, the Nutrition Section of the Arizona State Department of Health, Departments of Pediatrics and Family and Community Medicine of the University of Arizona College of Medicine, and a representative of the food industry.

By employing the Recommended Dietary Allowances for protein, the diet allows for individual taste and yet remedies a basic problem, namely, the excessive consumption of saturated fat and cholesterol. The concept of limiting protein intake to the Recommended Dietary Allowance is new to most consumers.

This concept is presented to the individual in the following manner. First, the importance of protein in the diet is stressed. Secondly, the amount of protein for the individual as stated in the Recommended Dietary Allowances is emphasized as adequate. Thirdly, the disadvantages of consuming excessive amounts of animal protein and thus animal products are enumerated as follows:

1. Many are associated with undesirably high intakes of saturated fat and cholesterol.
2. Undesirably rich sources of calories may be consumed, as many animal products are rich in fats.
3. This is a wasteful form of obtaining calories from an ecological viewpoint.
4. These animal foods are expensive from the financial point of view.

   Once the recommended daily dietary allowance for protein for each member of the family is presented, then the amounts of protein in the various foods are shown. For ease of calculation by the consumer, approximation of the protein content of these foods is made. Individualized dietary suggestions can then be offered. The protein quantities in the animal foods (dairy products and meats) have been averaged as follows: 8 ounces of milk and 1 ounce of cheese (average of 17 types) have 8 grams of protein; 1 ounce of meat has 7 grams of protein (an average of 54 meat types).

2. Obesity

---

### The Rhythm Method of Girth Control

The rhythm method of girth control is a phrase sadly described by Doctor Jean Mayer which is a grim cycle of lose a little, gain a little more.

---

Once upon a much simpler, and in many ways happier, time, fat was beautiful.

The reasons were many. Partly, Americans were closer to the farm, where plump animals won the blue ribbons and tilted the scales to bring home more money. Partly, fat meant affluence; the poor ate badly, and were further thinned by long days of toil. Partly, there were still many emaciating plagues of childhood, such as diphtheria, and fatter babies seemed to survive best.

Now all is changed. By the early 1950s the old attitudes had reversed. Almost everyone knew that fat was dangerous. Our culture was flooded with an awareness of fat, and with schemes and devices for disposing of it.

For some twenty years our fat-consciousness has grown steadily. We spend at least $100 million a year on weight-reducing plans and remedies. We read millions upon millions of books to tell us what to do about fat. We think and talk about it endlessly.

The result? A losing battle. The newest research indicates that one child in five is overweight. In our cities, about one-third to one-half of all adults are found to be obese. The United States is the only member country of the World Health Organization which has seen no increase in the life of its men in twenty years, and this fact is considered obesity-related.

The majority of seriously overweight Americans are in their 40s and 50s. For it takes most people time to build up big fat deposits, and after they do, they do not tend to survive very long. The death rate is half again as great among the obese. They are far more likely to develop heart disease, high blood pressure, diabetes, arthritis, kidney disease, and other problems. Overweight women have more trouble during pregnancy and bear fewer healthy babies. And they have more difficulty in conceiving at all.

Most people have at least an inkling of these facts. If they become fat, they fear the risks and they despise and blame themselves. Nutritionists are generally agreed that the majority make real, painful efforts to reduce. Yet studies show that only a small proportion of those who try to lose weight succeed in doing so and keeping it off; at best it would seem that no more than one or two of every ten dieters really accomplish very much.

## What is a Nutritionally Sound Reducing Diet?

A sound diet should follow the following guidelines:

Eat small servings from each of these food groups every day:

Milk—skim, buttermilk, or 2% modified
Meat, fish, or poultry, eggs
Vegetables
Fruits
Breads and cereals

## What is Your Desirable Weight?

| Height (without shoes) | Weight in pounds (without clothing) | | |
|---|---|---|---|
| | Low | Average | High |
| *Men* | | | |
| 5'3" | 118 | 129 | 141 |
| 5'4" | 122 | 133 | 145 |
| 5'5" | 126 | 137 | 149 |
| 5'6" | 130 | 142 | 155 |
| 5'7" | 134 | 147 | 161 |
| 5'8" | 139 | 151 | 166 |
| 5'9" | 143 | 155 | 170 |
| 5'10" | 147 | 159 | 174 |
| 5'11" | 150 | 163 | 178 |
| 6'0" | 154 | 167 | 183 |
| 6'1" | 158 | 171 | 188 |
| 6'2" | 162 | 175 | 192 |
| 6'3" | 165 | 178 | 195 |
| *Women* | | | |
| 5'0" | 100 | 109 | 118 |
| 5'1" | 104 | 112 | 121 |
| 5'2" | 107 | 115 | 125 |
| 5'3" | 110 | 118 | 128 |
| 5'4" | 113 | 122 | 132 |
| 5'5" | 116 | 125 | 135 |
| 5'6" | 120 | 129 | 139 |
| 5'7" | 123 | 132 | 142 |
| 5'8" | 126 | 136 | 146 |
| 5'9" | 130 | 140 | 151 |
| 5'10" | 133 | 144 | 156 |
| 5'11" | 137 | 148 | 161 |
| 6'0" | 141 | 152 | 166 |

Ronald Deutsch, *The Family Guide to Better Food and Better Health,* (Des Moines, Iowa; Meredith Corp., 1971) p. 124.

# A Day In Calories

Here is how the in-and-out flow of calories takes place during 24 hours. The subject is a typical college student, who combines sedentary and moderately active living. The intake and outgo of calories are shown on the arrows. Here a total of 3,400 calories is eaten and spent. Basal metabolism is included.

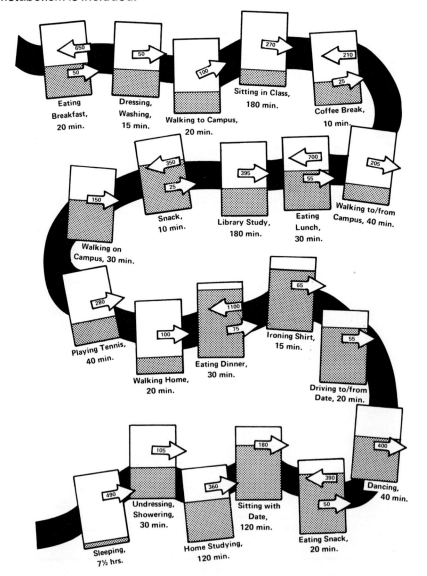

Ronald Deutsch, *The Family Guide to Better Food and Better Health* (Des Moines, Iowa: Meredith Corp., 1971), p. 131. Illustration by Diana Dennington Deutsch.

## Using Habits to Trim Your Weight

| Food | How Much to Omit | How Often | Loss Per Year |
|---|---|---|---|
| Butter or margarine | one pat | daily | 5 pounds |
| Average layer cake | half of one slice | weekly | 1½ pounds |
| Mashed potatoes | half a serving | twice weekly | 2 pounds |
| French fries | half a serving | twice weekly | 3 pounds |
| Medium-fried bacon | two slices | weekly | 1½ pounds |
| Ice cream soda | one | weekly | 5 pounds |
| Saltines | two instead of four | twice weekly | 1 pound |
| Whipped cream | two tablespoons | weekly | 1 pound |
| Oil-and-vinegar salad dressing | one tablespoon instead of two | twice weekly | 1½ pounds |
| Mayonnaise | one tablespoon | weekly | 1 pound |
| Bread or toast | one slice | daily | 6 pounds |
| Doughnut | one | weekly | 2 pounds |
| Pie | half a slice | twice weekly | 3½ pounds |
| Jam or jelly | one tablespoon | twice weekly | 1½ pounds |
| Scrambled egg | one | weekly | 1½ pounds |
| Sugar | one teaspoon | daily | 2 pounds |
| Rice | half a serving | weekly | 1 pound |
| Beer | 12-ounce can | weekly | 2½ pounds |
| Carbonated drinks | 8-ounce can | weekly | 1 pound |
| Whiskey | 1½-ounce glass | weekly | 2 pounds |
| Wine | three ounces | weekly | 1 pound |
| Most candies | one ounce | weekly | 1½ pounds |
| Most cheese | one ounce | weekly | 1½ pounds |
| Potato chips | 10 medium-size | weekly | 1½ pounds |

Excerpted from: Ronald Deutsch, *The Family Guide to Better Food and Better Health* (Des Moines, Iowa, Meredith Corp., 1971) p. 146.

Avoid or use very sparingly:

Fried foods

Fatty meat and fish (cut all visible fat from meat)

Gravies and cream sauce

Regular carbonated beverages and alcoholic beverages

Rich desserts and pastries, cookies, cakes, pies

Concentrated sweets (candy, jelly, jam, honey, molasses, and sugar)

## Iron-Deficiency Anemia

The normal adult hemoglobin value for males is 14 to 15 grams of hemoglobin per 100 milliliters of blood and for females is 13 to 14 grams per

100 milliliters. However, when iron levels are too low in the body, the hemoglobin level in the blood falls below these values, and the individual develops iron-deficiency anemia. The condition can be caused either by an inadequate intake of iron (nutritional anemia or by excessive blood loss (hemorrhage anemia). Persons most likely to have nutritional anemia due to iron deficiency are: young infants subsisting almost completely on milk, teenage girls (particularly teenage mothers), and women who have undergone closely successive pregnancies. However, others in the population also may develop this all-too-common deficiency condition. In many parts of the world where hookworm and other parasitic infections cause blood loss, iron-deficiency anemia is common.

Anemia can be prevented in most instances by careful attention to diet and by limiting blood donations to a frequency of not more than once every 2 or 3 months. When anemia has been diagnosed, it often is advisable to administer ferrous sulfate or other iron salts in the ferrous form. An elevated intake of ascorbic acid enhances the utilization of the iron.

## Uses and Abuses of Foods

An increasing number of Americans frightened by reports of the misuse of chemical fertilizers, pesticides, and additives are hurrying to buy "organic" foods. "Natural" food stores are multiplying daily, and conventional supermarkets now stock certain health foods. The health food industry is estimated to provide an income of over one billion dollars annually.

A positive aspect of the whole health food movement has been that more people have become aware that food and good nutrition can have an impact on one's health. On the other hand, however, millions of dollars have been spent by zealous, health-conscious Americans who have responded to misleading claims—who have not been able to separate fact from fiction, to be able to objectively examine statements presented by health food proponents or to know who to turn to for sound information are musts.

## Basic food myths

Four basic food myths, which occur in many different disguises, have been identified by the American Medical Association and the Federal

# Iron Content of Selected Foods

| | Amount | Iron (mg) |
|---|---|---|
| **Meat Group** | | |
| Beef, sirloin steak, lean | 3½ oz. | 3.9 |
| Veal loin chop | 3½ oz. | 3.2 |
| Pork loin chop, lean | 3½ oz. | 3.9 |
| Lamb loin chop, lean | 3½ oz. | 2.0 |
| Calf liver, fried | 3½ oz. | 14.2 |
| Bologna | 1 slice | 0.5 |
| *Poultry & Eggs* | | |
| Chicken, white meat | 3½ oz. | 1.7 |
| Egg | 1 med. | 1.1 |
| *Legumes & Nuts* | | |
| Kidney beans, cooked | ½ cup | 2.3 |
| Mixed nuts, oil roasted | 1 oz. | 1.0 |
| Peanut Butter | 2 tbsp | 0.6 |
| *Fish and shellfish* | | |
| Swordfish, broiled | 3½ oz. | 1.3 |
| Tuna, oil packed | 3½ oz. | 1.9 |
| Clams | 3½ oz. | 6.1 |
| Oysters | ½ cup | 6.6 |
| Shrimp | 3½ oz. | 3.1 |
| **Bread & Cereal Group** | | |
| White Bread, enriched | 1 slice | 0.6 |
| Whole wheat bread | 1 slice | 0.5 |
| Rye bread | 1 slice | 0.4 |
| Bran flakes | 1 oz. | 1.2 |
| Shredded wheat | 1 biscuit | 1.0 |
| Oatmeal | 1 cup | 1.4 |
| Corn grits | 1 cup | 0.7 |
| Rice, enriched, cooked | 1 cup | 1.8 |
| Macaroni, cooked | 1 cup | 1.3 |
| **Vegetables and fruit group** | | |
| *Vegetables* | | |
| Spinach, cooked | ½ cup | 2.2 |
| Beet greens, cooked | ½ cup | 1.4 |
| Peas, cooked | ½ cup | 1.6 |
| Lima beans, green, cooked | ½ cup | 2.1 |
| Potatoe, baked | 1 med. | 0.7 |
| *Fruits* | | |
| Prune juice | ½ cup | 5.1 |
| Prunes, cooked | 4 med. | 1.1 |
| Raisins | 1 oz. | 0.6 |
| Fig, dried | 1 med. | 0.6 |
| Grapefruit | ½ med. | 0.5 |

Data compiled and adapted from *Composition of Foods—Raw, Processed, Prepared,* Agriculture Handbook No. 8, U.S.D.A. 1963; *Nutritive Value of Foods,* Home and Garden Bulletin No. 72, U.S.D.A. 1971; and manufacturers' information.

Food and Drug Administration. Each one is compared with scientifically tested facts.

**Myth.** All disease is due to faulty diet. The proponents of this myth contend that certain chemical imbalances in the body are the cause of disease, and that these imbalances are directly due to improper or inadequate diet. Since it is impossible for the average person to eat an adequate diet, according to the myth, he must supplement it with whatever product is being sold at the time. The product in question usually contains a long list of ingredients, including those labeled as "mysterious substances as yet unknown to nutritional scientists."

**Fact.** Disease, by and large, is caused by many sorts of variation from normal states, such as inherited defects, and by any of a host of agents such as microorganisms and parasites. A large number of these causes of disease have no specific etiologic relationship to nutrients.

The few classic nutritional deficiency diseases such as scurvy, rickets, pellagra, kwashiorkor, and a small number of others, have been well studied by medical science. They are still a major health problem in some impoverished parts of the world, including sections of the United States (see p. 242). In such areas, the problem is usually one of a complex web of factors including politics, economics, social alienation, education, or rejection of middle class health values—not mere food availability per se.

**Myth.** Soil depletion causes malnutrition. People who believe this myth argue that the soil has lost its vitality from long overuse, and that crops grown on it are deficient in nutrients.

**Facts.** Both scientists and farmers have repeatedly observed that if a soil lacks minerals and other materials necessary for plant growth, the plant simply will not grow. Poor soil affects only the quantity of food grown on it, not the quality.

Fertilizing the soil significantly increases the yield, not the nutritive content, of the food grown on it. The kind of fertilizer used—commercial chemical mix or organic manure—makes no difference in the food's nutritional composition.

**Myth.** Food processing destroys the nutritive value of food. This myth is extensively promoted by food supplement exponents. They insist that such products as white bread and flour, refined cereals, canned foods, and even pasteurized milk are worthless or inferior because processing has removed their natural vitamins and minerals. They even lament that cooking causes further nutritive loss and advocate the use of raw foods, often liquefied in a blender. Some promote the sale of special cookware (at inflated prices) because they claim that certain utensils, especially aluminum, slowly poison the body.

**Fact.** Three false premises in this myth are refuted by scientific observations:

First, by and large, modern food processing methods are scientifically developed and highly controlled to preserve or restore nutritional values in foods. Processing times, temperatures, and quality are rigidly controlled in the canning and freezing of vegetables and fruits in order to preserve the nutrients that are present. Enrichment of grain products restores their major natural vitamin and mineral content. United States food enrichment laws in general have been a primary factor in almost eliminating deficiency diseases that were once prevalent in the American population. There is need; however, for still more rigorous study to meet the pressures generated by the rapidly changing food environment and socioeconomic problems.

Second, the nutritive qualities of vitamins and minerals as they occur naturally in foods do not differ from those that are synthetically produced in a laboratory and added to food. Categorically and unequivocally, a vitamin is a vitamin.

Third, aluminum is a trace element in the human body and widespread in nature. There is no evidence to indicate that these trace amounts are harmful, or that the amounts that may be ingested in food that has been cooked in an aluminum utensil significantly increases the total amount in the body.

**Myth.** The United States population suffers from widespread subclinical deficiencies requiring supplements of vitamins and minerals.

Many times in advertisements one hears or reads about "that tired feeling" or "tired blood" or vague aches and pains, for which the advertiser has blamed dietary deficiencies. The very vagueness of this myth makes it difficult to refute. It is particularly appealing to the anxious person who constantly worries about his health, and who fears that there must be something wrong with him which the doctors simply haven't been able to detect. Such a person accepts the claims of the vitamin or tonic salesman and purchases his product, perhaps because it provides the emotional support he needs. The vitamin is his placebo.

**Fact.** The word subclinical is a general, nonspecific term given to conditions for which there are no observable symptoms. It can be used in almost any context, depending upon the purposes of the user. It is therefore rather meaningless in itself, and if used by an irresponsible person it may be misleading. Moreover, every normal person occasionally experiences such vague feelings of fatigue due to any of a variety of life situations. Should such feelings persist, however, the patient should consult a qualified physician for a competent examination.

Is it possible for a vegetarian to obtain all of the necessary nutrients to maintain good health? It is possible, but somewhat difficult. Vegetarians may have deficient dietaries if they depend to a large extent on starchy foods, providing little protein, minerals and vitamins. Special care must be taken to include whole-grain cereals, legumes, nuts, and nut-like seeds as well as a wide variety of vegetables and fruits. This wide variety is necessary in order to be assured of an adequate intake of the more difficult to obtain vitamins (folic acid and vitamin $B_{12}$) and minerals (calcium and iron). Persons following vegetarian food patterns may be using one or more of the following four basic types of vegetarianism.

1. Lacto-ovovegetarian diets: All-vegetable diet supplemented with milk, cheese, and eggs. There would be no problem securing adequate protein with this combination.
2. Lactovegetarian diets: All-vegetable diet supplemented with only milk and cheese. Milk products add complete protein to this combination, and enhance amino acid values.
3. Pure vegetarian or vegan diets: All-vegetable diet without any animal foods, dairy products, or eggs. More careful planning is required to achieve combinations providing the necessary amounts of the essential amino acids. A deficiency of $B_{12}$ is a problem.
4. Fruitarian diets: Diet consisting of raw or dried fruits, nuts, honey, and olive oil. Potential inadequacy is greater here, although a classical California study describes a family of five observed over a five-year period with no health problems resulting.

## The Macrobiotic Diet

Macrobiotics is a food cult founded by a Japanese, George Ohsawa and based on the Oriental philosophy of Yin and Yang being the controlling forces over the entire universe. The word macrobiotics is from Greek and means the science of longevity and rejuvenation. The simple theory of the cult is that all foods should be eaten in proper balance and no medicine used; food prepared properly can cure all illnesses. Yang is characteristically extremely masculine; it includes red and yellow foods, meat, fish and eggs; and sodium (Na) is the most characteristic Yang element. Yin is extremely feminine; it includes blue and green foods; and Potassium (K) is the most characteristic Yin element. A ratio of 5:1, K:Na, or Yin:Yang is the most desired balance of foods. Macrobiotics includes seven possible diet combinations; the seventh is the most divine and includes only cereals and grain, foods that have a natural K:Na ratio of 5:1 and are intermediately between Yang and Yin extremes.

The macrobiotic cult is increasingly being practiced by teenagers and young adults; there are dangers of severe nutritional deficiencies inherent in the diets. Deficiencies in the diet are most likely to occur when the all-grain or vegetable and grain regimes are followed—vitamin C is the most common deficiency and calcium may be low. Protein is of a lower quality in grains, cereals and vegetables than in meat but by consciously combining foods high in different amino acids positive nitrogen balance and acceptable protein score can be attained.

## Faddy Reducing Diets

Down through the years, the low carbohydrate diet has popped up, disguised by various names as the Air Force Diet, The Drinking Man's Diet, Dr. Atkin's diet.

The rules of the diet have been the same: eat little, if any, carbohydrates. At the same time eat as much protein and fat-containing food as you like. And don't be bothered by the number of calories.

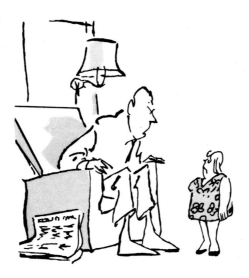

*"I warned you about those nutty crash-reducing programs, Martha."*

It is true that at first, weight loss is indeed rapid on a low carbohydrate diet—not, however, because of greater fat loss but because of a temporary loss in body water. It is also apparently true that many people who have been used to eating lots of carbohydrates lose their appetites when they suddenly cut way down. As a result they do lose weight, simply because their calories are restricted.

Once they get used to a low carbohydrate diet, however, their weight levels off or even goes back up.

Why are physicians and nutritionists concerned with the high-fat, low carbohydrate diets? Primarily because diets high in saturated fat (also cholesterol) promote elevation of the level of cholesterol in the blood and therefore increase risks of coronaries and other diseases of the heart and blood vessels—most particularly in men. Ketogenic diets also often increase the amount of uric acid in the blood, which poses a real hazard for gout-prone individuals. In addition, people on low carbohydrate diets tend to suffer fatigue very easily.

The secret of long term dieting is still the same: Moderation in the total amount of food you eat and increased walking and other forms of exercise to burn up more calories.

## Questions for Study and Discussion

1. What are the physiological functions of food?
2. What are the major nutrients required for growth and development?
3. Plan a menu incorporating the complete and incomplete sources of protein, utilizing both animal and plant sources of protein.
4. What are the functions of minerals in the body?
5. Distinguish between the fat and water soluble vitamins. What are the food sources of these vitamins and what functions do they perform in the body?
6. What is the transportation system for nutrients to all parts of your body?
7. Trace a hamburger and a glass of milk through the digestive system indicating what happens to the food.
8. Complete a three day record of the food you eat. Compare your record to the diet score table.
9. Plan a well-balanced meal utilizing foods from another cultural group.
10. Contrast the nutritional needs of a pregnant woman versus the teenager (12 to 18 years).

11. What are the cardiovascular disease risk factors? What foods are high in cholesterol?
12. Plan a nutritionally sound reducing diet. Check height and weight tables to determine your ideal weight.
13. What are the four basic food myths?
14. Select a popular family magazine containing a new reducing diet. Analyze the diet for accurate nutrient information.
15. Plan a week's food menu utilizing tables on inexpensive sources of various nutrients.

## References

Bogert, L.; Briggs, G. M.; and Calloway, D. H., *Nutrition and Physical Fitness.* Philadelphia: W. B. Saunders Co., 1973.

Deutsch, R. M. *The Family Guide to Better Food and Better Health.* Des Moines: Meredith Corp., 1971.

Friedman, G.; Yanochik, A.; West, N.; Goldberg, S.; and Bal, D. *Alternate Approach to Low Fat—Low Saturated Fat—Low Cholesterol Diet.* 6 (1974):8–10.

Kotschevar, L. *Food Service For the Extended Care Facility.* Boston: Cahner's Books, 1973.

Lappe, F. M. *Diet for a Small Planet.* New York: Ballantine Books, 1972.

Piltz, A. *How Your Body Uses Food.* The American Dairy Council, n.d.

Sebrell, W. H., Jr.; Haggerty, J. J.; and Editors of Life. *Food and Nutrition.* New York: Time Incorporated, 1967.

Stare, F. J.; McWilliams, M. *Living Nutrition.* New York: John Wiley and Sons, Inc., 1973.

White, P. L. *Let's Talk About Food.* Chicago: The American Medical Association, 1970.

Williams, S. R. *Nutrition and Diet Therapy.* St. Louis: C. V. Mosby Co., 1973.

Wilson, E. D.; Fisher, K. H.; Fugua, M. E., *Principles of Nutrition.* New York: John Wiley and Sons, Inc., 1959.

# 10

# Environmental Hazards and Man's Health

## General Concept

Modern technology has introduced a number of materials into the environment which are being found to be hazardous to human health.

## Outcomes

The student should be able to:
1. Identify the sources of various man-made pollutants
2. Explain their effects upon man
3. Offer suggestions as to how these pollutants can be controlled
4. Interpret his role as man to his environment

## Introduction

Many aspects of the environment which affect our health can be dealt with in a direct personal way; the use of alcohol, tobacco, or drugs ultimately reflects a conscious choice by an individual. But there is a growing variety of materials in our environment over which we have little direct personal control—sulfur dioxide, mercury, lead, radiation—but which have tremendous potential for personal injury because of their insidious-

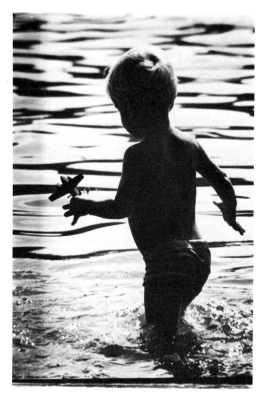

If water pollution control measures are not enforced soon, there will be few clean streams and safe recreational areas available to the public.

ness and ubiquity. Until quite recently most people were completely unaware of these environmental problems, despite their threat.

## The Air We Breathe

Because a typical person by breathing 580 million times in an average lifetime "processes" 8 million cubic feet of air, one major route of entry of environmental pollutants into our bodies is through the lungs.

One feature that ties all large and many not so large cities together is their chronic air pollution problem. The term "smog" has been used to describe this atmospheric pall, regardless of the nature of the pollution—which is perhaps unfortunate. For there are at least two major types of smog—sulfur dioxide smog and photochemical smog—each with different sources and ultimate effects upon people.

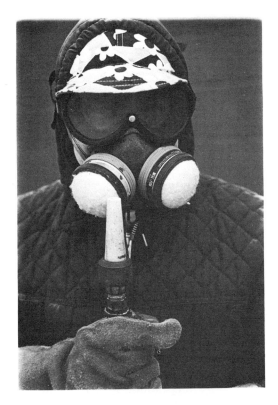

If air pollution control measures are not enforced, eventually man may have to resort to extreme measures to protect himself.

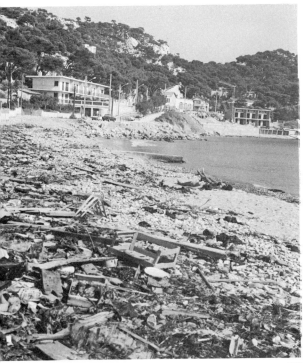

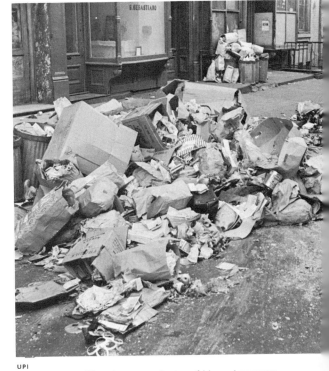

UPI     UPI

Man continues to pollute his water and shorelines.

Man, the contaminator of his environment.

## Runs in Nylons Caused by Acid in Soot

On March 10, 1952, in the neighborhood of Penn Station women discovered that their nylon stockings had suddenly developed runs. Macy's had three times as many returned as usual. The manager at Macy's had three pairs photographed only to find there were no snags; the threads had simply parted, causing as many as nine holes in one stocking.

The store consulted the House of du Pont, the sole manufacturer of nylon, and Clarence V. Ekroth who heads a chemical laboratory in Brooklyn and is a specialist in smoke.

The du Pont report stated that the problem had first occurred in Washington, D.C., in 1941, only two years after nylon hosiery had been on the market. By 1949 the problem hit Jacksonville, Florida. Accordingly, du Pont said that the running was caused by soot of a very special sort. The women in Jacksonville, for example, had all been in the area of the St. John's River when their stockings began to disintegrate. The moist and smokey air contained soot covered with sulfuric acid which was blown against the hosiery, thereby causing a chemical reaction of melting.

The next question put to Ekroth was "Why is there sulfuric acid on the grime?" He responded by stating, "Combustion of low grade industrial fuels produces sulfuric-dioxide and sulfuric-trioxide gases which are belched in quantity from factory and powerhouse chimneys thereby coming in contact with floating particles of dirt, ash, and the like in the air. On humid days these particles are, of course, covered with moisture, and the moment the gases and the moist particles meet —whango—they produce tiny specks of sulfuric acid."

"A nylon blouse," he continued, "is woven, and the threads are comparatively free from stress. The prospect of a young lady in an all nylon ensemble walking past a Con. Ed. smokestack on a sticky day and ending up in her skin is therefore unlikely, though charming." Still, Ekroth refused to rule it out; "It's a scientific possibility," he said.

*New Yorker* 28, March 29, 1952, pp. 25–6.

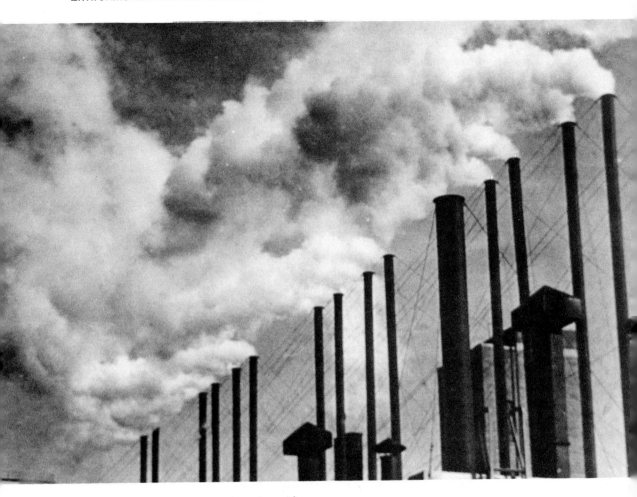

Smog is a combination of the words smoke and fog.

## Sulfur Dioxide Smog

Smog, a combination of the words smoke and fog, was originally used to describe the sulfur dioxide pollution in northern European cities such as London and Glasgow, cities which relied almost exclusively on coal as a source of heat. Coal contains 1 to 5 percent sulfur, which oxidizes to form sulfur dioxide when the coal is burned. As a gas, sulfur dioxide is not particularly dangerous or destructive, but in moist air it easily forms sulfuric acid, which is extremely corrosive to both people and materials.

Much of the fine ash (fly ash) produced when coal is burned goes up the chimney with the sulfur dioxide and absorbs sulfuric acid as it is formed from the sulfur dioxide. This fine dispersion or aerosol of sulfuric acid can then fall out on objects or, worse yet, be inhaled into the lungs.

The human respiratory tract is lined with cells which have cilia or tiny whips which beat 12 times per second in a series of wave-like motions which help the body to expel foreign objects that are inhaled. But there are substances in polluted air which so narcotize the ciliated cells that dust particles are no longer routinely expelled from the body. Sulfuric acid and other dangerous compounds can now contact the delicate membranes in the lungs across which the gas exchange so necessary to our well-being takes place.

Chronic exposure to sulfur dioxide smog, then, is particularly damaging to the lungs. Four of the most common respiratory ailments reported in cities with sulfur dioxide smog are bronchitis, bronchial asthma, emphysema, and lung cancer.

**Bronchitis.**  Overproduction of mucus associated with the failure of ciliary action in the bronchial tubes results in a hacking cough and shortness of breath. More than 20 percent of the men between 40 and 60 in Great Britain have chronic bronchitis.

**Bronchial Asthma.**  Respiratory membranes become oversensitized to foreign protein or other substances and swell, making it difficult to expel air from the lungs and causing wheezing and shortness of breath.

**Emphysema.**  The small subdivisions of the bronchial tubes, the bronchioles, constrict, allowing too much air to remain in the air sacs where gaseous exchange takes place. With the next breath they then become overinflated and in time collapse, reducing the gas exchange efficiency of the lungs and ultimately causing a severe shortage of oxygen in the body.

**Lung Cancer.** Carcinogens, substances that can cause cancerous cells to develop, are common in sulfur dioxide smog as well as cigarette smoke (see chap. 6). Inhaled particles containing carcinogens can greatly increase the probability of lung cancer.

## Photochemical Smog

Many cities in the United States, New York in particular, have a severe sulfur dioxide smog problem. But a more widespread problem in American cities is photochemical smog. For many years photochemical smog was thought to come from industry or incinerators but was finally identified with the internal combustion engine. Gasoline vapors from poorly sealed gas caps and carburetors, incompletely burned hydrocarbons from the exhaust manifold and tailpipe, together with carbon monoxide and nitrogen oxides enter the air whenever an internal combustion engine is in operation. If gasoline were a simple compound which burned cleanly to carbon dioxide and water, there would be no problem. But it contains tetraethyl lead to prevent knocking, ethylene dichloride and dibromide to prevent fouling by lead oxide, metal deactivators and anti-rusting agents, antioxidants, anti-icing compounds, detergents, lubricants—all of which contribute their share to the pollution problem. Furthermore, when this grisly mixture leaves the car it can react with sunlight to form secondary pollutants, PAN (peroxyacetyl nitrate), and ozone, not directly produced by the engine. The sunnier the climate, the greater the opportunity for sunlight to react with automobile exhaust and the greater the production of photochemical smog, as has been demonstrated by Los Angeles, Phoenix, and other cities in clear dry climates.

Photochemical smog tends to affect the upper respiratory tract, the eyes and nose, rather than the lungs, although ozone, a component of photochemical smog, can narcotize cilial action in the bronchial tubes and allow pollutant particles to enter the lungs.

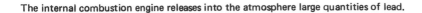

The internal combustion engine releases into the atmosphere large quantities of lead.

UPI

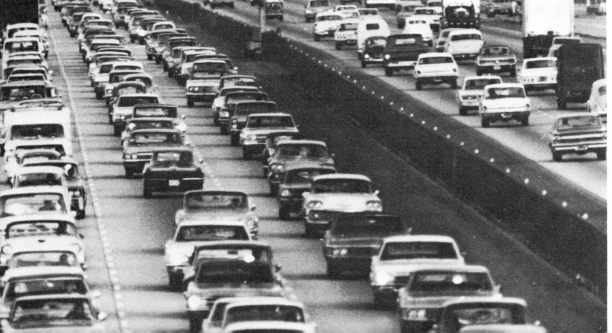

## Noise

The atmosphere bears not only particles and gases but sound waves, for technological "progress" seems to be inevitably accompanied by noise. By causing the constriction of blood vessels, the tensing of muscles, and the sudden release of adrenalin into the bloodstream, loud noise can lead to an increase in stress which first affects blood pressure, then the circulatory and nervous systems. For those people who already suffer from hypertension, heart disease, or various neuroses, noise may have a determining effect on their health.

Most urban noise is related to transportation and construction and although it is passively endured by urbanites, it need not be. There is no technical reason why noise must be an integral part of our culture. *All* sources of noise can be at least muted, and many eliminated altogether if proper insulations and mufflers are used and construction standards are established and enforced. What is required is not a technological revolution but the discovery by the average person that cities *can* be as quiet as suburbs if concern about noise is voiced and pressure applied through political channels.

## The Metals We Eat

### Lead

The internal combustion engine which generates photochemical smog ingredients also releases into the atmosphere large quantities of lead from the antiknock additive tetraethyl lead, as we have seen. Almost three million *tons* of lead have been released into the environment by automobiles since the use of tetraethyl lead began in 1923. Since lead has been recognized as a toxic metal from the days of ancient Greece, the wholesale release of large quantities into the air is of some concern. Normal lead levels in the bloodstream fall between 0.05 and 0.4 parts per million (ppm) and recognizable lead poisoning occurs at 0.8 ppm. The question that has been raised is whether the range 0.05 to 0.4 ppm is "normal" or whether this already reflects an increase from a past norm. If so, continued release of lead from gasoline is unconscionable. Although the recent decision by American automobile producers to retune their engines to burn unleaded gasoline was undertaken to prevent fouling of catalytic devices designed to reduce air pollution, rather than to deal with the problem of lead in the atmosphere, the end result should be a reduced contamination of the air with lead.

While we are all exposed to the hazard of atmospheric lead, the damage from this source if cumulative seems to lie in the future. More immediate is the ingestion of lead in paint, putty, and plaster. Interior paints contained lead pigments until 1958 when they were replaced by titanium compounds. But thousands of old, presently substandard houses and apartments were painted with lead-based paints for many years. As these dwellings deteriorate, paint and putty chip, flake off, and are eaten by children. Nearly 20 percent of one- to five-year-old children eat non-food materials, some out of simple curiosity, others because of an iron deficiency in the body which seems to be responsible for this behavior pattern called pica.

Lead poisoning can take one of two forms, symptomatic if the dose is massive, asymptomatic if the dose is small but steady. Lead is absorbed in a soluble form and initially deposited in various soft tissues of the body and so remains in equilibrium with the blood. Ultimately, soluble lead is voided in the urine, hence blood or urine analyses can determine the body burden of lead. However some lead is incorporated into bone tissue as insoluble salts which can be mobilized at times in children and returned to the bloodstream in a soluble form making treatment much more difficult. Symptomatic lead poisoning may include lower red blood cell production resulting in anemia, chronic nephritis leading to hypertension and failure of the kidneys, and behavior problems or convulsions resulting from nervous system impairment. Since these symptoms of acute lead poisoning are easily recognized and diagnosed, massive ingestion of lead can often be treated with little permanent damage. Asymptomatic lead poisoning is in a way more serious.

Of 1,000 children examined in Chicago ghettos, 70 were found to be suffering from asymptomatic lead poisoning. Perhaps as many as 50,000 children in the United States are suffering from this unrecognized form of lead poisoning. Since the children victimized are in a stage of rapid growth and development, permanent brain damage often results. In one group of 425 Chicago children found to have asymptomatic lead poisoning, 109 had sustained neural damage which led to permanent mental retardation.

Not only must all children exposed to leaded paint be examined as soon as possible to uncover all cases of lead poisoning, but leaded paints

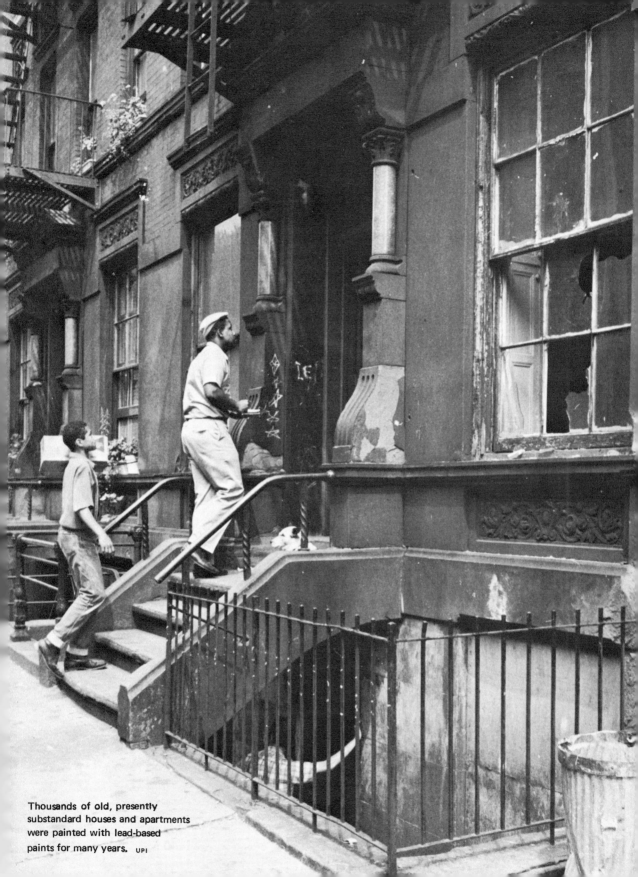

Thousands of old, presently
substandard houses and apartments
were painted with lead-based
paints for many years. UPI

must be removed from substandard housing units if the units themselves cannot be replaced. Until then, ghetto dwellers must endure the loss of lead-poisoned children, and the public at large the social cost of permanent retardation.

---

### Our Manic Environment

During the first six months of life a child receives deep and lasting effects from environmental influences. Since it is only in recent decades that pollutants everywhere have reached a peak, the worst effects of environmental pollution are yet to be seen in the next generation of children. Recent studies in England show that children raised in high pollution areas from the age of two or three show evidence of "permanent malfunction." In twenty or thirty years most of these children will have some type of chronic disorder.

Man will not become extinct but instead will adapt himself to progressively worse conditions. A child born into this polluted world will not have the chance to develop mentally and physically to his full potential. If we don't become actively alarmed by what our environment is doing to us, we will "witness something worse than extinction—a progressive degradation of the quality of human life."

Rene Dubos, "We Can't Buy Our Way Out," *Psychology Today,* vol. 3, no. 10, March 1970, p. 20.

---

## Mercury

While lead has been an environmental problem for thousands of years, mercury is a relatively new problem. People who have worked with inorganic mercury compounds, of course, often developed mercury poisoning —the expression "mad as a hatter" derives from the mental derangement of hatters who used mercuric chloride to treat the beaver skins once used to make men's hats. Inorganic mercury vapors are fat soluble and since nerve fibers are surrounded by a fatty sheath, mercury rapidly accumulates in the brain. Another problem associated with inorganic mercury poisoning is the rate at which sugar, protein, and salts are reabsorbed or secreted by the kidneys. The increasing use of inorganic mercury compounds which are dumped into the environment has resulted in episodes of mass mercury poisoning. In 1953, 52 people living near a vinyl chloride plant in Japan became ill from mercury poisoning; 17 died and 23 were disabled permanently.

Such examples of mass poisoning are certainly dramatic, but a much larger quantity of mercury enters the environment in the form of organic compounds. Organic mercury is especially effective in killing fungi and has seen increasing use in the past 20 years as a fungicide. Pulp mills have used large quantities of organic mercury to control microorganisms which might otherwise plug up machinery which is constantly being bathed with nutritious wood pulp. Release of mercury-treated waste water into lakes and streams has so seriously contaminated fresh water fish that people have been advised not to eat fish caught in the Niagara and St. Lawrence Rivers, and Lakes Champlain, Ontario, and Erie. Oceanic food chains have also been contaminated, leading to prohibitively high concentrations of mercury in some lots of tuna fish.

Another source of organic mercury in the environment is seed treated with mercury-containing fungicides. Pheasants in California in 1969 contained 1.4 to 4.7 ppm mercury, and a level of at least 1 ppm caused the cancellation of the pheasant hunting season in Alberta, Canada the same year.

Considering the widespread use of fungicides in the United States, it isn't surprising that many foods contain excessive quantities of mercury. The World Health Organization suggests a maximum of 0.05 ppm in food. But some food products that have been randomly sampled (besides tuna fish) contain considerably more than this—tomatoes, apples, eggs, and meat may have as much as 0.1 ppm. As with most poisonous substances, the question is whether these levels of environmental mercury are causing damage now or may prove to have a cumulative damaging effect in the future. Clearly we cannot afford the luxury of waiting to find out. Alternative fungicides either containing no mercury or a less toxic form must replace the broad-spectrum fungicides in use today. Industrial processing wastes must be decontaminated before being released into the environment. Once contaminated, food chains and the foods derived from them present the distinct risk of mercury poisoning, acute or chronic.

## The Biocide Spectrum

Fungicides containing mercury are just one of a large group of compounds, insecticides, herbicides, pesticides, which supposedly kill target groups of organisms. Unfortunately, all run quite wide of the mark and even when properly used may kill unintended organisms. Perhaps a better generic term for these materials might be biocide.

There are two major classes of biocides, organophosphates and organochlorines. Organophosphates, by interfering with the enzyme cholinesterase, allow nerve impulses to flow without interruption along the nervous system, leading to convulsions, paralysis, and death. Parathion and malathion are the two major organophosphates still in use today; although quite toxic to a broad spectrum of organisms, they are not very persistent. The most notorious of organochlorines or chlorinated hydrocarbons is probably DDT. The mode of action of the organochlorines is still uncertain, although the symptoms associated with acute poisoning, tremors, and convulsions suggest interference with the central nervous system. Organochlorines, while somewhat less toxic than organophosphates, are far more persistent. When first introduced, biocides seemed the answer to many of man's problems. The housefly and mosquito, with the diseases they transmit, appeared to be under firm control if not on the road to extinction. But after a few years unforeseen problems arose.

By 1948, 12 species of insects had become resistant to DDT; by 1957, 76 species were resistant; by 1967, 165. Not only were target organisms becoming immune, but beneficial organisms—the pollinating honeybee and a great number of desirable predators and parasites—were unintentionally killed by broad-spectrum biocides. Then it was found that many biocides were not readily attacked and broken down by microorganisms in the environment. After 15 years, half of the DDT originally present was still active. Although DDT is only slightly soluble in water it is readily absorbed by the bottom mud and by the fat bodies of microorganisms. This means that although only a few parts per billion may be found in water, as these are accumulated in the fat of living organisms, more DDT is released from the bottom mud. Through this mechanism, very small quantities of persistent biocides can be concentrated via the links of a food chain into potentially lethal doses. Mud at the bottom of Green Bay in Wisconsin contained 0.014 ppm DDT. Small crustaceans contained 0.41 ppm, fish were found to have 3 to 6 ppm, and herring gulls 99 ppm, which interfered with their reproduction. Apparently

many birds are similarly affected by DDT, which inhibits the production
of carbonic anhydrase, an enzyme that controls calcium metabolism in
birds. Eggs laid by severely contaminated birds have such a low calcium
content that they break easily. Reproduction in some populations of the
peregrine falcon, bald eagle, osprey, and brown pelican has virtually
ceased because of persistent biocide residues.

Of all the problems caused by biocides in the environment, biological magnification, the accumulation through food chains, seems to pose
the greatest threat to man, for we are uncertain just what effect body bur-
dens of persistent biocides may already be having or will have in the
future. There may be no effects, or effects that are too vague and general
to be connected to a particular biocide, or it may be that definite effects
will become evident in the future. In the 1920s a group of young girls
painted luminescent numbers on clocks in a factory. The paste contained
radium, which was considered relatively harmless, so the girls without
thinking pointed the tips of their brushes with their tongues. Thirty
years later the girls, now middleaged women, began dying of lip, tongue,
and mouth cancer.

Man as well as most other organisms has accumulated some biocides
in his body fat; the typical person in the United States averages about 8
to 10 ppm of DDT. While many people have certainly died from careless use or excessive exposure to biocides, at the moment there have been
no medically documented examples of death or even sickness from biocides when they have been properly used. A number of researchers however have found circumstantial evidence that suggests some links between certain biocides and various pathological conditions. Are biocides
so essential to be worth their potential risk to man's health? We have,
unfortunately, been so impressed with their effectiveness, convenience,
and cheapness that alternatives have been ignored. While huge quantities of biocides are used every year, there are relatively few pests against
which they are directed; one-third of all biocides used in agriculture are
employed to control the boll weevil. The concept of integrated control
holds much promise for reducing our present overdependence upon biocides. By using biocides sparingly and only when necessary, and avoiding
the broad-spectrum types, by using biological means of control and certain cultivation practices, the flood of biocides now polluting food chains
everywhere can be reduced to reasonable proportions, protecting not
only the elements of these food chains but ultimately ourselves.

## Food Additives

In addition to the mercury or DDT that we inadvertently consume in our food, there are other food contaminants, as well as materials intentionally added in the processing of many food products. While the Food and Drug Administration now protects the public from the crude and unsanitary contaminants and additives of the past—chalk in milk, for example—today's contaminants and additives are far more sophisticated and subtle in their effects.

## Antibiotics

Antibiotics have been in widespread use not only for humans but their livestock too. Cows are often treated with penicillin for various diseases. Indeed, it was found that chickens routinely fed antibiotics grew faster and heavier, yielding greater profit per unit time to the grower. To avoid contamination, treatment should be halted several days before marketing the animal or the product. But this isn't always done and people eating such contaminated products can be routinely exposed to antibiotics, encouraging the development of disease organisms resistant to antibiotics. Thus, when antibiotics are needed to combat diseases in humans, the drugs are no longer effective.

## Hormones

Another contaminant often found in meat products is the synthetic hormone stibestrol. When implanted behind the ear of a heifer, up to 15 percent faster growth utilizing 12 percent less food has been reported. Naturally the amount of this hormone ingested from treated beef is small, but then so is the concentration necessary to affect that fine balance between male and female that is maintained by hormones. Should excessive amounts of synthetic hormones be applied to livestock without allowing a sufficient period for absorption and metabolic breakdown, there could be side effects induced in an unsuspecting public.

## Additives

Pick up virtually any package in a supermarket and read the fine print—antioxidant, emulsifier, fortifier, extender, bleach, moistener, thickener

—the list goes on and on of substances intentionally added to food to improve its flavor, texture, color, or keeping qualities. Much of the fantastic variety of foods displayed in a large market is there only because of this array of additives.

Unfortunately, many additives which have been used for years have not had rigorous testing of their biological activity. Occasionally additives long in use are subsequently found to cause cancer in laboratory animals and are summarily withdrawn from the market—for example, the emulsifier, polyoxyethylene, and the sweetener, cyclamate.

While a case can be made for many additives that improve the keeping qualities of food or its taste, consistency, or texture, there is little rationale for coal tar dyes, which are still being used in many food products. Without nutritive or preservative function, coal tar dyes are used only to color foods to increase their esthetic appeal and salability. Since many of these dyes have been demonstrated to be cancer-producing or carcinogenic, closely related compounds are suspect. Much confusion exists as to which coal tar dyes are dangerous and which are not. The United States allows 15 dyes to be used and the English 30. But 9 of our acceptable dyes are banned in England and most of the 30 the English allow are banned in the United States! Perhaps the ingestion of *any* coal tar dye is unwise.

The greatest sources of additives in food are the so-called convenience foods, instant this, and ready that, which crowd the store shelves. The less work in preparation by the housewife, the more processing is required of the manufacturer; the more processing required, the more additives necessary to simulate the taste and texture of real food traditionally prepared. The end result may taste the same but the cost includes a long list of additives. Most of these may indeed be innocuous, but some have proven to be detrimental to health and more will surely be indicted in the future.

What can you as a consumer do? While there is no reason to panic and take refuge in wheat germ, yogurt, and carrot juice, neither should you limit your diet to neatly packaged convenience foods which are high in additives and low in nutrients and calories.

1. Whenever possible start from scratch—mash your own potatoes, whip your own cream, bake your own cake from flour, sugar, and whole eggs. It often takes little extra time to do this despite constant advertising claims to the contrary.

2. Learn to read the fine print on packaged food and avoid those which seem to consist of nothing but additives.

3. If you must include packaged TV dinners in your diet, serve them with a fresh salad and have fresh fruit for dessert.

As a consumer you are not as defenseless as you have been led to think. Selective shopping if thoughtfully done can more than make up for the excesses of impulse shopping which account for most of the sales of overprocessed and overpriced convenience foods.

## Radiation

Consideration of the materials in the air we breathe and the food we eat is not the whole story, for there is still one more environmental hazard that must be mentioned—radiation. There are three forms of radiation that are given off by radioactive materials: alpha particles, beta particles, and gamma rays. The first two have relatively low energy; alpha particles are stopped by a sheet of paper or human skin and beta particles penetrate only a millimeter or so into the body. But gamma radiation is far more powerful, easily penetrating lead and concrete and, of course, the human body. Regardless of the type of radiation, the dose received is measured in roentgens (r) or in some cases in rads, which are roughly equivalent to roentgens. The scale of injury from acute doses of radiation is fairly well known as is the mechanism. Below 25 r there is no measurable change. Between 25 and 100 r, the level of white blood cells drops but there are no external signs. From 100 to 300 r, radiation sickness is readily apparent, at 500 r 50 percent of a human population is killed, and at 1000 r *all* people die.

Radiation can act in two ways: it can interact directly with sensitive molecules like DNA or various enzymes, altering or destroying them, or it can ionize water molecules generating the exceedingly reactive free radicals OH· and H·. These then can inactivate metabolically important molecules. Since water is far more abundant than any other substance in living cells, its ionization and subsequent effect is the most important result of radiation on man. The tissues most sensitive to radiation are those in a state of rapid division, the hair follicle, gut lining, corneal epithelium, bone marrow, and gonads. Hence radiation sickness involves the loss of hair, nausea, vomiting, diarrhea, cataracts, drop in blood cell production, and sterility. Although many of these problems are reversible, drastic lowering of the white blood cell count so opens the body to normally innocuous diseases that death may result from a common cold, measles, strep throat, or pneumonia.

These dramatic effects result, of course, from acute exposure to radiation. Chronic or low level exposure is much more common and in a way more dangerous, because it is insidious and its expression is often delayed for many years. There is no lower threshold to radiation effects. Any radiation including normal background is potentially harmful, that is, able to cause mutations. Certainly evolution would not have taken place without this stimulus for change. But we should be extremely careful about adding significantly to the frequency of these occurrences, for most mutations are harmful.

There are two major sources of man-made radiation at large today: fallout and x-rays (similar to the naturally occurring gamma rays). While fallout from atmospheric atomic or hydrogen bomb explosions has been reduced significantly as a result of an international agreement banning such explosions, the rapid spread of nuclear power plants has to some extent recouped the loss.

Nuclear power plants produce three kinds of radioactive wastes: high-level fission products and contaminated materials which are contained and stored indefinitely; medium-level gases which escape from the core elements and are vented into the atmosphere; and low-level wastes which result from the neutron bombardment of impurities in the secondary cooling water. Ordinarily only the last two categories are of concern to us. The radioactive gases that leave the smokestack are the noble gases which, fortunately, decay in a few days' time. Of these gases, tritium is the greatest problem because hydrogen is a component of all organic compounds, hence a radioactive form of hydrogen can enter all forms of life in an endless variety of ways. The isotopes formed in the secondary coolant and released to the natural environment are in themselves not particularly dangerous, because of their dilution. But certain isotopes are differentially accumulated by aquatic organisms and passed on up the food chain so that a top carnivore such as ourselves might receive far more radiation than was present in the original effluent.

X-ray machines are at the same time less and more dangerous to man than fallout: less dangerous because many people are never x-rayed or have an option, while *everyone* is exposed to fallout; more dangerous because to those being x-rayed, more radiation is received with one shot than accumulates over several years of fallout exposure. The average x-ray exposure varies from about 0.5 r to 1 r per shot. If a number of photos are taken, the dose though usually localized can be considerable. While no one would seriously question the value of x-rays or their necessity in many instances, they are often routinely taken without sufficient justification, especially by dentists.

---

## Riding on Wastes

Every year, 100 million worn rubber tires and 26 billion nonreturnable glass bottles are discarded in the U.S. Disposing of them is a formidable problem, usually resolved by burning evil-smelling mountains of tires and burying tons of splintered glass. But there soon may be a neater and more practical solution: using the unsightly, troublesome waste products as construction materials in the 20,000 miles of highways that are built annually in the U.S.

In testimony before the Senate Committee on Public Works, Richard L. Cheney, executive director of the Glass Container Manufacturers Institute, called attention to an experimental product called "glasphalt." Developed at the University of Missouri, it uses finely ground glass granules to replace the rock aggregates now used as a construction material for highways. One 58-foot-long test strip of glasphalt pavement, outside the Owens-Illinois Technical Center in Toledo, has held up well during the worst winter in years; engineers reported virtually no cracking, rippling or holes in the surface and gave it a top rating for skid resistance.

At Texas A. & M., Research Engineer Douglas Bynum, 35, is testing his theory that the rubber in discarded tires might give asphalt added flexibility and more resistance to cracking. Test results showed that the powdered rubber increases asphalt's overall cohesiveness so that it does not split when roadbeds shift slightly or sink.

Best of all, Bynum says, there would be no foreseeable shortage of materials for the improved roads. Combined with asphalt, the old tires and bottles disposed of in 1970 could pave a freeway that would span the U.S. 23 times.

The long-term damage from weapons fallout has been reduced by international agreement, but standards for nuclear reactor emissions vary from country to country. Fallout generated from nuclear power plants should certainly be reduced as more plants come on line and perhaps eliminated altogether in the future, much as internal combustion engine emissions must be reduced and ultimately eliminated as the number of automobiles continues to burgeon. The radiation danger from x-rays can certainly be reduced by proper focusing which limits the area irradiated and by shielding which protects the rest of the body, particularly the gonads, from back scatter while the machine is in operation. Finally, the decision to x-ray or not to x-ray has to be taken far more seriously than it has in the past. Routine x-rays are as potentially dangerous as routine applications of persistent biocides or routine prescriptions of antibiotics.

When all the environmental hazards that man has generated are considered, one's initial feeling is paranoia or, worse yet, apathy. But there is much that the individual can do to protect himself. First he must be concerned, then informed, and finally activated, even if the action is only reading labels or refusing an unnecessary x-ray. All of the problems discussed in this chapter have solutions, most within the reach of current technology. What is necessary is a show of concern and interest on the part of individuals everywhere to assure that the proper solutions are found and applied. The responsibility is yours.

## The Energy Crisis

The energy crisis of 1973–74 jolted the average American, particularly when he found himself waiting in lines of twenty cars for any available gasoline. With a scarcity of heating fuel, the homeowner found himself turning his thermostat to a chilling 68 degrees. The further impact of the energy crisis hit the consumer in his wallet as prices of "necessities" escalated.

As a consequence, our society found itself in the midst of a dilemma best summed up by Bruce Netschert as:

We are currently witnessing one of those rare events in history when there arises a head-on conflict between a line of development in a society and a new social attitude. Consider these alternatives:

On the one side, we have a vigorous growth in energy consumption, closely related to a rising standard of living.

On the other side, we have a widespread public concern with preservation of the environment which has been translated into restrictive standards and regulations.[1]

We are forced, therefore, in the truest philosophical sense to determine what should be done to make living conditions in our society both technologically successful as well as humanely enriching.

The battle between those demanding increased energy availability and the environmentalists is demonstrated in a practical sense by the following:

... gas rates rise to reflect restrictions on offshore explorations;
... fuel oil prices rise to reflect the reduction in oil's sulfur content;
... coal prices rise to reflect the impact of the Coal Mine Health and Safety Act and restrictions on strip mining;
... electricity rates rise to reflect all of these things plus the cost of cooling towers and other environmental facilities.[2]

We may all find ourselves facing this dilemma on a personal level—we want our electric dishwashers and frost-free refrigerators, but we don't wish to endanger our environment and its resources. Are we willing to force a return to the usage of coal to feed our energy demands even though "coal mining creates acid mines drainage, earth subsidence, and wholesale destruction of landscapes in stripping operations"?[3] Are we so eager to keep our innumerable automobiles gassed that we can ignore the fact that "oil production carries the risks of massive marine pollution and the less-publicized problem of salt water from wells on land"?[4] The questions go on seemingly endlessly. Perhaps we can eventually find the Aristotelian mean, but meanwhile we must focus our energies and intellect dispassionately in seeking the solution. Although the problem may appear to be overwhelmingly complex and even insoluble, one can find some comfort in Norman Cousins' observation:

1. Bruce C. Netschert, "Energy Versus Environment," *Harvard Business Review* 51 (January, 1973):24.
2. *Ibid.*, p. 24.
3. Bruce C. Netschert, "Energy Versus Environment," *Harvard Business Review* 51 (January, 1973):26.
4. *Ibid.*, 26.

The American people may have lost their natural abundance, but they need not have lost their natural sense of adventure. The grand leaps of the creative intelligence and the resolute determination that pushed back the American frontier can now be put to work on the most magnificent research project of all time—creating a human habitat congenial not just to the human physical presence but also to the human spirit.[5]

## Questions for Study and Discussion

1. Contrast the effects of sulfur dioxide and photochemical smog on the body.
2. Why should we be concerned about contamination of food chains containing organisms of no direct interest to man?
3. Would you be willing to pay more for a lead-free gasoline?
4. What steps might you take to reduce the noise level of your community?
5. Because DDT seems to have no direct effect upon man, many have argued for its continued use in agriculture. Do you agree?
6. Have you ever analyzed your motivation in buying packaged foods? Are you attracted by the package, price, taste, convenience? Do you ever read the list of ingredients?
7. Do you have your teeth routinely x-rayed by a dentist "just to be sure"?
8. Have you ever thought about your increasing demands for electric power in terms of the sulfur dioxide, fly ash, or radioactivity that power generates?

## References

Burns, W. *Noise and Man.* Philadelphia: J. B. Lippincott, 1969.

Chisolm, J. J., Jr. "Lead Poisoning." *Scientific American* 224 (1971):15.

Cousins, Norman. "Survival Without Abundance." *Saturday Review/ World* 1 (1974):4.

Frye, A. *The Hazards of Atomic Wastes.* Washington D.C.: Washington Public Affairs Press, 1962.

Graham, F., Jr. *Since Silent Spring.* Boston: Houghton Mifflin, 1970.

Grant, N. "Legacy of the Mad Hatter." *Environment* 11 (1969):18.

Kohlmeier, L. M., Jr. *The Regulators, Watchdog Agencies and the Public Interest.* New York: Harper and Row, 1969.

Lapp, R. "The Four Big Fears About Nuclear Power." *New York Times Magazine,* February 7, 1971, p. 16.

5. Norman Cousins, "Survival Without Abundance," *Saturday Review/World* 1 (January 26, 1974):4.

Lewis, H. R. *With Every Breath You Take.* New York: Crown, 1965.

Lofroth, G. and Duffy, M. E. "Birds Give Warning. *Environment* 11 (1969): 10–17.

Longgood, W. F. *The Poisons in Your Food.* New York: Simon and Schuster, 1960.

Morgan, K. Z. "Never Do Harm." *Environment* 13:28–38.

Netschert, Bruce C. "Energy Versus Environment." *Harvard Business Review* 51 (1973):24–26.

Novick, S. *The Careless Atom.* Boston: Houghton Mifflin, 1961.

Novick, S. "A New Pollution Problem." *Environment* 11 (1969):2–9.

Patterson, C. C. and Salvia, J. D. "Lead in the Modern Environment." *Scientist and Citizen* 10 (1968):66–79.

Wagner, R. H. *Environment and Man.* New York: W. W. Norton, 1971.

Wise, W. *Killer Smog: The World's Worst Air Pollution Disaster.* Chicago: Rand McNally, 1968.

Woodwell, G. M., Wurster, C. F., Jr., and Isaacson, D. A. "DDT Residues in an East Coast Estuary: A Case of Biological Concentration of a Persistent Insecticide." *Science* 156 (1967):821–824.

# 11

# Human Sexuality: A Developmental Overview

## General Concept

Sexuality is the identification, application, and fulfillment of a masculine or feminine role in the society in which one lives.

## Outcomes

The student should be able to:

1. Understand that sexuality encompasses the psychological, intellectual, emotional, and possibly spiritual make-up of a male or female
2. Understand the principles involved with the emotional implications of the physical sexual drive
3. Feel a concern for planning a marriage and procedures for selecting a mate
4. Respect the opposite sex and the moral codes and behavior of others
5. Establish sound sexual behavior when dating, during engagement and throughout marriage.

   ". . . The sexual instincts of man do not suddenly awaken between the thirteenth and the fifteenth year, i.e., at puberty, but operate from the outset of the child's development, change gradually from one form to another, progress from one state to another, until at last adult sexual life is achieved as the final result from this long series of development."[1] Thus, Anna Freud, before a group of teachers forty years ago, described the concept of sexuality that dominates our thinking today.

Sexual behavior may be thought of as including only simple involvement of the sexual organs as in mating or reproduction or it may be thought of as including this aspect as well as the symbolic aspect— representative of being male or female as in masculine and feminine behavior. In order to encompass this totality of behavior, Kirkendall used the term *sexuality* to mean "a deep and pervasive aspect of one's total personality, the sum total of one's feelings and behavior not only as a sexual being but as a male or female."[2]

Expressions of sexuality, thus, go much beyond genital responses, and are subject to modification as a result of sexual learning and experience. Throughout the life of an individual, physiological, psychological, and sociological forces condition sexuality in important ways. Therefore, the adult pattern of sexual behavior represents a composite of many different maturational elements.

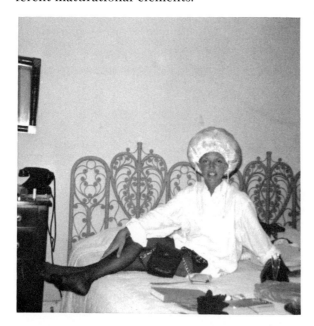

Women continue to struggle with their appearance and cosmetics in an attempt to express their identity and self-image.

1. Anna Freud, *Psychoanalysis for Teachers and Parents* (Boston: Beacon Press, 1935).

2. Lester A. Kirkendall, Isadore Rubin, "Sexuality and the Life Cycle" (SIECUS Discussion Guide no. 8, New York: SIECUS, 1969), p. 9.

## Sexuality in Infancy and Childhood

The turn of the century saw an awakening interest in sexuality and sexual learning among children. The most significant work of this period was Freud's theory of infantile sexuality, which directed the attention of the world to sexuality in early childhood and its importance for the future adult role. With the publication, in 1905, of his essay on *Infantile Sexuality,* Freud challenged the traditional view that children were essentially asexual. It was his contention that not only were children involved in sexual activity, but that this activity was an essential precursor and component in the development toward sexual maturity as a process of differentiation involving a series of psychosexual stages through which biology and culture conspired to focus adult sexual life onto appropriate sex objects and modes of gratification. This theory of psychosexual development was based on three assumptions: Sexual energy is a basic life force present from birth; ways of channeling this energy are learned so that one meets sexual needs through socially approved sex objects and modes of gratification; and finally, gender role learning itself occurs in an orderly series of psychosexual stages. This theory has formed the basis of modern psychiatric thinking.

Sexual socialization according to this theory occurs through the following stages: oral, anal, phallic, and genital. The first three stages, oc-

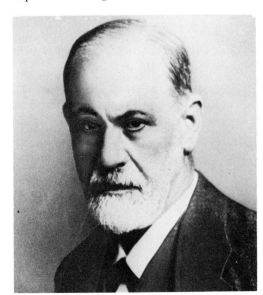

UPI

Sigmund Freud proposed the theory of psychosexual development.

curring in preadolescence, are usually referred to as the pregenital period. Although Freud admitted that little was known about this period,
he believed that two important developments took place during this
time. In the oral period (age zero-one) sexual energy is diffuse, and
gratification is obtained through the mouth by putting objects into the
mouth and by biting. Stimulation of the oral zone produces erotic pleasure. Since the infant is dependent on the mother for meeting oral needs,
she emerges as the first sexual object for both boys and girls. During the
anal period (ages one-three) the child is expected to control the plea-
sures obtained from defecation by regulating its occurrence. The mother
remains the love object for both boys and girls since she is still the one
who meets their needs and invokes discipline. Thus, during the pre-
oedipal period, the mother typically becomes differentiated out of the
universe as the love object for both boys and girls, and the pleasure zone
shifts from the alimentary orifices to the genitals. Since the genitals now
supersede other organs as the main source of bodily pleasure, this phase is
described as phallic. In the phallic stage (ages four-five) the boy com-
petes with his father for exclusive sexual possession of his mother. The
threat of castration by the father causes him to repress his incestuous desire for his mother and his hostility for his father. This is called the
Oedipus complex because it parallels the Greek myth of Oedipus who
killed his father and married his mother. In order to escape the consequences of this competition with his father, the boy lapses into the
latency period (ages six-twelve) and identifies with his father.

The dynamics of the girl's behavior in this period is less clearly
developed in Freud's writings, but she faces a similar dilemma. Her desire
to possess a penis, particularly her father's, and being denied it leads
her to develop penis envy; a complex comparable to the boy's castration
anxiety. As a result, she shifts to the father as a more adequate sex object
than the mother, and her complex culminates in a desire to be given a
child by her father. Since this wish is not fulfilled, the girl gradually
abandons it and finally resolves the complex by possessing a penis
through coitus in marriage. The desire to possess a penis and to bear a
child causes her to identify with her mother and prepares her for her
subsequent role in marriage and parenthood. Resolution of the Oedipus
complex by repression leads her to the latency period. Freud believed
that neither the period of the Oedipal conflict or the period of latency
occurred with the same intensity for females as it did with males.

The final step in this process is the move toward adult sexuality which is initiated by puberty; sexual urges emerge leading to the genital stage. In the genital stage, the adolescent seeks a love object outside the family and the chief sexual aim becomes full genital intercourse and reproduction.

The psychoanalytic theory of psychosexual development has been criticized from many sources, but the two most systematic sources of attack have come from learning theorists and anthropologists. The learning theorists believe that sexual learning, like any other type of learning, is simply a process of reinforcing socially approved behavior and punishing undesirable behavior. Anthropologists have attacked the idea that each of these stages, particularly the stage of the Oedipal conflict, is necessary to normal personality development. Their objections are based on studies of other societies in which very different patterns of psychosexual development seemed to occur.

Freud's general contention that children are not essentially asexual has been supported, however, by both anthropological and taxonomic data. Children, even in infancy, clearly respond to stimulation of the genitals and other erogenous zones of the body. Kinsey reported that orgasmic experiences occurred in infants and children throughout the pre-adolescent years. Numerous other studies attest to the actuality of childhood sexuality. Anthropological data demonstrate that children can respond sexually several years prior to puberty.

Current research has tended to move away from direct studies of infant and childhood sexual behavior. Sexuality has its roots in man's biological makeup, and the development of gender role or sex differences has become one of the main focuses of present research. Since the molding forces or socializing agents are the family and peer group (among others), sexuality is being pursued as a form of social development.

Social learning theorists, therefore, emphasize the fact that children learn about sex and sexuality in many ways. In the early years, beginning long before interpersonal communication reaches the verbal level, children acquire from their cultural milieu attitudes about their own sexuality. For example, one of these attitudes has to do with how people feel about their bodies and their bodily functions. With other children they often engage in exploratory activities—playing doctor or nurse, for instance, is a favorite game. Adults commonly frown on such activities. From parental reactions they often learn that some things and some behaviors are "bad" even to be talked about. From these experiences children often learn their first deep-seated feelings about sex.

## Unisex in the Laboratory

The man in the street has seen it happening for quite a while, but the psychologist in the laboratory is just beginning to confirm the fact: differences between men and women are indeed diminishing—or at least getting harder to detect.

In an article of the *Journal of Psychology,* Clinician Fred Brown of New York's Mount Sinai Hospital reports that people no longer respond to the well-known Rorschach ink-blot test the way they once did. One of the ten standard blots has long been helpful in spotting sexual difficulties. In the 1950's, 51% of patients who were shown the blot said that it looked like a male figure. That response was considered normal. As for the 39% who thought the blot resembled a female, they were suspected of homosexual leanings. The diagnosis applied to men and women alike.

Today, on the other hand, only 16% of those tested think the blot looks like a male figure; the percentage who sees it as female has risen to 51%. To Psychologist Brown, who based his conclusions on a careful study of 1,400 patients, the surprising reversal accurately mirrors a culture in which men have become more feminine and women more masculine than they used to be.

Why the change? Brown suggests that "society no longer rewards people for sexual individuality." Being male, he says, can mean being assassinated, as it meant for such strong male figures as John and Robert Kennedy. Or it can lead to death in the unpopular war in Viet Nam. Other anti-male influences, says Brown, are the belittling of fathers and husbands on TV, the blurring of sex distinctions in family life, and "a widespread cynicism about romantic love."

*Time,* September 6, 1971, pp. 48–9. Reprinted by permission of Time, Inc.

Psychoanalytic theory assumes that the acquisition of appropriate gender role behavior is imbedded in the resolution of the Oedipal conflict. The child identifies with the same sex parent, in order to escape the consequence of his incestuous desires, and this leads him to introject the characteristics and traits of that parent.

Learning theorists agree that gender role is not established at birth, but they believe that it is built up cumulatively through casual learning and explicit instruction. John Money, who has made extensive studies of this aspect of development, feels that the critical time for establishing gender role is from around eighteen months until about three or four years of age. It is necessary, however, to recognize that role behavior is learned and that instruction in role behavior begins with birth.

In the process of establishing gender role or, to use another common term, of establishing a sexual identity, the parents and others around the child play an extremely important part. By overt and covert communication they convey to the child what they consider to be appropriate role behavior. They do this through the words they use, the name they give the child, the way they treat and dress the child, the kind of games and toys they buy, the expectations they voice, the games they encourage, and their own example. In this way they give the child a concept of how he is to regard his own body and how male and female relate to each other.

The important contribution of early life experiences to later heterosexual attachments is universally recognized. Interaction between the child and his family lays the foundation for the development of mature sexuality. Carlfred B. Broderick, a leading researcher in sexual socialization, has hypothesized that three primary conditions are necessary in early childhood, to normal heterosexual development: (1) the parent or parent substitute of the same sex must not be so punishing on the one hand or so weak on the other as to make it impossible for the child to identify with him; (2) the parent or parent substitute of the opposite sex must not be so seductive, so punishing, or so emotionally erratic as to make it impossible for the child to trust members of the opposite sex; and (3) the parents must not systematically reject the child's biological sex and attempt to teach him cross-sex behavior.

He postulates a fourth factor as being a significant prerequisite to further heterosexual progress during the next stage of development. This is the necessity of establishing a positive conception of marriage as an eventual goal.

## Sexuality in Middle Childhood

Traditionally psychoanalytic theory regards middle childhood, (ages six-twelve, as the latency period in which the child's psychosexual life comes to a halt. However, psychoanalysts today agree that latency does not involve an absolute decline of sexual interest on the part of the prepubertal child, but a relative one at most. Social learning theorists refer to middle childhood as the school age or the gang age; the school age because the child is in school and the gang age because the peer group is of major importance during this period.

Current research findings indicate that sexual activity and curiosity do not stop during this period. The research of Broderick, for instance, has shown that, although there is a social segregation of the sexes in the middle grades which culminates at about age twelve, there is no period in which the majority of the boys and the great majority of girls are not interested in the opposite sex. There is a good deal of progress toward full heterosexual adjustment. This is shown by their conviction that they want to get married someday, by their reporting having a sweetheart, being in love, or having crushes, or liking love scenes in the movies.

Certain kinds of observed behavior can be interpreted as a continuation of sexual activity and experimentation. However, since sexual curiosity meets with adult disapproval, expressions of sexuality become secretive and camouflaged. Children at this age often exchange information through sex stories; they have a great interest in words having to do with sexual and excretory matters; they read dictionaries and consult pictures of the body wherever these can be found. Secretly, boys and girls do meet and compare anatomy; and when they have an opportunity engage in heterosexual play. Playing doctor or nurse continues to be a favorite game. Masturbation occurs secretly and with boys, perhaps, also in groups. During this period it is not uncommon for exchanges of genital manipulation and exploration to occur. What is learned in these situations is important; however, it is the context in which it is learned that is more important. The exchange of sexual information among children is clandestine and subversive, and the manner in which parents attempt to teach their children reinforces the learning structure. The admonitions of parents do not result so much in the cessation of either interest or behavior, but in their concealment and the provoking of guilt. The development of guilty knowledge occurs extremely quickly, and the children's world resembles a secret society keeping information from parents.

It is not uncommon, moreover, during this period for children to have a major attachment to a member of their own sex and to engage in mutual stimulation and exploration. For this reason, the stage has sometimes been called the "homosexual" stage. This concept is questionable, since there is no evidence that there is a homosexual stage through which all children must go. Available data support the belief that the prepubescent male has a high degree of sexuality. Kinsey found, for example, many boys in our society experience orgasm long before adolescence. Based on the limited data available it would seem that many infant males and younger boys are capable of orgasm, and it is probable that half or more of the boys in an uninhibited society could reach climax by the time they were three or four years of age, and nearly all of them could experience such a climax three to five years before the onset of adolescence.[3] In actuality, in our society, the majority of prepubertal boys experience some sexual play at about ten or eleven years of age. Usually the play is limited to manual exploration and various "doctor" games.[4]

The average prepubertal female is much less a sexual creature than the average prepubertal male. However, a small number (perhaps 4 percent) of females experience orgasm by three to five years of age.[5] About 16 percent of females experience orgasm by ten years of age, and about 25 percent by puberty. Most of this orgasmic experience occurs through masturbation. The ratio of preadolescent heterosexual sex play that reaches orgasm is thus about 7 to 1 for males and females.[6]

## Sexuality in Adolescence

Each period of development presents specific challenges. How an individual deals with these demands is influenced by his biological endowment, his previous life experiences, and the alternatives that his own culture makes possible at each stage of growth. It is difficult, therefore, to speak of universal characteristics of the adolescent period. Culture so influences the complexity of adolescence, that societies undergoing rapid change pose a wide range of problems for the late adolescent.

The onset of puberty arrives at different times for youth, ranging from nine-sixteen for girls and eleven-eighteen for boys. The average

3. A. C. Kinsey, W. B. Pomeroy, C. E. Martin, *Sexual Behavior in the Human Male* (Philadelphia: Saunders, 1953), p. 178.

4. *Ibid.*, pp. 167–73.

5. Lester A. Kirkendall, Isadore Rubin, "Sexuality and the Life Cycle," p. 187.

6. *Ibid.*, p. 110.

age is about two years earlier for girls than for boys. Current data suggest that the age of puberty has been lowering for both sexes over the past several decades. At this time, the child becomes adult biologically (able to reproduce the species); but it cannot be said that he is sexually mature. In our culture he now enters a stress period.

It is a stress period because biology has prepared him for heterosexual genital expression and yet our society traditionally denies and tries to repress this readiness by placing restrictive taboos on early sexual behavior. In some other cultures this experience is more freely available to him than in ours. Even though the median age for marriage is decreasing, there is still an average span of eight years during which our society acts in opposition to the biological urges of the adolescent. This span includes the most sexually active period in the life of the male. The pubescent male has already established his characteristic pattern of regular ejaculation.[7] Not surprisingly, masturbation becomes a central concern in early adolescence for males. The practice of masturbation is almost universal among males, but incidence varies slightly from group to group.

Unlike the male, the female does not experience a marked upsurge in the incidence or the frequency of orgasm at the onset of puberty. Most adolescent girls are sexually unawakened and do not reach a maximum of erotic interest and fulfillment until the mid-twenties or thirties. It is important to note here that these data refer to a generation of women born in the first third of the century. It seems likely that women who were born in the second third may well reach a maximum of erotic interest and fulfillment earlier in their lives.

Although for a variety of reasons masturbation has become the focus of many anxieties and fears, it is essentially a normal response to increased sexual development. It is, in fact, no less inevitable and no less a part of the psychophysical development of adolescence than is nocturnal emission, but it has been the subject of excessive and entirely irrational condemnation. A recent report, *Sex and the College Student*, formulated by the Committee on the College Student of the Group for the Advancement of Psychiatry, states:

Masturbation serves . . . a variety of purposes including different emotional needs at different stages of development for each person. The physical act is

7. A. C. Kinsey, W. B. Pomeroy, C. E. Martin, *Sexual Behavior in the Human Male*, p. 192.

# Sex Education: No Choice

We cannot return to or recapture an "age of innocence" regarding sex, if such an age ever existed. Yet those who argue against providing sex education for youth would appear to believe that an age of innocence still exists, and therefore we still have a choice between providing or not providing sex education.

Such a choice no longer exists. All of us are literally inundated with information, ideas, and attitudes about sex via television, movies, newspapers, paperback books, magazines and our peers. In view of the quantity of ideas and attitudes about sex readily available to youth, it is pointless to continue debating whether or not youth should receive sex education. They are! The crucial and reality question is: "Are we satisfied with the quality, the content, the accuracy and the value orientations of the ideas and attitudes about human sexuality which youth is now daily, if not hourly, receiving from current sources?"

Those who argue against providing adequate, competent education about human sexuality frequently reflect the worry that sex education will encourage permissive and promiscuous sexual behavior among young people. This worry does not accompany other areas of education. We do not assume, for example, that consumer education will encourage young people to be less wise or more foolish in spending money, but that it will aid them in exercising greater wisdom in the management of budgets and finances. Nor do we assume that physical education courses will immediately lead to abuses of the physical body. Nor do we assume that to provide driver education to the time youth may drive legally will increase the accident rate. In fact, we assume the opposite: the more education, the more respect for finances, the human body, and the car.

Clark E. Vincent, "The Pregnant Single College Girl," *The Journal of the American College Health Association,* vol. 15, May 1967, pp. 49–50. Reprinted by permission of the publisher.

importantly linked with conscious and unconscious fantasy. Altogether, in addition to the simple discharge of sexual tension, masturbation serves such purposes as the reduction of anxiety, expression of hostility, fantasizing of sexual experimentation, assertion of sexual identity in anticipation or recall. Masturbation also represents a response to difficulties being experienced in personal relationships by providing not only pleasure but comfort and re-assurance from one's own body.[8]

Parenthetically, it is interesting to note that many of the stigmata associated with masturbation are behind us, but tradition dies slowly and many children are still being told old wives' tales concerning the alleged effects of masturbation. This is unfortunate, for in early childhood mas-turbation might influence the child to accept his body as pleasureful rather than reject it as a source of anxiety. Society has progressed to the point where few parents punish their children for masturbating, but it is noteworthy that fewer still encourage it.

Most adolescents in our society are moving into some kind of hetero-sexual expression by the early teens. Actually, the age for moving into heterosexual activities is probably lowering, as the studies of Broderick and others show. The pattern of heterosexual expression seems, ordi-narily, to follow a definite sequence, moving through embracing and kiss-ing and light caressing, to the more involved stages with heavy petting to intercourse itself. Unmarried adolescents, of course, vary in the extent and rapidity with which they progress through this pattern. Some go through the entire sequence, while a few never begin until marriage.

According to Kinsey, masturbation is the most common mode of sexual expression for the adolescent male and heterosexual petting the second most common.[9] Premarital coitus is experienced by most males in our society—cumulative incidence of premarital coitus is 98 percent for the males who will never go beyond the eighth grade, 84 percent for those who will finish high school, and 67 percent for those who will be college graduates.[10] Ultimately, according to Kinsey, 58 percent of fe-males masturbate.[11] However, the frequency of masturbation among this

8. Group for the Advancement of Psychiatry, *Sex and the College Student* (New York: 1965), p. 71.

9. A. C. Kinsey, W. B. Pomeroy, C. E. Martin, *Sexual Behavior in the Human Male*, p. 397, pp. 537–39.

10. A. C. Kinsey, W. B. Pomeroy, C. E. Martin, *Sexual Behavior in the Human Fe-male* (Philadelphia: Saunders, 1953), pp. 549–52.

11. *Ibid.* pp. 137–40.

We are "sex saturated" in the ugly exploitive aspects of sex.

58 percent is much less than for the male. Heterosexual petting experience is common among females, with 90 percent of all females,[12] and nearly 100 percent of those who marry having had some heterosexual petting experience. Premarital coitus occurs for about half the females in our society, but usually only in the year or two prior to marriage.[13]

## Sexuality in Adulthood

The personal experience of growing up as a sexual creature has meaning only with respect to the society in which the individual lives. Our particular society happens to be curiously ambivalent concerning sex. In the aspects of sex that are good and warm and constructive, and in our frantic search for a more meaningful and fulfilling experience, we are "sex starved," whereas we are "sex saturated" in the ugly exploitive aspects of sex. We have, on the one hand, a rigid set of specifications intended to regulate and generally restrict sexual behavior in the course of life. On the other hand, we are subjected to intensive stimulation via private conversation, movies, magazines, advertising, and so on. The net result tends to be an extraordinary preoccupation with sex coexisting with a generally negative attitude toward sex and sexuality, particularly in the young. Compromising and reconciling of the divergent biological, psychological, and sociological pressures associated with sex is a problem that must be dealt with throughout most of life.

In adulthood, heterosexual expression is inevitable among a certain large portion of the people. A wide variety and many combinations of sexual patterns exist. Some will achieve heterosexual adjustment; others will rely on masturbation and homosexual activities. Some may come close to a renunciation of overt sexual expression, and those who have made a heterosexual adjustment will have a variety of patterns of sexual behavior. According to Kinsey,

There is no American pattern of sexual behavior, but scores of patterns, each of which is confined to a particular segment of society. Within each segment there are attitudes on sex and patterns of overt activity which are followed by a high proportion of the individuals in that group; and an understanding of the sexual mores of the American people as a whole is possible only through an understanding of the sexual patterns of all the constituent groups.[14]

12. *Ibid.,* pp. 234–37.

13. *Ibid.,* p. 330.

14. A. C. Kinsey, W. B. Pomeroy, C. E. Martin, *Sexual Behavior in the Human Male,* p. 329.

## Sexuality in the College Student

The college student is confronted with many dilemmas. Biologically, he is mature and ready for sexual experiences, including mating and marriage; but the cost and rigors of study force the student to postpone or divert the orderly progression of adult expression of sexuality through marriage. Men and women pursuing college studies often become painfully aware of the contradictions in themselves and their society. They postpone marriage to pursue a profession, yet want to experience sexual fulfillment now. The student is expected to control his destiny but finds he cannot regulate his sexual drives. The student is often torn between the well-nigh insatiable demands of burgeoning physical potentialities

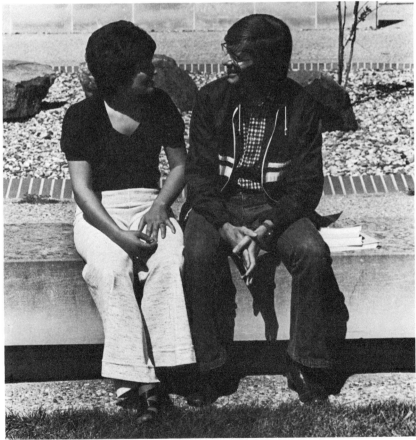

For many students increased experience with their heterosexuality is a lonely and painful search in a vital area of life.

and the frequently confused and contradictory ideals which society presents. Whether the student's tendency is to be traditionally moralistic or violently rebellious, he simply cannot shed the inhibitions and restrictions placed on him by parents, churches, and college administrations. Even less can he ignore the economic structure of our civilization. The best he can do is to understand the facts, gain some perspective on the alternatives which are open to him, and then try to act with integrity.

Another dilemma is created by the fact that the college is a community in itself. The usual social controls of parents, churches, and the home community are questioned in the classroom by the scientific study of man, his behavior and his ideas. At the same time, from the peer group of fellow students there emerges an informal social order and culture which attempts to meet the needs of the students. Very often this social order becomes an all-pervasive cultural pressure that establishes and maintains the centrality of sex in the thinking of the student. Frequently, too, this college community encourages the student to abandon the controls established by his parents and their community.

Mary Calderone cites, as an example of this, an experience she had when, following a formal presentation at a women's college, she talked confidentially with a group of freshmen. They told her that while they felt that they could cope with the pressures put on them by their dates, which they expected and understood, what they did not know how to meet was the pressure exerted upon them by their own upperclassmen to conform by having sexual intercourse.[15] Thus, we see that the peer group pressure to engage in and be considered competent in sexual intercourse drives both boys and girls further, at times, than they feel ready to go.

Another dilemma is the challenge of simultaneous emotional and intellectual development. It has been suggested that from a developmental point of view the four years of college come at the worst possible time in the schedule of biological and emotional development. For many individuals, the internal thrust toward emotional and sexual maturity collides in an abundance of apparently undirected energy with the demands of intellectual discipline or the social requirements of an orderly college community. Society expects of the college student that he simultaneously complete emotional, sexual, and intellectual development and that he meet radically increased standards of

15. Mary Calderone, "Sexual Energy—Constructive or Destructive?" *Western Journal of Surgery, Obstetrics and Gynecology* 71:275 (Nov.–Dec., 1963).

achievement. Not all students can so schedule their biological progression to fit this external demand.

One dimension of the student's sexual dilemma has only been widely recognized since the publication of Kinsey's *Sexual Behavior in the Human Male*—namely the fact that men attain their greatest sexual capacity in their late teens. Kinsey's studies showed that "teenage boys are potentially more capable and often more active than their 35-year-old fathers."[16] It is ironic that although the sex life of the average college student has no formally recognized existence in our society, the average male student is experiencing higher frequency of orgasm, with a greater variety of modes of response, than are his teachers. And he grows up in a society which not only fails to acknowledge its own sexuality, but blames the younger generation for sexual nonconformity, which is almost inevitable in our culture and is frequently exaggerated and misrepresented.

In our culture the expression of sexuality is restrained by a variety of complicating factors—some inseparable from our civilization, others entirely irrational, and most frustrating to the growing man. The fulfillment of sexual relations in marriage is an economic impossibility for those who have an interest in higher education. On the other hand, religious sanctions and social conventions either morally condemn or legally prohibit all but one sexual outlet. Nocturnal emissions are the only generally acceptable outlet in conventional Western society by which the young man can find relief from sexual pressures.

It is the college student, and particularly the male student, who epitomizes for the general public the breakdown in public morality. The first newsletter of the Sex Information and Educational Council of the United States (SIECUS) set forth as its general aim "to establish man's sexuality as a healthy entity . . . to dignify it by openness of approach, study and scientific research, designed to lead toward its understanding and its freedom from exploitation." The Council then went on to express concern over the failure of much discussion to get at the real issues involved and to point out that "favorite scapegoats are the college students whose widely publicized behavior has given rise to an epidemic of tongue-clackery among adults, all of whom are beyond college age."[17] Certainly there is a great deal of irresponsible sexual activity on every campus; but what are the facts about this public image?

16. *Ibid.*, pp. 219–22.
17. "Sex Education" (SIECUS Discussion Guide no. 1. New York: SIECUS, 1965), p. 5.

## Can "Shotgun Weddings" Succeed?

Love cannot be forced. It was formerly the practice among social agencies to compel the man responsible for a girl's pregnancy to marry her. They no longer do so because experience has shown that the man harbors a deep and permanent resentment against the woman for forcing him into matrimony. This resentment is shown in various acts of hostility and neglect which create an unwholesome environment for the child. The impulse to marry must originate from an inner compulsion to join with the person of one's choice. Even in those situations where the man offers to marry the pregnant woman it is best to probe into his reasons. If he seeks marriage in order to lessen his guilt feelings, the outlook for marital happiness is unfavorable. Forced marriages almost always continue in an atmosphere of bitter resentment in which one or the other of the partners feels cheated and imprisoned. Marriage should be a bond between two people who love each other, rather than a shackling together of two individuals who were momentarily driven together by compelling biological cravings.

Fred Brown and Rudolf T. Kempton, *Sex Questions and Answers*, 2nd ed. (New York: McGraw-Hill Book Company, 1970), p. 40. Reprinted by permission of the publisher.

In the first place, Kinsey found that whereas about 70 percent of the total male population engaged in coitus at least occasionally between the ages sixteen and twenty-five, the corresponding figure for males who go beyond the twelfth grade was only 48 percent—about one-third less.[18] It is probably certain that both of these figures have increased since Kinsey did his research, and also that the gap between the educational levels has narrowed. But, even so, some of Kinsey's comments on the discrepancy between college students and other young men are highly relevant. He pointed out: "The mother who is afraid to send her boy away to college for fear that he will be morally corrupted there, is evidently unaware of the histories of the boys who stay at home. Moreover, nearly half of the

18. A. C. Kinsey, W. B. Pomeroy, C. E. Martin, *Sexual Behavior in the Human Male,* pp. 248–49, 347–48.

males who have intercourse while in college had their first experience while they were still at home, before they started college."[19] Furthermore, the college student is likely, if he does have intercourse before marriage, to engage in it far less frequently and with fewer companions than his contemporaries in the lower educational groups; and he is far less likely ever to visit a prostitute. Furthermore, he points out that a good many college males "never have premarital intercourse with more than the one girl whom they subsequently marry, and very few of them have premarital intercourse with more than a half dozen girls or so."[20]

Why do college students have such an undeserved reputation for excess? Undoubtedly, the reputation is due in part to the descriptive imagination of the student, who for reasons of prestige or pure egotism translates his intentions and desires into actuality for the benefit of fraternity members or the kids back home. Another element contributing to the impression of sexual promiscuity among students is the practice of heavy petting, frequently in public or semi-public places. Among lower educational groups, manual genital stimulation is widely regarded as a sign of perversion, whereas it is often accepted among college students as a substitute for actual coitus. The general population, observing these activities of students, concludes that they are not only "oversexed" but that they find relief in undesirable and obscene practices.

The reasons underlying the student's relative restraint are varied and complex. Surely, the economic factor enters the picture. The student knows that an accident leading to forced marriage would put an end to his academic career. Moreover, the whole cultural pattern of sexual relationships in the upper educational level requires more romantic preliminaries to intercourse, which are both time consuming and expensive.

The student is very often far more deeply imbued with the distinctive Judeo-Christian respect for virginity than he would like to admit. He may publicly dissociate himself from the antisexuality of much church teaching, but he finds it far less easy to free himself from ingrained assumptions about sexual practice. Among educated young men and women, the influence of religious tradition on sexual standards is considerable, and more so than among the less well educated. It seems a truism that while today's students may convince themselves intellectually that sex is good, they seem to feel almost as guilty about sex for sex's sake as did their predecessors.

19. *Ibid.,* p. 347.
20. *Ibid.,* p. 349.

What about the sexual revolution? In 1929, there was still a profound gap between the sexual practice of many parents and that of their children. This is no longer true today. There is indeed still a gap between the professed public morality of the adult world and that of the college student, but there is surprisingly little difference between their respective sexual histories. The Kinsey reports have made clear that, although today's student is undoubtedly more ready to boast about and defend his sexual emancipation, his father actually enjoyed—though more discreetly—a very similar sexual freedom. The precise forms of sexual outlet have changed. There is more petting to orgasm and less visiting of prostitutes today.

In the 20 years since Kinsey gathered the material for his book *Sexual Behavior in the Human Male,* there has certainly been an increase in the percentage of students engaging in intercourse. But the real change came with the generation born between 1900 and 1910, who were in their teens just after World War I. Since then, there has been a progressive trend toward justifying sexual freedom, or rather a progressive repudiation of the need to justify one's natural inclinations. The overt sexual behavior of today's student, the public and dramatic representation of sex,—all approximate much more closely to what actually goes on in private or semi-private. But the actual practice of this generation is very little different from that of those who graduated 40 years ago. Kinsey found:

The increase in the incidence of premarital coitus, and the similar increase in the incidence of premarital petting, constitute the greatest changes which we have found between the patterns of sexual behavior in the old and younger generation of American females. . . . Practically all of this increase had occurred in the generation that was born in the first decade of the present century, and therefore, in the generation which had most of its premarital experience in the late teens and in the 1920s following the First World War. The later generations appear to have accepted the new pattern and maintained or extended it.[21]

The message conveyed by college students in their demands in the sexual area is misread if it is seen only as a defense of the pursuit of pleasure. Under the guise of asking for sexual freedom, the student may be concerned with such fundamentals as identity, relatedness, and security. Those students whose sexual activity goes more or less unnoticed

21. A. C. Kinsey, W. B. Pomeroy, C. E. Martin, *Sexual Behavior in the Human Female,* pp. 298–99.

probably represent a large middle group who handle their sexual life privately and without its being an apparent problem to themselves or to others. Their activities may include intercourse or they may be limited to petting, but in any event do not come to the notice of authorities. It is well worth noting that promiscuity characterizes only a few individuals on each college campus, although these cases, frequently inflated by publicity, are often conspicuous. For the majority of students, increased experience with their heterosexuality is a lonely and painful search in a vital area of life which many adults are unable to discuss comfortably.

Sexual relationships serve many functions. For the girl, even a brief sexual intimacy may provide a temporary sense of being wanted; she may assume that nothing else she has to offer would be of equal interest to her partner. This feeling may be based on a low self-esteem; or it may, in fact, be true. A more neurotic pattern is apparent where the individual uses sexual intimacy to handle feelings of depression, emptiness, and dependency. The importance of this kind of relationship lies only in seeking a sense of closeness as a temporary haven against loneliness and other anxieties. Compulsive sexual activity usually represents an unresolved conflict and an attempt to relieve anxiety, rather than a simple pursuit of pleasure. Behavior that has an exaggerated sense of urgency often serves a defensive purpose not recognized by the individual.

Young men and women attempt to express and confirm identity through physical intimacy, and sexuality is employed toward this end in various ways. The range extends from demonstrations of aggression, prowess, and dominance to more complex modes of interaction in which the mutuality of the relationship between two people is the major aspect of self-fulfillment. Although pride in conquest is commonly attributed to boys, it also excites many girls. When sex is used solely to prove power and dominance, sexual expression can veer in pathological directions.

The need of men to confirm their sexual capacity has long been recognized. Sexual proficiency and the achievement of satisfaction by women have also been recognized as important, but it is currently a matter of intense concern among young women. Sometimes both partners behave as though the adequacy and self-esteem of each was dependent on whether or not the woman achieves orgasm or even on whether their orgasms occur simultaneously. This sort of exaggerated emphasis not only can create undesirable tension in the sexual act itself, but can devalue important satisfactions in other areas of the relationship as well.

## Summary

Sexuality is a deep and pervasive aspect of one's total personality, the sum total of one's feelings and behavior not only as a sexual being, but as a male or female. Adult sexuality represents a composite of sexual learning and experience, and can be most meaningfully understood when it is related to the rest of personality development at the particular phase of the life cycle under consideration. This, in turn, must be seen in terms of earlier and subsequent biological and psychological development.

The integration of the biological drive of sexuality into the personality presents special problems to today's college student. His sexual drive makes imperative demands, while society restricts opportunities for sexual expression. His problems have to do with the search for identity, the search for masculinity and femininity; and the search for understanding of himself and his society.

## Questions for Study and Discussion

1. Are femininity and masculinity determined by the individual or the society and environment in which he lives?
2. What characteristics do you look for in a date? In a marriage partner?
3. Are premarital relations determined by the length of courtship?
4. What are the advantages and disadvantages of premarital relations?
5. Should college students live together or marry while in college?
6. What do you think is the purpose of an engagement period? Is it necessary?
7. Is there a double standard since the sexual revolution?
8. Do you think the era of Puritanism will return someday?
9. How do the mass media contribute to the sexuality of an individual?
10. If sex is only a part of a complete relationship with a person, why has all the attention and controversy arisen?

## References

Broderick, Carlfred B. "Sexual Behavior Among Pre-adolescents." *Journal of Social Issues* 22 (no. 2), 6–21 (April, 1966).

Calderone, Mary. "Sexual Energy—Constructive or Destructive?" *Western Journal of Surgery, Obstetrics and Gynecology* 71:227–77 (Nov.-Dec., 1963).

Freud, Anna. *Psychoanalysis for Teachers and Parents.* Boston: Beacon Press, 1935.

Ford, Cellan S., and Beach, Frank A. *Patterns of Sexual Behavior.* New York: Harper and Brothers, 1951.

Group for the Advancement of Psychiatry. *Sex and the College Student.* New York: 1965.

Johnson, Warren R. *Human Sex and Sex Education.* Philadelphia: Lee and Feberger, 1963.

Kinsey, A. C., Pomeroy, W. B., Martin, C. E. *Sexual Behavior in the Human Female.* Philadelphia: W. B. Saunders, 1953.

Kinsey, A. C., Pomeroy, W. B., Martin, C. E. *Sexual Behavior in the Human Male.* Philadelphia: W. B. Saunders, 1953.

Kirkendall, Lester A., Rubin, Isadore. "Sexuality and the Life Cycle" (SIECUS Discussion guide no. 8). New York: SIECUS 1790 Broadway, 11019, 1969.

Kirkendall, Lester A. *Premarital Intercourse and Interpersonal Relationships.* New York: Julian Press, 1961.

Money, J. "Anomolies of Sexual Differentiation." In Broderick, C. B. and Bernard, J. (Ed.), *The Individual, Sex and Society,* a SIECUS Handbook for Teachers and Counselors. Baltimore: The Johns Hopkins Press, 1968.

Sex Education, (SIECUS Discussion Guide no. 1). New York: SIECUS, 1965.

# 12

# Planning Your Family

## General Concept

The patterns and problems of family planning are in a constant state of change.

## Outcomes

The student should be able to:

1. Explain the basic principles of the process of ovulation and conception
2. Understand the terminology used in the explanation of the male and female reproductive systems
3. Describe the various means of contraception
4. Understand the data on the safety and effectiveness of contraceptive devices and techniques
5. Explain the more common conditions which may lead to infertility or modify fertility in the male and female
6. Understand how to improve the prospects for achieving a pregnancy that is wanted
7. Understand the procedures for correcting infertility in the male and female

## An International Imperative

According to British scientist and novelist C. P. Snow, "Many millions of people are going to starve to death before our eyes. We shall be surrounded by a sea of famine involving hundreds of millions of human beings." This grim prediction is based on existing factual data concerning our present and projected population statistics. If the world population continues to grow at its present rate, there will be twice as many people—more than seven billion—by the year 2000—only twenty-nine years away.

Within the United States alone, at present rates, our population is expected to grow 50% to 300 million by the year 2000. As President Nixon has stated, to accommodate these 100 million new Americans we'd have to build a new city of 250,000 persons—the size of Tulsa or Dayton or Jersey City—every thirty days for the next twenty-nine years.

In the burgeoning nations of Asia, Africa, and Latin America, the number of people is increasing three times faster than the food to feed them. The result: three and a half million people—most of them children—will starve to death this year.

Whereas family planning cannot by itself solve the plagues of modern mankind such as pollution, poverty, or hunger, it can be an invaluable tool in buying us time for planning and technology to catch up with the population.

Overpopulation, It's Everybody's Problem, pamphlet (New York: Planned Parenthood Association, 1970).

## Contraception

The human female produces, on the average, 400 mature egg cells in a lifetime. The egg cells which do mature are derived from thousands of primordial cells found in the ovaries which are potential egg cells. The human male produces up to 120 million sperm cells per cubic centimeter, or about 500 million sperm cells per ejaculation. Multiplying this by the number of ejaculations per week or month or year gives us numbers that are astronomical and almost beyond belief.

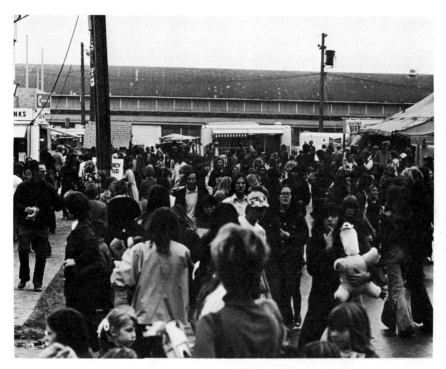

In recent times, the problem of overpopulation of the earth has become acute.

Since human females ovulate about once a month and the period of **gestation*** in the human is nine months, it is possible for one woman to have one child per year or as many as 30 to 40 children in a lifetime. The number of children that one human male could father has never been computed, but undoubtedly the figure is extremely large. Considering such possible excesses, is it any wonder that man has been and continues to be concerned with the problem of overpopulation and contraception?

In recent times, the problem of overpopulation of the earth has become acute. Population increases are tremendous and yet the production of food has not increased proportionately. In the face of increased poverty and hunger in the world, a limitation on the number of people born each year has become a necessity. Such limitation is complicated by religious, racial, nationalistic, and moral issues, but it is becoming more and more the general opinion that the prevention of an unwanted preg-

*Note: Any term that appears in **boldface** is defined in the glossary at the end of this chapter.

nancy is justifiable. Therefore every couple (or individual for that matter) should have the necessary knowledge to so plan their lives that they have as many or as few children as they desire.

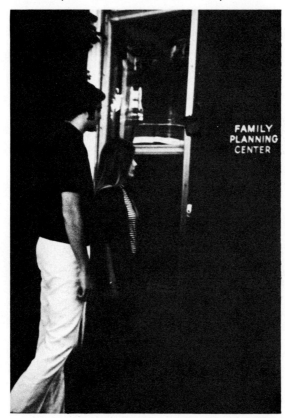

Local family planning centers are springing up throughout the country to assist couple's family planning needs and to provide medical advice counseling.

Man's early attempts to achieve contraception were crude, and it has been only recently that our knowledge of anatomy and physiology has led to more effective techniques. We can surmise that at first there was only the simple expedient of abstinence. One of the earliest references to contraception is made in the Old Testament where it is stated that semen should not be allowed to fall to the ground during intercourse. This probably alludes to coitus interruptus (the withdrawal method). In the New Testament, Paul speaks often about the benefits of celibacy. Without a doubt, he had some listeners.

The introduction of foreign bodies into the genital tract in order to achieve contraception is of ancient origin. Egyptian camel herders in-

troduced a small stone into the **vagina** or **cervix** of their camels to prevent undesired pregnancies. Many years ago, native girls in the Carib-
bean Islands used an ordinary sea sponge, tied to a string, as an intra-
vaginal tampon, a contraceptive technique that must have developed
through trial and error. In the early nineteenth century the gold stem
**pessary** and the coil of German silver wire became popular. These were
foreign bodies placed in the **uterus** on a more or less permanent basis.
From these our present-day intrauterine device (IUD) has developed.

The modern development of the rhythm system depended upon the
complete understanding of the menstrual cycle and **ovulation.** The use
of vaginal douches or washings is also a modern technique. With the per-
fection of thin latex rubber, the condom or sheath was developed and
has been a widely used contraceptive in the twentieth century. The
development of the diaphragm, spermicidal creams, jellies, and foams,
followed soon by the pill has all been in our generation.

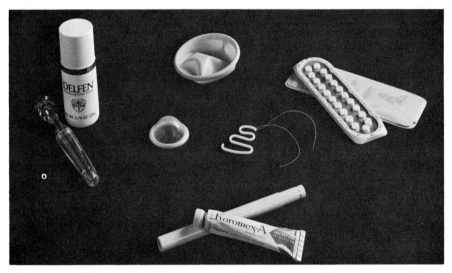

Various types of birth control measures: chemical foam, condom, diaphragm, the IUD, the
oral contraceptive pill, and a tube of vaginal jelly.

Lastly, we should not forget that there are surgical procedures that
insure contraception. Among these are operations such as hysterectomy
(removal of the uterus) and tubal **ligation** in the female and **ligation**
of the **vas deferens** (vasectomy) in the male.

## The Pill

"The pill" is by far the most effective contraceptive ever devised by man. The contraceptive pill is a combination of **estrogen** and **progestin** (the synthetic form of **progesterone**), two hormones normally present in the female. Hormones are substances secreted by the **endocrine** glands, the glands of internal secretion. Since hormones are transmitted through the blood stream, they can reach all parts of the body easily. It is true that the hormones used in the pill are synthetic, but this in no way makes them different. Therefore it is to be emphasized that estrogen and progestin are not foreign to the human female. The human female is constantly subjected to the effects of these hormones throughout her active sex life.

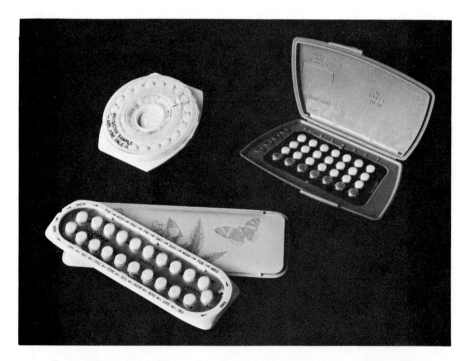

Types and containers of the combination and sequential oral contraceptive pills.

The production of estrogen and progesterone is controlled by the **pituitary gland** (attached to the base of the brain) through the **gonadotropic hormones** produced by it. One of these hormones is called the

**follicle stimulating hormone** (FSH) and another is called the **luteinizing hormone** (LH).

After puberty there is a constant interplay between these hormones and the glands from which they are derived. For instance, if there is a small quantity of estrogen in the blood stream, the pituitary is stimulated to produce FSH. If there is a large quantity of estrogen in the blood stream, the production of FSH is inhibited.

At the time of **menses,** in an ordinary cycle, the amount of estrogen in the blood stream is low and the pituitary gland is stimulated to produce FSH. The FSH excites the **ovary** to produce a mature **follicle** from a primary follicle. The mature follicle consists of an egg cell enclosed in a cyst-like compartment filled with fluid. The fluid contains follicular hormone or estrogen.

At ovulation the follicle ruptures, expelling the egg into a cavity near to the fringed end of the **Fallopian tube,** through which the egg passes on its way towards the uterus. At the site of the ruptured follicle, a small blood clot (corpus hemorrhagicum) forms which eventually will become the **corpus luteum.** At the time of ovulation, LH is produced by the pituitary gland and LH stimulates the growth of mature corpus luteum, which now produces both estrogen and progesterone in large quantities.

If the egg becomes fertilized and embeds itself in the wall of the uterus, the tissue formed by the already developing fertilized egg also has the ability to produce LH. This LH causes the corpus luteum to develop further and thereby produce more estrogen and progesterone. In the presence of all this estrogen, the pituitary gland is inhibited in its production of FSH, and therefore, during a pregnancy, no new mature follicles are formed and ovulation does not take place.

The fact that in the presence of large amounts of estrogen and progesterone no FSH is formed—and therefore no ovulation—has led to the development of the contraceptive pill. In the first pill, relatively large doses of estrogen and progestin were used. As time passed and experience with the pill increased, smaller and smaller doses were used, with apparently no change in efficacy. At present, most pills contain about 1 mgm. of progestin and 0.05 mgm. of estrogen. Ovulation definitely does not occur with this therapy and therefore it is 100 percent effective.

There are about 24 different pills on the market today and their differences are minimal. There are two basic patterns in their use. The one is called the combined pill and the other is called the sequential pill.

In the combined pill, both estrogen and progestin are given continuously for 20 or 21 days. Then there is a discontinuance of the pill for 7 to 8 days and the pills are begun again for another 20 to 21 days. This process is repeated again and again. In the interim, when the pills are not taken, a bleeding usually occurs (but may not) which simulates the menses but it is not a true menses. Usually the blood flow is less copious, the number of days of bleeding are fewer, and there may not be the usual cramps and discomfort that some women experience with menses. This is called a withdrawal type of bleeding. Since the withdrawal bleeding does not always appear, many physicians disregard it completely. Some patients take the combined pill for 21 days, stop for 8 days, and recommence the pill for another 21 days, not taking the bleeding day into account at all.

In the sequential pattern, estrogen alone is given in the early stage of the cycle and estrogen and progestin are given in the later stage of the cycle. The idea behind this is that a more normal or usual bleeding will occur in the interim between cycles.

The merits of each pattern should be discussed with a gynecologist and his judgment should prevail in deciding which pattern to use. Both the combined pill and the sequential pill are effective contraceptive devices.

Any woman who desires to be on the pill should consult with a gynecologist and have a thorough gynecological examination before the pills are taken. Every six months to a year she should be reexamined. The continued use of the pill must then be reevaluated in the light of any change from the normal that may be found. Whether or not a **"Pap" smear** is needed should be determined by the gynecologist.

The taking of the pill is not without some drawbacks. Sometimes there are side effects which can be disconcerting. These, however, occur relatively infrequently.

About 95 percent of the U.S. women between the ages of 18 and 28 take the pills with no ill effects. Occasionally there is some nausea. This is usually temporary and often disappears within the first month of therapy. Persistant nausea may necessitate changes in therapy. Sometimes there is a weight gain with concomitant swelling of the ankles. As in pregnancy, there may be an accumulation of sodium in the body and a resultant fluid retention. Limitation of fluid and salt intake is essential for these patients if they are to continue on the pill. One of the most common side effects in this age group is a **vaginitis.** The vaginitis presents itself as a discharge which itches and burns. The cause may be a change in the PH or acidity of the vagina with an associated invasion of parasitic fungi. Continued treatment under the guidance of a gynecologist will usually clear up the condition. The pill need not be discontinued. Rarely, changes in the cervix appear which may require biopsy and treatment. Unusual blood clotting (phlebitis and pulmonary embolism) is rare in this age group unless the women have had **varicosities** and pregnancies before being placed on the pill.

In the 28- to 38-year-old group of women, the side effects mentioned above are more common. This group of women must be watched carefully for **cervical lesions.** All cervical lesions should be thoroughly investigated, with "Pap" smears and biopsies, and if benign should be treated strenuously until they disappear. Proper treatment will be instituted if the lesion is not benign. Women in this age group must also be watched carefully for varicosities, phlebitis, and all the associated complications. Discontinuance of the pill is advisable in all questionable cases.

In the 38- to 48-year-old group, the side effects are most common. In addition to the other side effects, tumors of the **body of the uterus** have to be watched carefully, as they may increase in size rapidly in the presence of large doses of estrogen. Most gynecologists are reluctant to prescribe the pill to women in this age group.

Much has been said about the connection of the pill with the formation of blood clots (**thrombophlebitis** and **pulmonary embolism**). Women who are not on the pill can develop thrombophlebitis and pulmonary embolism, but it is true that women on the pill develop the conditions more frequently. It is stated that the death rate from pulmonary embolism is 1 in 30,000 women who are on the pill. But one should equate this with the maternal mortality rate which is 3 to 4 in 10,000 pregnant women and with the death rate in criminal abortions which is 1 in 1,000. It is far safer to take the pill than to face the risks involved in a pregnancy or abortion. Physicians are constantly dealing with risks whether they are prescribing contraceptive pills or aspirin, and the statistics concerning the pill are within the satisfactory range.

Scientific investigation in the field of contraception is a never-ending process. There is a constant search for newer and safer methods. A "morning-after" pill is being investigated. If large doses of estrogen are given to a woman within a day or two of an unprotected exposure, pregnancy will be prevented. Some investigators claim that this works every time. However, since massive doses of estrogen are used, the technique may be useful for one time but should not be used repeatedly.

A new pill containing progestin alone is getting a good deal of publicity. The most recent thinking is that progestin alone can prevent pregnancy without interfering with ovulation and the normal menstrual cycle. Estrogen, the cause of the side effects previously mentioned, is not used in this pill. However, until a better method is found, the present estrogen-progestin pill is very satisfactory.

## The IUD

In the last century an intrauterine device called the gold stem pessary was developed in Europe. It consisted of two prongs and a button with an opening in it. The gold stem pessary was placed inside the uterus with the two prongs pointed toward the top or fundus of the uterus and the button pressed closely to the cervix. The opening allowed the menstrual flow to pass freely into the vagina. At regular intervals the pessary was removed, inspected, and replaced.

We do not know how it worked, but it is thought that its mere presence interfered with the **nidation** (implantation) of the already fertilized egg. Another theory is that it set up a chronic inflammation of the Fallopian tubes with subsequent obstruction.

Most gynecologists were convinced that the complications ensuing from this method did not warrant its use. In this country there are some women who have had the pessary inserted by European physicians. Several of the patients would come to me for regular gynecological examinations and for reinsertion of the pessary. The last pessary I saw was embedded in the wall of a uterus which had to be removed because of persistent severe uterine bleeding.

A similar device which developed in Europe was the German silver wire coil which looked like a miniature coil spring. This was placed inside the uterus on a permanent basis. It worked in the same manner as the gold stem pessary. Neither of these devices gained popularity in this country.

In the last few years, a plastic IUD has been developed in this country. The only difference between this IUD and the older forms is in the materials used. The plastic material is less irritating and better tolerated than the metals formerly used. The plastic devices are made in various shapes and are placed inside the uterus by a physician. The most common shapes are a double coil or a loop.

The IUD should never be inserted by anyone but an experienced physician to avoid perforating the uterus and the subsequent consequences of such an accident. Before insertion, the IUD is straightened by pulling it back through a plastic canula, which is in the shape of a straight tube. The canula is flexible and can pass through the cervix either anteriorly or posteriorly according to the curvature of the cervical canal or the position of the body of the uterus. The IUD is pushed forward into place at the same time as the canula is withdrawn. The IUD will then resume its original shape while it lies in the uterus. Then that portion of it that extrudes from the cervix is treated as follows. If it is a firm plastic tail, it is broken off at one of the notches, leaving only a small piece of plastic extruding from the cervix. If the end is a string of plastic, it is left lying free in the vagina. The patient should be able to feel either one of these to ascertain that IUD is still in place. Very few husbands have complained about feeling these objects during the act of intercourse.

As with the earlier metal forms, we do not know exactly how the plastic IUD works. It is effective, but not as effective as the pill.

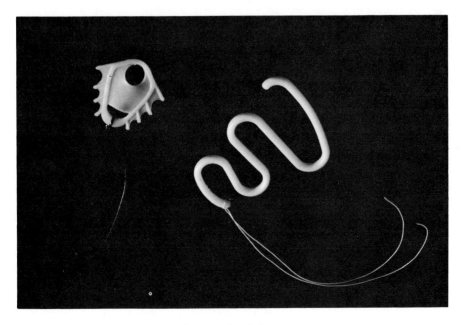

Intra-uterine devices.

There are complications associated with this technique:

1. There have been reports of many pregnancies resulting even with the IUD in place.
2. The IUD can get lost in the uterus and then must be retrieved by a surgical procedure similar to a dilatation and evacuation of the uterus.
3. IUD's have been known to fall out without the knowledge of the patient.
4. They have been the cause of much intermenstrual bleeding.
5. They have been the cause of an inflammation of the membrane of the neck of the uterus with erosions of the cervix.
6. They have been the source of pelvic inflammatory disease.

Nevertheless, in some countries the IUD is the method of choice as it is inexpensive, can be applied easily to large numbers of women, and eliminates the discipline of taking daily pills. It is a good method where the control of the over-all birth rate is important and where some failures are not important.

In the United States women do not seem to be interested in over-all statistics. They are interested in obtaining 100 percent effectiveness, if at all possible, in their individual cases. Various studies have been made of the American women who use contraceptives. In one clinic, where the women were on a high socioeconomic level, 60 percent used the pill, 28 percent used the diaphragm, 11 percent used the IUD, and 4 percent used other methods. In another clinic where the women were on a lower socioeconomic level, 60 percent used the pill and 40 percent used the IUD.

The IUD has been a boon to the woman with many children, a crowded home and no privacy, who is so preoccupied with household duties and children that she may forget or find it inconvenient to take the pill or make use of a diaphragm or foam.

## The Diaphragm

With the advent of the pill and the IUD, the diaphragm has lost some of its popularity. For certain selected patients it is still an extremely effective method of contraception.

The diaphragm consists of a round spring covered with rubber and a dome of rubber simulating a cap. When placed in the vagina correctly, it covers the cervix and becomes a mechanical barrier between the outside and the inside of the uterus.

It is necessary that each patient be examined carefully by a gynecologist and that a proper fitting be made. The diaphragm varies in size from 65 to 90 millimeters in diameter. The size does not depend on the diameter of the vaginal orifice but depends more on the elasticity of the vaginal walls. The diaphragm folds together and can be introduced

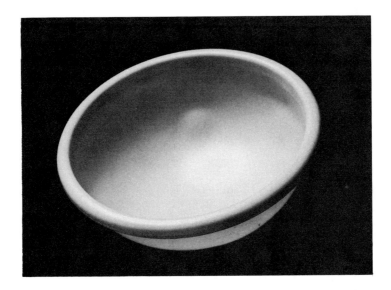

The diaphragm.

through the vaginal orifice easily. After a proper fitting, the patient should be instructed by the gynecologist himself until she becomes proficient in its use, even if many visits are required.

The two main types of diaphragm are a flat spring or a crescent-shaped one (in the flexed position). The crescent-shaped diaphragm is an improvement over the flat spring. It seems to be easier to introduce and to place correctly.

A contraceptive jelly is used with the diaphragm. Some jelly is placed in the cup-like concave portion of the diaphragm and some is placed along its rim. This is done just before insertion of the diaphragm into the vagina. The diaphragm may be inserted hours before an expected exposure. The male, therefore, is not required to use anything during intercourse. The normal course of events takes place with the foreplay changing to the act itself with no interruptions.

After intercourse the diaphragm is allowed to remain in place for six hours. The theory is that the acidity of the vagina will kill the sperm in that time. However, to make absolutely certain, after six hours a vaginal **douche** is taken with the diaphragm in place. The diaphragm is removed and a second douche is taken. This insures removal of all possible spermatic fluid from the vagina. The diaphragm is then washed, dried, powdered, and put aside for the next use.

This method precludes that there be only one intercourse within the six hours mentioned. Multiple exposures lessen the efficacy of this method.

The effective use of this technique requires a well-disciplined, sophisticated woman. If a woman feels that this method is too bothersome, she should be advised against using the diaphragm. This method should not be used by those women who for some reason might forget to insert the diaphragm or who have no time, patience, or privacy.

The method works best for those women who have never had a vaginal delivery of a baby. In these women, the diaphragm fits better and does not move out of its fixed position. After a vaginal delivery of a child many women have some relaxation of the tissues surrounding the **urethra** and this does not allow for the diaphragm to stay in place. Following a delivery of a child, the patient should be re-fitted, and a careful evaluation of the vagina and urethra should be made before allowing the patient to resume use of a diaphragm.

Once a diaphragm is correctly fitted, it can be used for years without replacement if it is cared for properly. After removal and washing, the diaphragm should be checked for perforation. Careful drying and powdering will prevent the deterioration of the rubber.

Because contraceptive pills or the IUD cannot be used in every case, the diaphragm remains as a good alternate method of contraception.

## Foams, Jellies, and Creams

The efficacy of this group of contraceptives depends mainly on the action of their chemical constituents. They all contain **spermicidal** substances. Many sources claim that this group of contraceptives is as successful in its results as the diaphragm. In any case, if the use of any of the previously

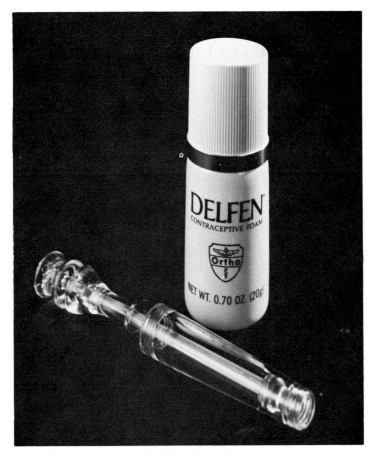

Contraceptive foam.

discussed contraceptives is not feasible for any reason, then one of the chemical spermicidal foams should be used.

The foams are easy to apply. The container and the vaginal applicator come together in a kit. Directions are included and are easy to understand. Foam is introduced into the vagina before intercourse takes place. The container is shaken. The vaginal applicator is placed over the opening of the container, tilted slightly, and the applicator fills with the foam. The vaginal applicator is separated from the container, the open end of the applicator is introduced into the vagina, and the plunger is depressed. In this position the applicator is removed and the foam remains in the vagina.

Jellies and creams are also applied with a vaginal applicator. The jellies and creams come in tubes. The vaginal applicator is applied to the end of the tube after the cap is removed. The tube is squeezed, allowing the jelly or cream to enter the applicator. The applicator is removed from the tube and the open end of the applicator is inserted into the vagina. The plunger is depressed. In this position the applicator is removed from the vagina, leaving the jelly or cream in the vagina.

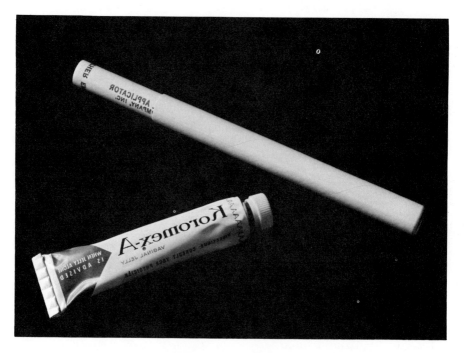

**Vaginal jelly with applicator.**

The advantage of this method is its ease of application. A prescription is not necessary to buy the materials. This eliminates the necessity of physical examinations and the need to obtain parental permission, and in many ways leaves the situation in the realm of privacy that some women want.

This method requires that there be only one exposure per given period, as in the case of the diaphragm. The percentage of success can be increased to almost 100 percent if the male uses a condom at the same time that the female uses one of the chemical spermicides.

## The Condom

The condom is a rubber sheath worn by the male during intercourse. It is placed over the erect penis, as one would put on a finger cot or glove. The advantage of this method is that the spermatic fluid which collects at the end of the condom is withdrawn completely from the vagina at the end of the sexual act.

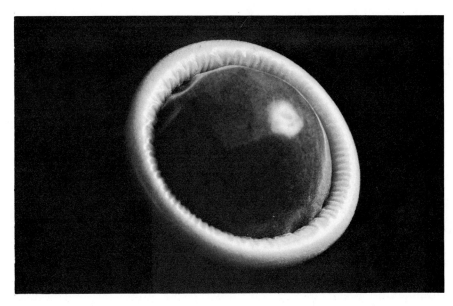

Condom.

Many men complain that their sexual sensations are dulled by the condom. There is available a moist type of "skin," as it is called, which is very thin and should not interfere with the male's pleasure and sexual excitement.

Most men can and will use the condom if it is necessary, although some men will not use the condom under any circumstance. With a little self-discipline, the average male can become adept at this method so that it can be very successful.

Granted that there is a very occasional imperfect condom containing small perforations which will allow **spermatic fluid** to escape, most of the failures in this method are caused by human errors. The condom can be torn as it is put on by the nervous, inexperienced male who is flustered and embarrassed. The condom can be lost in the vagina when it slips off the penis at the time of withdrawal, especially if the male waits too long and allows the penis to become flaccid. A simple check by the male before withdrawal will ensure that the condom is still there and both the condom and penis can be withdrawn at the same time.

A certain amount of cooperation and sympathy is required from the female. One young woman told me that her sex partner refused to wear a condom after she had laughed while he was putting it on, telling him that it all seemed too funny for words.

If the condom is used by the male and the female uses a spermicidal form of contraceptive, the percentage of success increases to such an extent as to rival the best methods known.

## The Withdrawal Method or Coitus Interruptus

This is an ancient form of contraception, referred to in the Old Testament. With dedicated people it has been a successful technique over the years. It is widely used in countries where the church or state bans the use of mechanical or chemical contraceptives. It is useful in situations where the materials for contraception are not available, either temporarily or permanently.

The technique calls for the male to withdraw the penis from the vagina just before ejaculation occurs and to cause the semen to fall away from the female. It is a good idea for the male to be ready to catch the seminal fluid in a handkerchief or similar tissue. At any rate, the seminal fluid should not be allowed to splatter in the vicinity of the **vulva** of the female.

It is possible for the female to get pregnant if seminal fluid is deposited in the general area of the vaginal orifice. During ovulation, thick strands of stringy alkaline mucous are often seen at the cervix, coming through the vagina and extruding from the vulva. It is not impossible for the sperm cells to travel up this ladder of mucous and get into the uterus and tubes, escaping meanwhile, the acidity of the vagina. There have been several pregnancies resulting from cases where there was no penetration of the vaginal orifice at any time.

The main cause of failure in this technique is that there is a small quantity of mucous extruded from the penis before the main flow at the time of ejaculation. The small pre-ejaculatory mucous secretion contains sperm cells and these can be the cause of a pregnancy. Of course, failure results if the timing is lost and ejaculation occurs intravaginally.

In many cases this technique allows only the male to reach a climax, the female being disregarded completely. This can be a real disadvantage. In the optimum form of this technique, the male waits until the female has an **orgasm** and then allows for his own ejaculation. This requires a great deal of discipline and dedication.

In spite of all the disadvantages, **coitus** interruptus is still satisfactory for many couples.

## The Rhythm System

This system is based on the idea that ovulation occurs 14 days before the expected menstrual period and that the ovum has a limited life span. It also depends on the assumption that ovulation occurs only once in any cycle. It again assumes that the sperm cell has a limited viability in the female genital tract. These four conditions are all variable and for that reason not too much dependency can be placed on this method. But it can still work if certain conditions are met and certain rules are followed.

The female involved should have a very regular period. Whatever the cycle is, be it 28 days, 31 days, or 35 days, it can be proven that ovulation occurs 14 days before the menses. For example if a woman has a 28-day cycle, ovulation will occur on the 14th day, counting the first day of the menses as no. 1. If a woman has a 35-day cycle, ovulation will occur on the 21st day of the cycle. We can assume that the time of greatest fertility will be on the day of ovulation. If intercourse is avoided for 4 days before ovulation and 4 to 5 days after ovulation, it is possible to avoid pregnancies.

For a woman with a 28-day cycle, the schedule would be as follows: Intercourse may be allowed until the 10th day of the cycle. Abstinence should be maintained from the 10th to the 19th days. Intercourse may then be allowed from the 19th day to the end of the cycle. Necessary adjustments should be made for the longer or shorter cycle.

There are many pitfalls in this method. Ovulation may not occur as planned. There are times when the most regular of women will even miss a complete cycle, upsetting the whole schedule. Ovulation may occur twice in one month. (Fraternal twins, which develop from two separate eggs, are evidence that this does occur.) Another pitfall is the dependence on the sperm to die within a few days. We do not really know how long the sperm live in the female genital tract. Another problem is that too many people have been misinformed about the details of this method. For example, some have been taught to avoid intercourse on the day of ovulation only.

This method cannot be officially recommended by gynecologists. We can only teach the theory behind it and the precautions to be followed if any couple insists on using the method.

## Douches

The use of postcoital douches as a contraceptive is mentioned only to be condemned. It cannot be very effective. The vaginal douche only washes out the vagina. None of the fluid used in the douche enters the cervix or uterus. Since sperm cells are found deep in the cervical canal within minutes following intercourse, they would be beyond the reach of any douche.

For those who are in a situation where an unprotected exposure has occurred, the female would be well advised to take a douche as quickly as possible.

## Operations Insuring Contraception or Sterility

**Tubal Ligation.** This operation involves an abdominal approach to the Fallopian tubes or salpinges. The abdomen is entered in the same manner as for any exploratory operation. The peritoneal cavity is entered and each of the tubes is isolated and identified. Then one of the various common procedures is followed for tying the tubes and dissecting away the section of the tube between the ties. The operation has all the risks associated with any abdominal operation requiring anesthesia.

It is often done in conjunction with or following another operation. Women who have had two or more Caesarean sections are often given the choice of having a tubal ligation at the time of their next Caesarean section. Tubal ligations are sometimes done following plastic operations on the bladder, rectal, or vaginal tissues. This is done to prevent further pregnancies which might lead to the breakdown of the primary operation.

A tubal ligation is sometimes permitted in the case of a woman who has had seven or eight children and for whom all forms of contraception have failed. Tubal ligation has been allowed by the courts for certain mental cases in which the individual was considered not mentally responsible for her actions.

**Ligation of the Vas Deferens in the Male (Vasectomy).** The ligation of the spermatic duct in the male is a much simpler operation than its equivalent in the female (tubal ligation). It is done through a simple skin incision in the scrotum and may be done under local anesthesia. In this operation the vas deferens is cut in order to prevent the sperm cells that are formed in the **testes** from reaching the urethra, so that the spermatic fluid will not contain any sperm. This operation in no way interferes with potency or the ability to complete the sex act.

Physical complications are few, but the psychological effects following such operations are many and varied. Many men become depressed and feel that they have become less masculine.

**Hysterectomy.** There are many abnormal conditions in the female that necessitate a hysterectomy or removal of the uterus. Removal of the uterus produces sterility and menstruation will no longer occur. The operation is usually performed by an abdominal approach, but in selected cases may be performed vaginally.

Most often the ovaries are left in place in the younger woman. If the ovaries are left in, **menopausal** symptoms will not occur and there will be no evident change in the female physically or sexually. If the ovaries are removed with the uterus, hormones can be used to counteract any menopausal symptoms which might occur.

A review of all the methods discussed should prove that there is a method of contraception for all persons seeking it. Under the guidance of a gynecologist, the most suitable method for each individual can be found.


## Infertility


According to the laws of Moses, of ancient Rome, and of Mohammed, a sterile marriage was a mark of divine displeasure. In ancient Rome sterility was regarded as an offense against the state and ample cause for divorce. The burden of barrenness was usually borne by the wife. There are still some individuals who believe that only the wife can be responsible for sterility in a marriage, but it has been shown that the husband is responsible for the difficulty in one-third to one-half of the barren unions. In all cases, infertility is a problem for the *two* people in the union and should be studied from that standpoint. Sometimes an infertile couple may become divorced, remarry, and each may have children with a different mate.

---

### Homeless Children

In this imperfect present, homeless children are scattered around the world like throwaway bottles. The first World Conference on Adoption and Foster Placement was held in late September of '71. In this country the Federal government says at least 60,000 children need homes. Of those, 40,000 are non-white. The Child Welfare League of America thinks there are more: perhaps 80,000 non-white, plus 110,000 in foster homes and institutions who haven't been placed in permanent adoptive homes because they're in legal limbo or handicapped or too old to be wanted. On the orphan circuit you're a geriatric loser if you've hit kindergarten.

Anywhere between 60,000 and 190,000 children, then. Nobody knows for sure. Americans keep computerized tabs on credit ratings and airline seats; they publish nationwide litter lists describing the age, sex and physical characteristics of thoroughbred puppies. But no one keeps comprehensive count of this hidden nation of children who need permanent homes and parents. No one even mentions the 10,000 to 20,-000 babies of mixed blood who've been sired by Americans in Vietnam and have little hope of adoption in the U.S.

What is known is that there are nearly 2.5 million children under 18 in the United States today who are adopted. There were about 171,000 legal adoptions in 1969, the latest year for which statistics are available. Slightly fewer than half of these children were adopted by stepparents or relatives, the rest by persons unrelated to them. Only 19,000 of these adoptions involved minority children. As Billie Holliday used to sing: "God bless the child who's got his own, who's got his own . . ."

Excerpt from Joseph Morgenstern, "The New Face of Adoption," *Newsweek,* September 13, 1971, p. 66. Copyright Newsweek, Inc. 1971. Reprinted by permission.

About 10 percent of all U.S. marriages are barren. In addition, there is an equal number of couples who have only one child (the so-called "one-child sterility"). If we include all the women who habitually abort, then the number of couples who are unable to have children is indeed very great.

Detailed investigations of infertility should not be considered until a couple has tried for a full year to initiate pregnancy. Fertile couples often require that amount of time.

In the vast majority of childless marriages, it is the wife who first consults a physician about her inability to become pregnant. On the first visit to the physician, the wife is examined and a general physical examination and pelvic examination are performed. Certain routine laboratory tests are ordered. Unless there is a specific reason to believe that the wife is totally incapable of conception, the husband is asked to submit himself for examination at this time. Many men are reluctant to undergo examination because they feel that if they are potent, they must be fertile, not knowing that many potent males are infertile. If the husband can be convinced that a complete examination is important and necessary, he is sent to a urologist. It is expedient to make all these investigations a joint effort between the urologist and the gynecologist.

The husband's aptitude for inducing pregnancy is primarily determined by a careful and complete review of his past health record, an inquiry into the marital habits, and a thorough physical examination. The final index is the evaluation of the semen.

## Evaluation of the Semen

Spermatic fluid should be correctly collected for evaluation. Seminal fluid has been found to be stable enough for analysis, provided that it is not contaminated and that it is collected in a clean, dry, wide-mouthed bottle, equipped with a cork stopper. Under no circumstances should a condom be used to collect sperm because the condom has been found to have spermicidal properties. The bottle used for the collection of sperm should be dry, since water itself is spermicidal. When seminal fluid comes in contact with a solution less concentrated than itself, the sperm will swell and die.

A three-day period of abstinence is advised before collecting the seminal fluid in order to obtain the best possible count. Repeated, frequent coitus tends to lower the number of sperm cells in subsequent ejaculations. Coitus interruptus (withdrawal and discharge in the container) or masturbation with discharge into the container will usually produce a good sample. The bottle is labeled and the time of collection is specified. The specimen should be delivered to the examiner within two hours of collection. It is carried in an inner pocket and protected from the possible extremes of outside temperature.

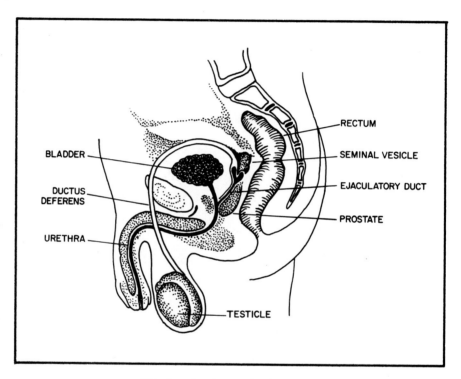

Side view of male reproductive system.

**Appearance and volume.** The fresh ejaculation is a white opalescent mixture of a gelatinous character. There are tapioca-like bodies in the sperm which are liquified within three to fifteen minutes. At the end of that time, the overall appearance of the seminal fluid is changed and it is more translucent. The volume of the seminal fluid is important. The average amount of fluid ejaculated is about four (4) cubic centimeters, but it may be as much as 6 or 7 cc. or it may be very little. The importance of a good seminal pool in the vicinity of the cervix has been stressed. If the cervix is well bathed by the seminal pool, pregnancy is more likely to occur. The seminal fluid whose PH is 7.8 is also important in buffering the vaginal PH which is 3.5 to 5.0. Normal amounts of semen are desirable in obtaining this buffering action.

**Motility.** In order to impregnate the **ovum,** the **spermatozoa** must pass through the entire female genital tract. Fertilization usually occurs in the Fallopian tube and only the most active sperms are likely to succeed in completing this long journey. The motility of the sperm cell (and therefore its longevity) is greater within the female genital tract than it is in the spermatic fluid itself, as the female genital tract supplies a nutritive environment for the sperm. In any sperm analysis, the motility of the sperm cells is recorded as the number of active cells seen through the microscope in high power field and the cells are graded as to the degree of activity.

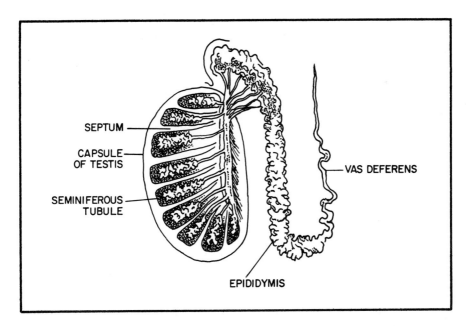

Diagram of a portion in male reproductive system.

**The sperm cell count.** The average cell count in highly fertile men is about 120 million sperm cells per cubic centimeter or about 500 million sperm cells per ejaculation. The likelihood of conception parallels the cell count and as the cell count decreases the chances for successful impregnation becomes progressively less. There is no evidence to indicate that any one figure can be established below which conception is impossible. Pregnancies become fewer in number when the cell count is below 60 million per cc.

There is a definite relationship between the number of abnormal cells and infertility: the greater the number of abnormal cells, the greater the incidence of infertility.

When the sperm count falls below 60 million per cc. and the abnormal forms are about 18–20 percent or more and the motility of the sperm is greatly impaired, infertility becomes more frequent. The sperm analysis varies considerably in any one individual. Poor health, fever, fatigue, and sexual excesses seem to cause changes which result in a poor analysis. A long vacation away from a city, outdoor exercise, and general good living with few excesses have often resulted in improvements in the sperm analysis.

Some of the more common conditions which may lead to infertility or modify fertility in the male are:

1. Congenital factors
2. Inflammations and infections
3. Operations
4. Trauma
5. Habits, fatigue, anxiety
6. Irradiation
7. Diet
8. Marital habits
9. Impotence
10. Endocrine imbalance and faulty spermatogenesis

## Congenital Factors

Undescended testes is a common condition. Ordinarily, both testes are found in the **scrotal sac** at birth. Occasionally, the testes are in the **inguinal canal** at birth, but can easily be lowered into the scrotal sac. In some cases, the testes are not easily lowered into the scrotal sac, but are hidden in the inguinal canal or in the abdomen. Most often, these testes will descend into the scrotum spontaneously, if a reasonable amount of time is allowed. If descent does not take place by the time the child is a year old, an operation for the condition should be considered. The operation should be done very early in life, for infertility usually results if the condition remains uncorrected until after puberty.

Congenital absence of any of the ducts leading from the testes to the urethra will result in **azoospermia** (absence of sperm).

## Inflammations and Infections

Inflammations of the urethra, prostate gland, or any of the accessory ducts will lead to **oligospermia** (low sperm count) or to an increase in the viscosity of the seminal fluid which will interfere with fertility.

Gonorrhea, with its urethritis, prostatitis, and epididymitis has long been a cause of infertility. The various ducts can be occluded by this infection, either because the lumen itself may be occluded or because of the adhesions formed in the periductal tissues. Direct chemical treatment (as with silver nitrate) of the urethra may occlude the vas deferens as it enters the urethra.

Mumps in an adult is a very dangerous infection as it is often complicated by an infection of the testes (orchitis) with degeneration of the testes and interference with **spermatogenesis.**

Advanced genital tuberculosis with complete degeneration of the testes produces lesions that do not respond to treatment.

## Operations

Operations on the inguinal canal, such as repair of a hernia, may lead to damage to the vas deferens or interference with the circulation to it and to the testes, thereby causing infertility.

Of course, vasectomy produces sterility.

## Trauma

Injuries to the testes can cause **hemorrhage** into the testes or torsion of the testes with gangrenous degeneration and subsequent infertility.

## Habits, Fatigue, Anxiety

Constant fatigue, anxiety, and overwork are not beneficial to general health and testicular tissue, just as other body tissue reflects depressed states. If the fertility index is low and no organic disease is found, a program for weight reduction, balanced diet, exercise, and restricted use of alcohol, tobacco, and drugs would lead to better general health and an improvement in seminal analysis.

## Irradiation

Exposure to x-ray and to radioactive substances may cause marked degeneration of testicular tissue, with marked reduction in the number of sperm cells produced. There are many situations where x-ray technicians and workers in laboratories are under constant exposure to radioactive substances. People in these occupations have a greater chance of becoming infertile.

## Diet

Diet is mentioned since many people are on reducing diets and it is possible that some of the fad diets lack essential vitamins A and E and proteins essential to fertility.

## Marital Habits

An account of the patient's marital life is of immense importance since it can sometimes indicate the cause of infertility. Years of marriage with incomplete entry have been noted and coitus without ejaculation over the entire duration of a marriage has occurred.

Infrequent intercourse may lessen the chance of intercourse occurring on the day of ovulation. Excessive intercourse leads to low sperm counts and relative infertility.

## Impotence

Impotence and premature ejaculation should be noted as possible causes of infertility and treatment should be vigorous, as there may be physical or psychological factors present.

## Endocrine Imbalance and Faulty Spermatogenesis

Endocrine imbalances involving the pituitary gland may result in poor spermatogenesis (formation of sperm). **Testosterone** is influential in developing the secondary sex characteristics (such as masculine voice,

# What Is Artificial Insemination?

Artificial insemination is the introduction of sperm cells into the female by instruments rather than by sexual intercourse. In cases in which the husband is able to produce sperm cells but, due to impotence or abnormal structure, is unable to place them in the vaginal tract, artificial insemination may seem desirable. In cases in which the number of sperm in the husband's semen is too low to result in conception, the placing of his sperm within the cavity of the uterus, instead of being deposited in the vagina during coitus, often leads to fertilization. In these cases, in which the sperm is that of the husband, the man is as truly the biological father of the child as though it were conceived as a result of sexual intercourse.

In other cases, where it has not been possible to obtain from the husband sufficient living cells for this purpose, or where there are hereditary reasons for not using them, sperm cells can be supplied by a donor selected by the physician. The donor is not known to the couple, and the couple is not known to the donor. It is as impersonal as the use of blood from a blood bank. The woman in this case is the mother of the child in every sense, but of course the child does not inherit any genetic qualities from the husband. While this idea is distasteful to some persons, others prefer to have a child in this way rather than remaining childless or adopting one. The legal status of such a child has not been finally decided by the highest court, but a number of decisions in the lower courts have ruled that the child produced in this way is legally the child of both the husband and wife. To make it entirely certain that the child's rights are protected, it might be well to adopt the child officially.

Fred Brown and Rudolf T. Kempton, *Sex Questions and Answers,* 2nd ed. (New York: Mc-Graw-Hill Book Company, 1970), p. 165. Reprinted by permission of the publisher.

hair distribution, size of penis) and it improves the sex desire. Large amounts of testosterone depress spermatogenesis. The use of thyroid clinically has been shown to improve spermatogenesis.

## Examination of the Female

After the husband has been examined, a complete physical examination of the wife is performed. The attempt is made to eliminate the possible presence of any chronic disease that may in any way interfere with fertility. Such diseases or conditions might include **anemia,** blood abnormalities, cardiac disease, mental disease, pulmonary disease, diabetes, nutritional disorders, renal diseases, venereal diseases, congenital defects, and neoplasms (tumors). If any of these conditions exist, corrective measures should be instituted.

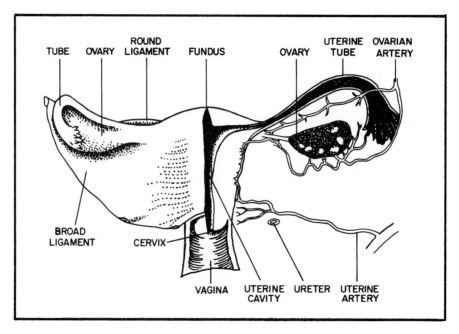

Female reproductive system. The left side shows the tube in natural relationship to ovary. The right side is a diagrammatic section.

A pelvic examination should then reveal any physical abnormalities in the genital tract. The complete absence of vagina, ovaries, or uterus has occasionally been seen. In such cases, absolute sterility exists and cannot be alleviated.

It is now important to determine whether ovulation occurs. A biopsy near the end of the cycle (just premenstrual) should show a secretory type of mucous membrane if ovulation has occurred.

Another method of ascertaining whether ovulation occurs is the use of basal temperature curve. It has been noted that the presence of progesterone in the body has an effect on the heat center in the brain and that body temperatures are higher than when progesterone is not present.

If a woman were to take her rectal temperature every morning before arising from bed and record it on a graph paper, a curve would be

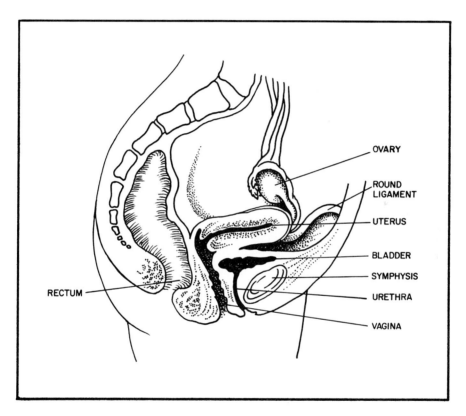

OVARY

ROUND
LIGAMENT

UTERUS

BLADDER

SYMPHYSIS

URETHRA

VAGINA

RECTUM

Sagittal section of the female pelvis and reproductive organs.

formed which would show whether ovulation occurred and when it occurred. A graph with the temperature reading as the vertical axis and the days of the cycle as the horizontal axis will reveal the following: that the temperatures are relatively low in the first half of the cycle (proliferative phase), but as soon as ovulation occurs and progesterone is present, the temperatures rise to a new level and return to the lower level only after the next menses.

A typical graph is as follows:

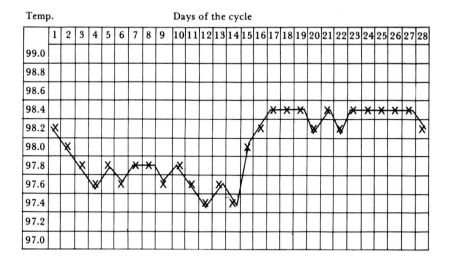

In this graph, day 14 is the day of ovulation. The day of temperature change and the two phases of the cycle are very distinct.

The biopsy and the basal temperature curve should reveal whether ovulation occurs and should indicate the day of ovulation. Ovulation always occurs 13 to 14 days before the expected menstrual period.

The basal temperature chart also happens to be a good pregnancy test, provided that the temperatures are taken continuously over a longer period of time. If pregnancy occurs, ovulation will be noted on the graph, the menses will not appear when expected, and the rectal temperatures will stay at the higher levels and go even higher. This is a very accurate test and has been proven time and again.

When ovulation has been confirmed, the patency of the Fallopian tubes is to be investigated. (The tubes should be open [patent] to allow the sperm and fertilized egg to pass through easily.)

Endocrinologically, a woman is a fine balance of all the hormones constantly present in her body. Any modification will result in an imbalance and resultant poor function. Hormonal imbalances can produce all sorts of menstrual disturbances. Hormone imbalances may cause infertility by interfering with ovulation. A good endocrine study is necessary if there are no positive findings in an investigation of infertility.

Infertility in the female can be corrected by: (1) Surgical procedures, such as the removal of tumors, the dilatation of stenosis of the cervix; the replacement of a retroflexed uterus; (2) the use of hormones, such as gonadotropic hormones, estrogen, progesterone, thyroid; (3) special procedures, such as opening blocked tubes with tubal insufflation, **artificial insemination.**

Infertility is very complex and requires thorough investigation and treatment. It has been stated that contraception is no longer a serious problem; the real problem in gynecology is infertility.

## Glossary

**Adhesions:** bands of tissue formed in the abdomen between the various organs.
**Anemia:** lack of red blood cells or hemoglobin.
**Anlage:** pre-cursor, i.e., original cells or tissues.
**Artificial insemination:** the mechanical placing of sperm cells into the female genital tract, usually into the cervix of the uterus.
**Azoospermia:** a complete lack of sperm cells.
**Body of the uterus:** the larger, pear-shaped portion of the uterus, as distinguished from the neck or cervix.
**Broad ligaments:** the connective tissue extending from the side of the uterus pelvic wall.
**Cervical lesion:** inflammatory growth found in the cervix.
**Cervix:** the neck of the uterus.
**Coitus:** sexual intercourse.
**Corpus luteum:** the yellow body found on the ovary at the site of ovulation.
**Douche:** a technique for washing out the vagina.
**Dyscrasia:** abnormality.
**Endocervicitis:** an inflammation of the inner lining of the cervix.
**Endocrine:** relating to the glands of internal secretion.
**Estrogen:** a hormone found in the ovarian follicle.
**Fallopian tubes:** tubes extending from the inside of the uterus to the abdominal cavity near the ovary (also called salpins, *pl.* salpinges).
**Fibrinogen:** substance found in the blood which is necessary for clotting.
**Follicle:** the cyst-like structure in the ovary containing the mature egg.
**Gestation:** pregnancy.
**Gonadotropic hormones:** hormones which are stimulating to the gonads or sex glands.
**Hemorrhage:** extensive loss of blood.
**Hypogonadism:** a condition in which the sex glands are poorly developed.
**Imperforate hymen:** a condition in which the vaginal opening is covered completely with hymenal tissue.
**Inguinal canal:** an opening in the lower abdominal wall through which the spermatic duct passes.

**Ligation:** the operation of tying, especially arteries, veins, or ducts, with some form of knotted ligature.

**Menopause:** the cessation of menses, usually occurring in the late forties or early fifties in most women.

**Nidation:** the implantation of the fertilized ovum into the wall of the uterus.

**Menses:** the regular monthly bleeding experienced by women.

**Oligospermia:** a diminution in the number of sperm cells.

**Orgasm:** the complex combination of spasms occurring at the height of sexual excitement.

**Ovary:** the female sex gland, found in the pelvis, which produces eggs.

**Ovulation:** process by which an egg is freed from the follicle.

**Ovum:** egg cell.

**"Pap" smear:** a technique for examining tissues for cancer cells, named after Dr. Papanicolaou.

**Pessary:** appliance or suppository placed in the vagina or the cervix.

**Pituitary gland:** an endocrine gland found at the base of the brain.

**Progesterone:** one of the female hormones.

**Progestin:** synthetic progesterone.

**Pulmonary embolism:** a condition in which a freed blood clot settles in one of the pulmonary blood vessels.

**Scrotal sac:** loose area of skin in which the testes are located; scrotum.

**Sedimentation rate:** time taken for red blood cells to settle in a test tube (part of a laboratory test).

**Seminal fluid or semen:** fluid ejaculated from the male which contains sperm cells.

**Seminiferous tubules:** tubules found in the testes in which the sperm cells are formed.

**Spermatocyte or spermatozoon** (*pl.* spermatozoa): sperm cell.

**Spermatogenesis:** the formation of sperm cells.

**Spermicidal:** having the ability to kill sperm cells.

**Testes:** male sex glands.

**Testosterone:** male sex hormones.

**Thrombophlebitis:** inflammation of a vein with clot formation.

**Urethra:** Urinary canal leading from the bladder to the outside of the body.

**Uterus:** muscular organ found in the pelvis of the female in which the fertilized ovum develops.

**Vagina:** the elastic canal leading from the uterus to the outside of the body.

**Vaginitis:** an inflammation of the vagina.

**Varicosities:** enlarged, dilated veins.

**Vas deferens:** the spermatic duct.

**Villus** (*pl.* villi): hair-like projections extending from the fertilized ovum which contain blood vessels. Through the villi, the embryo gets its nourishment from the uterus.

**Vulva:** female external genital organs.

**Vulvitis:** an inflammation of the female external genital organs.

## Questions for Study and Discussion

1. What bearing does the problem of overpopulation have on contraception?
2. Is it important in planning a family that the matter be more choice than chance?
3. What is the historical significance of contraception?
4. What effects has the birth control pill had on modern society?
5. From a physical health standpoint how safe is contraception in general? Specifically, how safe is the pill, the IUD and the diaphragm?
6. What is meant by the statement "the real problem in gynecology is infertility not contraception"?
7. What procedures might a sub-fertile couple follow in order to enhance the possibilities of conception?
8. What possible psychogenic problems might be encountered by a couple experiencing infertility?
9. What other avenues are open to infertile couples desiring children?

## References

Consumer Report. *Family Planning.* Mount Vernon, N.Y.: Consumers Union of the United States, Inc., 1966.
Dalrymple, Willard. *Sex is for Real: Human Sexuality and Sexual Responsibility.* New York: McGraw-Hill, 1969.
Fluhmann, C. Frederic. *The Management of Menstrual Disorders.* Philadelphia: W. B. Saunders, 1956.
Hamblen, E. C. *Endocrinology of Woman.* Springfield, Ill.: Thomas, 1949.
Hotchkiss, Robert Sherman. *Fertility in Men.* Philadephia: Lippincott, 1944.
Jones, Kenneth L., Shainberg, Louis W., and Byer, Curtis O. *Sex.* New York: Harper and Row, 1969.
Siegler, Samuel L. *Fertility in Women.* Philadelphia: Lippincott, 1944.

# 13

# Pregnancy, Childbirth, and Abortion

## General Concept

Human conception is one of nature's greatest achievements.

## Outcomes

The student should be able to:
1. Understand the developmental stages of the ovum, embryo, and fetus
2. Explain the maternal changes during pregnancy
3. Explain how a pregnancy is diagnosed
4. Comprehend the nature and importance of prenatal care
5. Understand the medical usage of the term abortion
6. Explain in general, the various kinds of abortion

## Pregnancy, Labor, Delivery

The birth rate in the United States fluctuates widely. There have been long periods in our history when the birth rate was 17 births per 1,000 population. After World War II, the rate increased to 26 births per 1,000 population. A so-called "population explosion" was forecast for

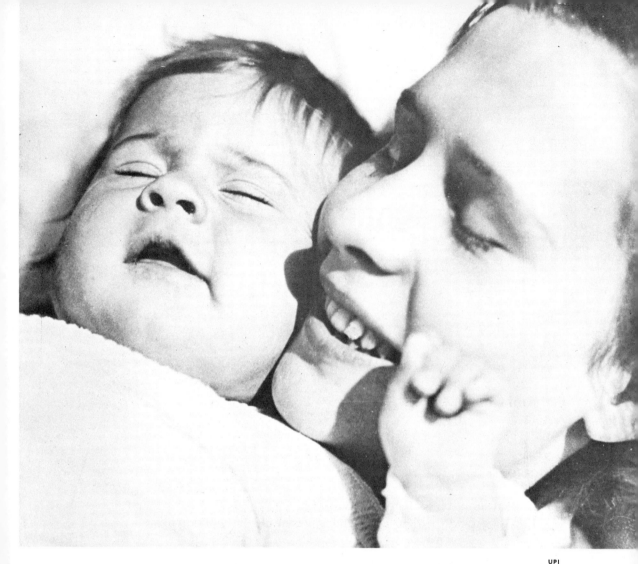

UPI

Contrary to all expectations, the birth rate has been decreasing during the last decade.

the 1960s and 1970s but, contrary to all expectations, the birth rate has been decreasing during the last decade. One of the explanations is that 6 million women are using the contraceptive pill.

In spite of our high figures for spontaneous and induced abortions, 80 percent of all pregnancies reach term and are delivered as live babies.

## Development of the Ovum and Embryo

All pregnancies start from the one-celled ovum. We have already stated that ovulation occurs 14 days before the expected period. Under the stimulus of follicle-stimulating hormone secreted from the pituitary gland, the follicle matures and its cyst-like structure is filled with follicular fluid under pressure. The follicle approaches the surface of the ovary, which thins out considerably, and finally the follicle bursts, allowing the follicular fluid and the ovum to escape. The ovum is picked up by the Fallopian tube.

The exact mechanism by which the ovum enters the tube is not known, but movements at the end of the tube have been noted and it can be assumed that the ovary and the tube are in close approximation to each other at the time of ovulation. There are cilia in the tube, and their constant motion creates a sucking action which draws the egg into the tube. The cilia and the muscular action of the tube drive the egg down the tube towards the uterus.

Fertilization usually occurs in the tube. Unlike the ovum, the sperm cell has motility of its own. It can travel 2.7 mm. per minute and it has been estimated that the sperm can reach the ovum in the tube within 65 to 75 minutes after ejaculation.

Both the sperm and egg must be specially prepared for fertilization so that each has 23 chromosomes in its nucleus rather than the 46 chromosomes normally present in tissue cells. When fertilization occurs, hundreds of **spermatocytes*** surround the ovum, but only one spermatocyte breaks through the surface of the ovum and enters it. The tail portion of the sperm soon degenerates, leaving the head or nucleus to fuse with the nucleus of the ovum. This fusion forms a new nucleus containing 46 chromosomes. The new cell is a fertilized ovum, a new individual, completely different from either parent cell from which it was derived. This new organism is called a zygote for about the first three weeks; from the third to the fifth week it is called an **embryo;** it is called a **fetus** from the fifth week until delivery.

## Development of the Fetus

The embryo develops so that by the third week the head folds appear, the double-chambered heart is noted, visceral arches appear, and the limbs make their appearance.

By the end of the fourth week, the embryo has increased greatly in size, being 7.5 to 10 mm. in length, and the rudiments of eyes, ears, and

*Note: Any term that appears in **boldface** print is defined in the glossary at the end of this chapter.

nose make their appearance. The first traces of all the organs have become differentiated by the end of the first month.

By the end of the second month, the embryo is called a fetus. It is 2.5 cm. in length, the head has become disproportionately large, the extremities are now more developed, and the external genitalia make their appearance.

At the end of the third month, the fetus is 7-9 cm. in length, the centers of ossification appear in the bones, and the fingers and toes become differentiated. The external genitals are beginning to show sexual differentiation. A fetus aborted at this time may make spontaneous movements inside the amniotic sac.

By the end of the fourth month, the fetus is from 10-17 cm. long and weighs 120 grams. External genitals definitely reveal the sex.

By the end of the 20th week, the fetus varies from 18-27 cm. in length. The skin has become less transparent.

By the end of the 24th week, the fetus varies from 28-34 cm. in length and weighs 634 grams. The skin is wrinkled, fat is found under the skin, and the head is still disproportionately large. A fetus born at this time will attempt to breathe, but almost always dies.

By the end of the 28th week, the length is 38 cm. and the weight is 1,200 grams. The entire body is thin and the skin is covered with a cheesy material (vernix caseosa). A fetus born at this time moves energetically and cries with a weak voice. Usually, it cannot survive, but occasionally one will under expert care.

At the end of 32 weeks, the fetus is 46 cm. long and weighs 1,900 grams. Children born at this time may survive if cared for properly.

At 36 weeks, the fetus is 46 cm. long and weighs 2500 grams. Children born at this stage have a very good chance of survival, but expert care is needed.

**Full term** is reached at 40 weeks. The length of the fetus is 50 cm. or 20 inches and weight is 3,200 grams or 7 lbs. The skin is smooth and the whitish, cheesy material (vernix caseosa) is spread over the entire surface. The head is usually covered by hair. The fingers and toes have well developed nails which project beyond their tips. In males, the testes are usually in the scrotum; in females, the **labia majora** are well developed and hide the rest of the genitalia. The eyes are an indeterminate gray color and it is impossible to predict their final color.

The head of the baby is very important, as the essential feature of labor is a process of adaptation between it and the bony birth canal

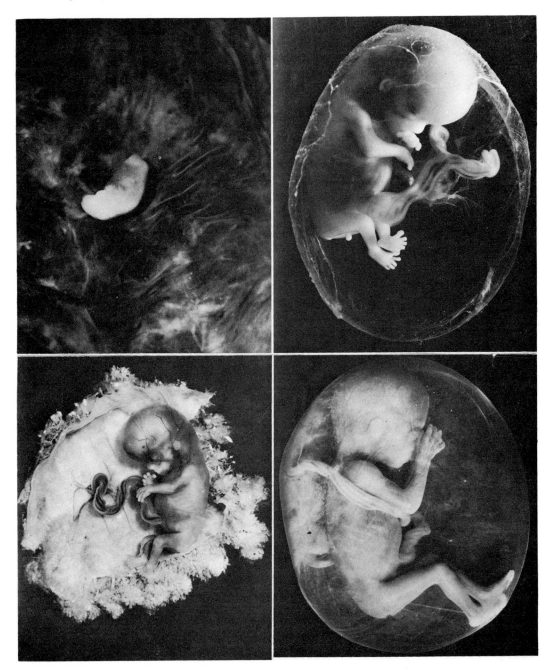

Four stages in human development. Upper left, 1 week; upper right. 2 months; lower left, 3 months; lower right 4 months. (R.H. Albertin photos.)

through which it must pass. The bones of the skull at term are well formed but are not firmly united and are separated by spaces called sutures. The head is thus very malleable and can change shape in order to adjust to the birth canal.

## Maternal Changes During Pregnancy

At 16 weeks gestation, the uterus is felt about 4 finger breadths above the pubic bone, at 20 weeks it is felt just below the umbilicus, and at 24 weeks, slightly above the umbilicus. At 28 weeks, it is felt 3 finger breadths above the umbilicus; at 32 weeks, 3 finger breadths below the end of the breast bone. At term, particularly with first babies, the uterus sinks down and assumes the position found at 32 weeks.

The uterus grows in size, but only by the enlargement of each individual muscle fiber, some fibers getting to be about 11 times normal size. After delivery of the baby, the uterine muscle fibers return to their normal size.

There is also a **vascularity** and **hypertrophy** of skin and muscles in the area. With the enlargement of the uterus, the skin overlying it is subject to considerable tension and it spreads to form scar tissue called "stretch marks" or striae of pregnancy. Sometimes the recti muscles of the abdominal wall separate under the tension of the growing uterus.

There are various changes in the pigment of the skin during pregnancy. There is a condition where brownish patches appear in the skin of the cheeks. This is called cloasma or "the mark of pregnancy." The nipples become more pigmented and the midline of the abdomen becomes darker.

During pregnancy there are marked changes in the breasts. In early pregnancy there is a tenseness and tingling in this region. After the second month, the breasts begin to increase in size, due to the enlargement of the milk-producing glands. The nipples become larger, more pigmented, and erectile. After the first few months, a thin yellowish fluid (colostrum) may be expressed from them. Stretch marks may appear in the skin of the breasts.

The average weight gain in a woman during a pregnancy is about 20-24 lbs. Of this, about 15 lbs. has to do with the baby and the changes during the pregnancy. The remainder has to do with water retention. During a pregnancy there is a retention of the sodium ion in the tissues with subsequent water retention. In extreme cases, the retention of water and sodium is so great that it may result in one of the greatest complications of pregnancy: eclampsia or **toxemia** of pregnancy.

The basal metabolic rate is elevated during a pregnancy.

Protein is stored in the body during the gestation.

Iron and calcium are constantly transferred into the fetus and a lack will occur in the mother if the iron and calcium are not replaced.

The blood volume increases greatly during pregnancy and reaches its maximum about the seventh month. Pregnant mothers with rheumatic heart disease have to be watched carefully in the seventh month and sometimes go into cardiac failure due to the increase in blood volume. Bed rest and treatment with digitalis may be necessary in such cases. Both the red blood counts and hemoglobin diminish as the pregnancy progresses. This may be due, in large part, to the increased blood volume.

The thoracic cage broadens and the heart shadow changes. The cardiac output is increased during the pregnancy.

Mild degrees of mental disturbances are noted in most pregnant women. Many women have pronounced changes in disposition and are cranky. Some become excitable, morose, or morbid, and in some a true psychosis develops.

## Diagnosis of Pregnancy

The diagnosis of pregnancy is most often easy to make after the pregnancy has been established for a few months. The enlargement of the uterus and the absence of menses are evident to the expectant mother. The positive sign is hearing the fetal heart beat, the second is noting fetal movement, and the third is seeing fetal bony parts on x-ray. Unfortunately, these positive signs appear relatively late.

Some probable signs of pregnancy are the enlargement of the abdomen; changes in the shape, size, and consistency of the uterus; changes in the cervix; and positive hormonal tests for pregnancy.

At about six weeks gestation, the uterus is slightly enlarged, soft, beginning to assume a globular shape, and there is a marked softness above the cervix (between the cervix body of the uterus). The cervix develops a characteristically bluish discoloration at this time. At this stage, a hormonal pregnancy test may be useful. These tests are not usually positive until the menstrual period is about 10 days to 2 weeks late. The Ashheim-Zondek test (rat test), the Friedman test (rabbit test), and the frog test have all been used. The most recent successful test

## Smoking and Pregnancy

The old bugaboo with which parents tried to frighten their children away from smoking by saying it would "stunt your growth" is true, especially when applied to the smallest children. A study of over 2,000 English women by Dr. C. R. Lowe found a significant connection between the number of cigarettes smoked by a mother and the weight of her baby at birth. The babies of heavy smokers weighed the least of all the children studied. Children of moderate smokers came next on the scale, and children of non-smokers weighed the most. It is known that tobacco smoke will constrict blood vessels, thus it is reasonable to assume that each time an expectant mother smokes a cigarette, the baby's blood vessels will constrict. Therefore if twenty or more such constrictions occur daily during pregnancy, the child will have a reduced amount of oxygen reaching the tissues, consequently affecting his growth.

Ashley Montagu, *Life Before Birth* (New York: The New American Library, Inc., 1963), pp. 53–4.

is an agglutination test on sensitized animal red blood cells which clump together in the presence of a product of progesterone. The test is called the Ortho-Gravindex test.

Many women make the diagnosis of pregnancy on themselves when there is a cessation of menses, tender, sensitive breasts, morning sickness, and, later on in the pregnancy, when they can feel the baby move.

## Estimated Date of Delivery

The pregnancy usually takes 280 days or 10 lunar months. It is customary to estimate the expected date of confinement by adding 7 days to the first day of the last menstrual period and counting forward 9 months or back 3 months. This is only an approximation and can be as much as 3 weeks off. Since ovulation occurs 14 days before the expected period, then the expected date will be later in those women who have a longer cycle.

## Prenatal Care

Pregnancy should be considered a normal process. However, the changes in the mother are so great and varied that at times it is difficult to differentiate between health and disease. Occasionally, pathological conditions appear insidiously in a pregnancy and may be mistaken for normal occurrences. It is therefore necessary to keep the pregnant woman under strict observation during the pregnancy or she may develop conditions which might threaten her life or her baby's life.

The drop in the maternal mortality rate is related to improvements in **prenatal** care. At present the rate is about 2 to 4 maternal deaths per 10,000 live births. Two decades ago the mortality rate was five times that. The common causes of death in child bearing are hemorrhage, puerperal infection, and toxemia of pregnancy. A pregnant woman should be under the care of an obstetrician throughout her pregnancy and should consult with him at all times when there is any vaginal bleeding, severe headache, or swelling of the legs. It is true that many symptoms are only temporary, but whether the symptoms are of any consequence or not should be decided by the obstetrician.

On the expectant mother's first visit to the obstetrician a medical history is taken and a complete physical examination is done to rule out any disease or condition that might interfere with the pregnancy. She is examined vaginally and a diagnosis of pregnancy is made, if possible. A complete blood count, urine analysis, a serology test for syphilis, and Rh and blood typing are tests which are taken early in pregnancy.

The patient is then instructed as to diet. An attempt is made to keep the weight gain during pregnancy to around 20 lbs. The diet should be a well-balanced one with necessary minerals. Most obstetricians also supplement the diet with a capsule containing vitamins, iron, and calcium.

The pregnant woman should do a normal amount of exercise. However, she should not do strenuous exercise or engage in sports with which she is not acquainted.

The pregnant woman becomes constipated easily and, if this becomes a problem, mineral oil or milk of magnesia may be taken.

Intercourse is allowable if it is not painful to the expectant mother or if there is no vaginitis. A severe Monilia albicans or Trichomonas vaginalis infection may not clear up until intercourse is discontinued.

Today, proper maternity garments can be obtained easily and supports of all kinds for the breasts and abdomen are available. For those women who wish to feed their babies by breast, a supportive bra is usually all that is necessary during the pregnancy. A gentle massage of the nipples with lanolin may be advisable in the last month of the pregnancy.

We are a country of people on the move and the question of travel is one that arises frequently during a pregnancy. For those who have no history of frequent abortions, we have allowed long trips when they were necessary and with no apparent ill effects. At the same time, long unnecessary trips should be avoided. There is no reason to increase the chances of a calamity occurring.

## The Birth Canal

Many women fear that they may not have a large enough pelvis for delivery. At the first examination, an evaluation of the size of the pelvis can be made. However, since babies differ greatly in size, a true evaluation of the size of the baby and the pelvis should not be made until the last month. In the last month, x-ray pelvimetry can be performed and an accurate estimate of the pelvis can be made. In general, in the normal female the birth canal is like a curved tube through which the baby's head, its largest component, has to pass. In women who are having their first babies (**primigravida**), the baby's head usually descends into the pelvis in the last month of the pregnancy. When it does this, it can be assumed that the baby's head fits easily into the pelvis. However, descent of the baby's head into the pelvis sometimes does not occur until the onset of labor.

## Fetal Position

In the uterus the fetus assumes a posture with the head slightly flexed, the back rounded, and the arms and legs folded under the fetus to form a compact mass. However, the fetus does not stay quietly in one position. It is freely movable and arms and legs have a wide range of motion. However, the fetus must adapt itself to the walls of the uterus and the abdomen and, when these are firm, the motion of the fetus is limited to some degree.

The long axis of the baby can be either longitudinal or transverse in its relation to the mother. In 99 percent of all cases the fetus will assume the longitudinal relationship. The longitudinal attitudes are two: either the head is down, pointing to the pelvis or the feet or buttocks are down. The baby is said to have a cephalic (head) presentation when the head is pointing down. If the buttocks are pointing to the pelvis, the baby is said to have a breech presentation. About 95 percent of all pregnancies are head presentations, about 4 percent are breech presentations, and only about 1 percent are transverse presentations.

If **x-ray pelvimetry** is needed in the last month, the x-ray will also show the attitude of the baby in relation to its mother (longitudinal or horizontal), the presentation (head or buttocks first), and the exact position.

## Labor

By *labor* is meant the series of processes by which the mature or almost mature products of conception are expelled from the mother's body. Childbirth, travail, accouchement, confinement, and parturition are other words used for labor. The word delivery refers to the actual birth of the baby. Labor consists mainly of uterine contractions that are regular, that last 45 to 60 seconds, and that cause the changes in the uterus and cervix which are necessary to effect the delivery of the baby.

There are contractions of the uterus throughout the entire pregnancy which are not labor. They are called Braxton-Hicks contractions and they are characterized by being haphazard and not regular. They do not last 45 to 60 seconds and they are ineffectual, causing no changes in the cervix. Near the end of the pregnancy the Braxton-Hicks contractions can be very annoying, because they may simulate labor contractions. Many women are admitted to the hospital in "false labor" as a result of these contractions.

The first stage of labor starts with the first true contraction of labor and ends with the complete dilatation of the cervix.

The second stage of labor starts with the complete dilatation of the cervix and ends with the expulsion of the baby.

The third stage of labor starts with the birth of the baby and ends with the delivery of the placenta.

The actual start of labor has to be estimated, as the process is a gradual one and comes on slowly, and cannot be pinpointed to any one minute. Most often, the contractions of early labor are about 20 minutes apart and slowly become more frequent. When they are occurring about 8-10 minutes apart, labor can be definitely established. There may be a show of mucous or blood with these contractions.

The contractions should be obvious and last 45 seconds to a full minute. Many women experience pain with the contractions, but some do not. Therefore, "labor pain" is being used less frequently as a synonym for the contraction of labor. Most women do not realize that they are in labor until a few hours have passed. Surely there is no need for sedation in the early part of the first stage of labor.

When the contractions are 8-10 minutes apart, strong, and definite, it is time to call the obstetrician who will then admit the patient to the hospital. On admission to the hospital, she will be examined rectally or vaginally by the obstetrician and observed to confirm the fact that she is really in labor. (The rectal examination is specifically mentioned, because up to this time most examinations on the patient have been vaginal.)

Having been found to be in labor, the expectant mother is then prepared for delivery (prepped). The rectum should be empty and an enema is given. The pubic hair is shaved and the **perineum** cleaned. A urine specimen is tested for albumin. The fetal heart is examined with a stethoscope and the labor is then allowed to progress.

The cervix dilates during the first stage of labor. Under the force of the contractions of the uterus, the long thin cervix becomes widened at its upper end, assuming the shape of a cone. Slowly the walls of the cone flatten, leaving only the opening at the bottom. Still under the effect of each contraction, the opening in the cervix slowly becomes wider and wider until its diameter reaches about 10 cm. At this moment, the cervix is considered fully dilated.

The fetal membranes may be bulging through the opening at this time. Sometimes they rupture spontaneously, but most often they are ruptured by the obstetrician before delivery of the baby. A woman should not remain at home waiting for the membranes to rupture. Too many young women have been erroneously advised by their friends to wait until the membranes are ruptured before going to the hospital. If the fetal membranes should rupture early in labor, the obstetrician should be called. At the time of rupture, a certain amount of amniotic fluid escapes. This is called the "breaking of the bag of waters." A woman near term should be prepared for this and should not be frightened. A show of blood has been mentioned, but if there should be hemorrhage in the first stage of labor, the diagnosis of placenta previa (low implantation of the **placenta**) must be entertained. Quick attention is needed and the obstetrician should be informed immediately.

After full dilatation, the baby's head starts its descent through the pelvis. If the patient is a primigravida (a woman pregnant for the first time), the head may be well down in the pelvis at this time, further descent occurs and the **caput** (head) presents itself at the perineum. In the latter part of the first stage and early part of the second stage of labor, sedation may be needed to relax the perineal muscles and the cervix and to allow the mother to more easily push with each contraction. Sedation has been minimized and today only enough is used to sedate the mother. The dosages are carefully gauged not to affect the baby. During all of this, the contractions have continued at regular intervals, but the intervals now are much closer and may be coming every two minutes.

When the caput (baby's head) shows at the perineum, the baby is ready for delivery. The patient is now taken to the delivery room and is prepared, as for a sterile surgical procedure. She is covered with sterile drapes after all skin areas are treated with soap, water, and antiseptics. The obstetrician and his assistants then scrub their hands and don sterile operating room gowns and wear caps and masks, as for a surgical procedure. At this point, some form of **anesthesia** is needed because the pain of the baby's head coming through the perineum is extreme. An incision in the perineum (an episiotomy) is usually necessary at this time also and this requires anesthesia.

Under the necessary anesthesia, an **episiotomy** is performed and the baby is delivered by the obstetrician, with various maneuvers that are part of his art.

After the baby is delivered, the umbilical cord is clamped in two places and cut between the clamps. This frees the baby completely from the mother. The baby is now attended to by the obstetrician (or pediatrician, if one is present). The mouth and nose are suctioned to free the passages of mucous and some oxygen is given, if necessary. The baby usually breathes spontaneously and, in a short time, cries vigorously. The cord is tied close to the baby's abdomen. The eyes are treated with silver nitrate or an antibiotic to prevent infection.

The obstetrician returns to the mother and attends to her. A sample of blood is taken from the umbilical cord routinely in some hospitals and kept for 4 days, just in case some studies are necessary. Studies on the cord blood are always necessary in the Rh negative mother. The placenta is then delivered, examined to see if it is complete, and put aside.

A hormone is then given to the patient and an inspection of the genital tract is made. Cervical tears are repaired; vaginal tears are re-

## Breast Feeding

It is interesting to note that breast feeding has not been popular in the United States during the past 30-40 years, although it appears to be reviving slightly in the 70's. Many new mothers claim they cannot breast feed, yet upon investigation, very few women are found who, for physiological reasons, cannot breast feed. It appears rather to be a problem of attitude and/or lack of knowledge. One reason for a poor attitude toward breast feeding may be the close association that has developed between a woman's breasts and her sexuality. Breast size and shape have, since World War II, become increasingly important to attractiveness and sexuality. One need only remember the popularity of the flat-chested look of the flapper, 1920's era, to realize that breast size has not always implied sexuality. In fact, in most primitive societies, the breast is left exposed since the primary function is feeding rather than sexual arousal. Because of the association between the breast and sexuality, some girls are afraid that breast feeding will ruin their figure, thus decreasing their sex appeal. In reality, this very rarely happens. Sometimes the girl may think that the normal maternal feelings of warmth she experiences during breast feeding are only sexual in nature, thus leading her to feel guilty. . . .

Frank Cox, *Psychology* (Dubuque, Ia.: Wm. C. Brown Company Publishers, 1970), p. 69.

paired; the episiotomy is repaired. If all the bleeding is controlled and the patient seems to be in good general condition, she may be sent to the post-partum recovery room, where she is watched for a reasonable length of time. She is then returned to her room.

If all goes without any complications, most women are up and about in 24 hours and are discharged from the hospital after 4 or 5 days. During her hospital stay, the mother is carefully observed for the presence of infection. Today, with the proper use of antibiotics, many infections have been eliminated.

It takes 10 days to 3 weeks for the episiotomy wound to heal. There will be a discomfort until healing is complete. Most women will have a bloody discharge at first and a lighter discharge later, which will continue for a few weeks. It take 6 weeks for the uterus to become fully involuted (to return to its original size). Breast feeding causes the uterus to involute more quickly. Breast feeding may delay the first menstrual period after the baby is born, but it may not prevent ovulation or a pregnancy. If a woman does not breast feed, the menses may appear any time from 6 to 12 weeks after delivery.

## Some Complications of Pregnancy and Delivery

### Abnormal Deliveries

We have now discussed the normal spontaneous delivery with an episiotomy. However, this does not account for all the deliveries.

About 20 percent of all the primigravida require a low forceps delivery. This means that even after the baby's head passes through the bony canal, the soft tissues of the perineum may hold it back and it may be necessary to guide the head through the perineum with **obstetrical forceps** after an episiotomy is performed. This is, in the hands of a good operator, a simple and gentle procedure for the mother and the baby.

In about 8-10 percent, low mid-forceps are necessary to effect the delivery because the forces of labor are poor, or the baby's head does not fit well in the pelvis, or the position of the head in the pelvis does not allow for the normal progress of the delivery. This type of delivery may be difficult and should be attempted by only the well-trained obstetrician.

Approximately 4 percent of the deliveries are breech presentation and this type of delivery requires a trained obstetrician.

Twins are a special situation and also require special attention because the second twin is most often in an abnormal position of presentation.

### Rh Factor

In this century, 85 percent of the population is Rh positive and 15 percent is Rh negative. We have come to recognize that **erythroblastosis**

**fetalis,** a condition found in the fetus, is a direct result of the Rh factor and the **antigen**-antibody reaction induced by it.

The "Rh" is derived from the fact that the Rhesus Macacus monkey was used in the experiments leading to the discovery of the factor. Individuals who are Rh positive have in their blood cells a **lipoprotein,** the antigen. The Rh negative individual does not contain this protein. If Rh positive blood is injected by transfusion into the Rh negative individual, a reaction is set up which results in the creation of anti-Rh antibodies. We knew that such transfusion reactions were existent even before the Rh factor was discovered.

Applying this new knowledge, we have come to explain how erythroblastosis fetalis occurs. If an expectant mother is Rh negative and the father of the baby is Rh positive, it is possible that the baby is Rh positive. If, by any chance, some of the baby's blood (while still **in utero)** should enter the mother's blood stream, this would act like a transfusion of Rh positive blood into an Rh negative person. Rh positive **antibodies** then could be formed in the blood stream of the mother and, since antibodies cross the placental barrier with ease, they would attack the baby's Rh positive blood, destroy it, and set up the condition known as erythroblastosis. It is unusual to see this condition in a woman's first pregnancy, however.

The theory today is that the exchange of blood occurs at the time of the first delivery, when the placenta is delivered in the third stage of labor. At that time, antibodies are formed and these antibodies create the problem in the next pregnancy. Not every Rh negative mother encounters this problem.

Recently, there has been developed a gamma globulin derived from Rh negative individuals who have already been sensitized against Rh positive blood. When this globulin is given to an Rh negative woman at the time of delivery of the first baby, it will give her a temporary immunity against Rh positive blood and thereby suppress the formation of antibodies. The globulin acts for only a few weeks and therefore this procedure would have to be repeated following each subsequent delivery. If antibodies are already present, either from a previous pregnancy or transfusion, the globulin will not work.

In the case of an Rh negative mother, Rh typing, and antibody studies are made early in the pregnancy and at regular intervals during the pregnancy. The father is also studied. If he is Rh negative, there are no problems. If he is Rh positive, an attempt is made to ascertain whether

---

## The Preemie

When a baby is born prematurely, it may be unable to suck or swallow properly. A soft plastic tube is inserted into its throat so it can be fed at frequent intervals. The premature baby also may be unable to provide defense against the much cooler temperatures outside its mother's body. A six-month fetus lacks the layer of fat that normally develops later to serve as insulation. It may not be able to move its skeletal muscles, such as in kicking, to generate body heat. And it may lack a properly developed temperature control device in its nervous system.

Eventually, the preemie acquires its natural layer of insulating fat and loses its wrinkled appearance. It may double its weight in a single month and will have adjusted to its new environment by the time that a larger, full-term baby is beginning the crisis of birth.

*The Miracle of Life*, booklet (Chicago: American Medical Association, 1967), pp. 18–19. Reprinted by permission of the American Medical Association.

---

he is a combination of Rh positive and Rh negative (heterozygous). If he is, the baby will have a 50 percent chance of being Rh negative. If the baby is Rh negative, there is no problem.

If no antibodies are present in the mother during the pregnancy and immediately following, she is given Rhogam (the **immune globulin**). If antibodies present themselves and the baby is affected, it may be necessary to deliver the baby at 38 weeks gestation and to study the baby quickly. If there is a positive Coomb's test (for the presence of erythroblastosis), a low hemoglobin, a low red blood count, the presence of erythroblasts (immature red blood cells), the baby is given an exchange transfusion with Rh negative blood. Many affected babies are too badly injured in utero and may die in utero or soon after delivery.

For those mothers who already have antibodies and who have a history of erythroblastotic babies, there is one solution: artificial insemination with an Rh negative donor. For the Rh negative mother with no antibodies, there is great hope in the Rhogam treatment.

## Toxemia of Pregnancy

We have already stressed prenatal care as being important in preventing some of the calamities that occur in pregnancy. One of these conditions is called toxemia of pregnancy or eclampsia. The extreme case, which usually occurs in the last month of pregnancy, is associated with a large gain in weight; swelling of the ankles, legs, back, face and hands; an elevated blood pressure; and albumin in the urine. Severe eclampsia terminates in convulsions, coma, and even death. During the convulsion, the baby may die in utero. The condition is stabilized as quickly as possible with sedation and anti-hypertensives and the uterus is emptied as quickly as possible.

This condition is not sudden in its onset. It comes on slowly and the signs are there for the obstetrician to see (therefore, the necessity of frequent prenatal visits in the last two months of the pregnancy). Pre-eclampsia (the toxemia as it exists before the convulsive seizures) has to be treated forcefully, either ambulatory or in the hospital when necessary. Frequently, termination of the pregnancy is indicated, either by induction of labor or by **Caesarean section.**

Today, eclampsia and pre-eclampsia are seen less frequently in private practice. The condition is most prevalent in the clinic patient who presents herself for her first prenatal visit late in the pregnancy.

## Premature Separation of the Placenta

This condition also creates a crisis in a pregnancy. The condition most often occurs in the last 4-6 weeks of a pregnancy, but may occur sooner. The characteristic symptom is a sudden hemorrhage from the vagina with no labor. There is a painful uterus, but no contractions. Any hemorrhage in the last three months of a pregnancy must be investigated.

When the hemorrhage occurs, the patient is transferred as quickly as possible to a hospital, where blood is available for transfusion. Hemorrhage cannot be treated at home. On admission to the hospital, blood is made available and the patient is examined by her obstetrician. If the diagnosis is confirmed, he will probably empty the uterus by Caesarean section, replace the blood loss by transfusion, and often obtain a healthy baby and a happy mother.

If the separation of the placenta is complete, the baby's circulation is separated from the mother's and the baby will die in utero.

Occasionally, due to the hemorrhage behind the placenta, blood seeps into the uterine musculature, leading to a condition which does not allow the uterus to contract well and only leads to more uterine hemorrhage. Such a uterus sometimes must be removed to save the mother's life.

Premature separation of the placenta often brings the most serious complications in obstetrics.

## Placenta Previa

Ordinarily, the fertilized egg implants itself high in the uterus and the placenta forms in that area. On rare occasions, the ovum implants itself low in the uterus near to the cervical opening. When labor starts, the placenta separates from the dilating cervix, exposing large uterine vessels (sinuses), and hemorrhage ensues. The condition is associated with the rhythmic contraction of labor.

In the face of hemorrhage, the patient is transferred to the hospital where blood is made available. In this situation, it is possible to deliver the patient vaginally, if the placenta is only partially covering the cervix. The skill and training of the obstetrician will be greatly needed in these cases. The uterus is emptied either by a vaginal delivery or by Caesarean section and the blood is replaced by transfusion.

## Induction of Labor

It has been known for a long time that the posterior lobe of the pituitary gland secretes a substance, pituitrin, which has the capacity to cause contractions of the uterus. However, the extract which was made from the posterior lobe also had a component, pitressin, which caused an elevation of the blood pressure. Any elevation of the blood pressure is dangerous in obstetrics and may precipitate toxemia. Therefore, pituitrin was not used freely before or during labor, but was used only post-partum.

When the active contractive substance pitocin was isolated and found to be free of pitressin, it was used more freely to induce labor. At present, a synthetic pitocin called syntocinone is used very often to induce labor. It is usually given as an intravenous infusion, in the form of a solution in dextrose and water.

There are many situations in obstetrics where an induction of labor may be necessary. There is the post-mature baby, the toxemias of pregnancy, Rh negative mothers with antibodies, the diabetic mother, the low-lying placenta with moderate bleeding, to name a few.

When patients live a great distance from the hospital, it is sometimes wise to admit them near term and induce labor in order to prevent an unattended delivery, which could be dangerous for the mother or the baby.

At no time should the induction be accomplished for the convenience of the obstetrician or the patient. There are enough complications in obstetrics without looking for more of them.

## Abortion

The term abortion means detachment or expulsion of the ovum before the stage of viability. In general, the fetus is not viable before the 28th week of gestation. To the laymen, the term abortion often suggests illegality, in contradiction to the word miscarriage. In medical usage, however, it has no such implications. The word miscarriage is not a medical term.

### Spontaneous Abortion

In general abortions are either spontaneous or induced. Spontaneous abortions are those that occur unintentionally. Spontaneous abortions are frequent in the United States, but the exact statistics are difficult to obtain. Hospital figures do not represent conditions of private medical practice, because only complicated cases of spontaneous abortion are sent to the hospital. Many women who have completely spontaneous abortions never consult a physician. Some abortions occur early and pass under the diagnosis of delayed or profuse menstruation, while other abortions are deliberately concealed. However, estimates have been made that about 10 percent of all pregnancies in the United States end in spontaneous abortion.

The abortions usually occur in the first three months of the gestation, most frequently in the first month. An abortion is called an early abortion if it occurs before the 22nd week and a late abortion if it occurs between the 22nd and the 28th week of the gestation. Any mishap after the 28th week and before term is called a premature delivery.

In general, the causes for spontaneous abortion may be classified as *intrinsic* or *extrinsic*. Defective ova and spermatozoa are an intrinsic cause of spontaneous abortion. Since very few unfertilized eggs have ever been seen and studied, we cannot know how often defective ova occur. It is well known, however, that defects are frequently seen in the ova of other species. Human spermatozoa have been studied extensively, and abnormal forms have been found. Men with abnormal spermatozoa are most often sterile, but it is possible that an ovum might be fertilized by one of the abnormal sperm cells and the product of such a fertilization might well be defective. The most common cause of abortion is some malformation of the fertilized ovum, which, if carried to term, would produce an abnormal child. Spontaneous abortion is sometimes a blessing in disguise.

There are many extrinsic factors which interfere with the nutrition or health of the developing fetus. Virus infections have a predilection for the fetus. They have the ability to pass through the placental barrier and attack the fetus directly. Any virus infection in the mother may cause death of the fetus. If a mother is very sick in the early months of a pregnancy with high fever, cough, and general malaise, it is not unusual for her to abort spontaneously. German measles is another cause of damage to the fetus. Some fetuses die in utero as a result of this infection, but many go on to term and develop abnormalities with which they can survive.

Drugs of all kinds may damage a fetus. Thalidomide has gained world-wide notoriety by its effect and it may be possible that some drugs like LSD will be found to have serious effects on the growing fetus.

In any early pregnancy, any excesses of drugs, alcohol, cold, heat, trauma, exertion, or infections can be a cause of damage to the fetus. Pelvic infections in the mother, such as gonorrhea, tuberculosis, or a previous **post-partum** infection may affect an ovum.

A uterine fibromyoma, the so-called fibroid of the uterus, is a common cause of spontaneous abortion. If the tumor invades the cavity of the uterus, it will not allow a pregnancy to develop. **Ovarian** tumors or **cysts** may cause abortion by pressure, by irritating the uterus, or by interfering with the circulation of the uterus.

If the uterus is retroflexed, abortions may result. Ordinarily, the uterus is **anteflexed**. This means that the body of the uterus points towards the front of the abdomen. Some women have a uterus whose body is bent over and points towards the rectum. This is called a **retroflexed uterus,** a condition which is usually congenital, but which may be acquired later in life following pregnancies. Usually a pregnant retroflexed uterus assumes the anteflexed position spontaneously as the pregnancy progresses, but if there should be adhesions holding the uterus down and it becomes incarcerated in the hollow of the sacrum, abortion may follow.

There is a condition which is called incompatent internal **cervical os** which is caused by injury to the cervix (the type of injury that could follow an abortion or dilatation of the cervix). In such cases, repeated abortions occur. The cervix, having been traumatized, remains patulous (expanded, open) at the internal cervical os (orifice). As the pregnancy progresses to the fifth month, the cervix opens further and further and allows the fetal membranes to protrude from the cervix. When they protrude far enough, they will rupture, allowing the fetus to be aborted without any labor. The condition can be relieved by an operation to repair the cervix.

Some spontaneous abortions are due to a decrease in the amount of the corpus luteum hormone, progesterone, after the eightieth day of pregnancy and a simultaneous lag in the production of this hormone by the placenta. In such cases, progestin (the synthetic hormone corresponding to progesterone) may have to be given to the patient to decrease the sensitivity of the uterus and to prevent contractions of the uterus.

Endocrine imbalance in the mother may also be a cause of abortion.

The use of drugs such as quinine, castor oil, and ergot may be the cause of abortion.

X-ray to the lower abdomen may affect a fetus.

Heavy exercise may cause abortion, but the ovum must have a low vitality for this to be a factor. Some women who work as hard as men until the day of confinement are not subject to abortion.

Operations in the pelvis will often bring on an abortion.

General anesthesia can be a cause of abortion.

Major auto accidents and falls may cause abortion.

The symptoms of spontaneous abortion are usually clear. After a period of amenorrhea (absence of menstruation), during which pregnancy may or may not have been recognized, the patient will have some bleeding associated with cramps. The cramps become more severe and resemble labor pains. The cervix will dilate slowly and finally the entire ovum will be expelled. The size of the ovum will vary according to the period of gestation. Following the expulsion of the fetus and placenta, the uterus will contract down and bleeding will become minimal and may stop completely. All cramps may stop. If the events occur as described above, the abortion is called a complete abortion.

Sometimes, however, only a portion of the ovum is extruded from the uterus and placental tissue can remain attached to the wall of the uterus. If such is the case, we are dealing with an incomplete abortion. The bleeding may become more profuse and even take on the aspects of severe hemorrhage. Such cases should be moved to a hospital, where an examination should reveal that some of the products of gestation are still in the uterus. If the condition was a spontaneous abortion, it can be assumed that the patient is not infected. A blood count and temperature reading will bear this out. The patient is typed and cross-matched, and blood is obtained to be ready for transfusion at a moment's notice. The patient is taken to the operating room and the uterus is emptied. Ergotrate, pitocin, or a similar substance for contracting the uterus is administered and blood is given by transfusion, if needed.

Complete recovery from such an episode may be slow and require much supportive treatment. The complications of even a spontaneous abortion can be many or none at all. Most women have spontaneous abortions without any after effect. There are some, however, who develop infections of the uterus, tubes, or broad ligaments with resultant distortions of the tubes and perhaps even sterility. Some women have a poor endometrium following the abortion and may have abnormal menses. Chronic anemia and general poor health may also be complications.

## Ectopic or Tubal Pregnancy

The symptoms of tubal pregnancy sometimes resemble those of the spontaneous early abortion. Tubal pregnancy is caused by some factor which interferes with the normal progress of the fertilized egg through the tube to the uterus.

**Salpingitis** (inflammation of the Fallopian tubes) is the common cause of tubal pregnancy. Due to the infection, a maze of crypts and blind passages form in the lumen (interior) of the tube, which do not allow the egg to pass through. Infection of the tubes is often followed by adhesions on the tube which, when they contract, cause distortion of the tube. The distortions do not allow the fertilized egg to pass through. Repeated induced abortions may be followed by salpingitis and subsequent tubal pregnancy.

The fertilized egg remains in the tube and continues to grow. It invades the wall of the tube with its **trophoblastic cells** and these cells enter blood vessels and cause hemorrhage. Unlike the uterus, the tube has no thick **endometrium** in which the egg can imbed itself. Soon the wall of the tube gives way, ruptures, and allows much blood to escape into the peritoneal cavity. The ruptured tubal pregnancy is one of the classic crises met in medicine.

Before rupture, the symptoms may be a missed period (**emenorrhea**) and there may be nausea or vomiting, an occasional cramp-like pain, and some slight spotting. These could be the symptoms of an early intrauterine pregnancy threatening to abort spontaneously.

When the tube ruptures, the symptoms are classic: amenorrhea, followed by spotting for some days, and then, a sudden severe lower abdominal pain, associated with a feeling of weakness or faintness, actual fainting, nausea or vomiting, some more vaginal bleeding which may resemble the menses, pain in the rectum, shock and collapse (the symptoms of shock being the fainting, pallor of skin, cold wet perspiration, chilly extremities, no pulse or a weak pulse, unconsciousness). The patient looks exsanguinated (bloodless). Anyone confronted with a situation like this should immediately seek the help of a physician or a hospital.

The treatment for such a condition is surgical. The surgery should be done as soon as possible in a situation where blood, by transfusion, can be replaced as quickly as possible. The mortality rate in such a condition is high.

## Therapeutic Abortion

We have already stated that abortions are either spontaneous or induced. The **therapeutic** abortion is an induced abortion which is performed because of some disorder that concerns the mother or the fetus.

In the past, the laws of the various states were such that a therapeutic abortion was allowed only if the condition demanding the therapeutic abortion would damage the mother's life. The various state legislatures have been appealed to constantly concerning change and liberalization of the abortion laws.

In the last few years, we have seen some of these changes take place. Many states now have laws which allow a therapeutic abortion if the mother's life or health is in jeopardy or if there is sound reason to believe that the fetus will be abnormal. A broad definition of the word "health" is being used. The mother's health can include physical, mental, and social conditions. Most physicians generally agree that an abortion is justified if a woman's life or health is threatened. This would include many diverse medical conditions, from heart disease to mental disease. Internists and psychiatrists have to be consulted and, if the medical indications are present and the hospital's conditions are fulfilled, most gynecologists would not object to performing the operation.

We now know that many situations arise which may lead to an abnormal child. We are generally agreed that a therapeutic abortion is indicated if there is reason to believe that the fetus will be abnormal. We know that Thalidomide and German measles have caused abnormal development of the fetus. The conditions which are detrimental to a developing fetus are changing almost every day. It was recently reported that LSD can cause chromosomal changes in the individual using the drug, as well as in the fetus which may be present in her uterus. This new possibility for an abnormal fetus has created another indication for therapeutic abortion.

The operations for therapeutic abortion are no different than those ordinarily used to empty the uterus of the products of gestation. In the early stages of a pregnancy a simple **dilatation and curettage** is performed, under anesthesia, with all the precautions necessary for such an operation. The cervix is dilated and the fetus and its accompanying membranes are gently removed with ovum forceps. The remainder of the tissue is removed with a **curette.** This procedure is best done in the first two to three months of the pregnancy. In the fourth month of the pregnancy it is usually too dangerous to perform a dilatation and curettage, as the risk of cervical or uterine perforation is very great. In the fourth month, it is wise not to interfere with the pregnancy, but to wait until the fifth or sixth month and then to induce premature labor by injecting saline solution into the uterine cavity after rupturing the fetal membranes.

Neither of these procedures is without its dangers. Perforations of the cervix or uterus may occur even in the hands of good physicians. The mortality rate for therapeutic abortion is about 1 percent. Therefore, therapeutic abortion is not to be taken too lightly.

## Illegal Abortion

The criminal or illegal abortion is an induced abortion. It falls into the category of being illegal or criminal because no medical reasons can be found to justify the abortion. Most women who seek to have a pregnancy terminated have already seen a physician. He has probably established the fact that a pregnancy exists and has gone into the possibilities of a therapeutic abortion. Since the laws vary considerably from one state to another, there is no one solution to the problem. The physician can only outline what the rules are in his locality. If a therapeutic abortion is not feasible in one area, the woman may go to another area where such cases are approached more liberally.

If all attempts fail, the woman may next try to abort herself. She will inquire of her friends or at a drug store for some drug that might bring on a delayed menstrual period. In the past, women have used quinine and castor oil to bring on a menses and every rural community has had its favorite **abortifacient** concoction: tansy tea, parsley, juniper, and others. Ergot is used extensively for this purpose.

The use of abortifacients goes far back in the history of man. The Oath of Hippocrates, taken traditionally by all physicians at the time of graduation from medical school, includes an admonition to all physicians that they should in no manner ever prescribe or give abortifacient drugs to a woman. Yet every ancient tribe or clan had its witch doctor, medicine man, or midwife, a person who was very powerful in the community because of his or her ability to eliminate unwanted pregnancies. Some of this was based on prayer, incantation, and magic words, but it is surprising how often there was real pharmacology behind the magic.

This type of magic still exists today in some cultures. While in Trinidad in the British West Indies, I learned about the Mammaloi (the female voodoo midwife) who sold love potions, spells called *abeahs*, and a magic potion to bring on delayed menses. The magic potion was made by collecting the leaves of certain flowering vines at certain times of the year. A tea or brew was made from the leaves and the necessary magic words were added. Although the Mammaloi was unaware of it, she collected the leaves at a time when an ergot-producing fungus was present on them. It was this ergot in the tea which was the effective ingredient.

Women have also attempted self-induced abortion by introducing foreign bodies into the uterus. The slippery elm stick, **bougies, catheters,** and many other strange and bizarre substances have been used. Many years ago I remember seeing one woman who had self-induced an abortion with an old fashioned shoe hook. On removing the instrument, she had lacerated the cervix badly. The resultant bleeding was very heavy and she sought medical aid. Extensive repair of the cervix was required to control the hemorrhage.

It is possible that in some cases drugs and other crude methods may work to produce abortion, but the percentages are low and the time wasted on some procedures only prolongs the agony experienced by these women. Most women seek the help of an abortionist when early preliminary methods fail.

The number of women who are aborted illegally in the United States every year is not known. There is a great deal of secrecy attached to this procedure and most women will not discuss it publicly. It has been estimated that about one million women a year are aborted illegally. It has also been stated that anywhere from 10–20 percent of all pregnancies are aborted illegally. Knowing that 10 percent of all pregnancies abort spontaneously, we can then say that at least one out of every five pregnancies in the U.S. is lost by abortion—spontaneous or induced.

Surprisingly, most women seeking illegal abortions are married. They already have the desired number of children in their family, and an additional child would become a terrible burden. These women may be the victims of a rhythm system that did not work or they may have become pregnant because of the failure of one of the less successful contraceptive measures. In a surprising number of women, contraceptives are not used at all. In this era of frank discussion and knowledge there is no excuse for the married woman who does not use a contraceptive device to avoid an unwanted pregnancy. Planned parenthood applies especially to married couples who already have their desired number of children, and such couples should seek all the help they can find.

A number of women seeking the help of abortionists are unwed mothers whose pregnancies are unwanted due to the social stigma attached.

When the unmarried woman gets pregnant, she can get married and have her baby, she can have the baby and put it up for adoption, she can keep it herself, or she can seek out an abortionist.

One of the questions most frequently asked of a gynecologist is how to obtain the services of a good abortionist. In all fairness, he must answer that he does not know, because abortionists are always moving from one place to another. If the legitimate physician refers a patient personally, he is implicated and becomes an accessory in the eyes of the law. He cannot afford to do this, for he might lose his license to practice medicine.

Most people find abortionists by word of mouth. One friend refers another. Pharmacists, beauticians, barbers, hotel help, and taxi drivers know more about this than the average physician. Recently, groups of religious leaders have organized committees for investigating undesired pregnancies. These men are dedicated to the idea that the present laws concerning abortion should be changed. Since the existent laws are not just in their opinion, they will investigate each particular applicant and, if they think that there are good socioeconomic reasons for terminating the pregnancy, they will refer the applicant to a physician who is willing to perform an abortion under these circumstances. In this way, they hope to avoid the tragic complications that often result from these operations.

In the past, it was the midwife or the physician who was the operator. Today it might be anyone. Many nonprofessional people with no knowledge of anatomy, physiology, or operative techniques are attempting procedures that would frighten some of the best-trained gynecologists. This type of abortionist is not really trying to empty the uterus of the products of gestation. He is attempting to start the abortion and he hopes that the uterus will complete the abortion on its own.

A common procedure is to thread an ordinary rubber catheter through the cervical canal and to push it into the uterus, in the hope that it will interfere with the pregnancy by rupturing the **fetal membranes** or interfering with the circulation of the fetus, thereby causing death to the fetus, which in turn will cause the patient to empty the uterus spontaneously. Packing the cervix and uterus with gauze, introducing solutions and pastes into the uterus, and introducing metallic instruments are other methods. All of these procedures are dangerous, and perforations of the uterus, hemorrhage, and pelvic infections frequently result. Rarely does one of these procedures result in a complete abortion. Most often an incomplete septic abortion results and these patients are among the sickest we ever see.

A gynecologist should be consulted at this point and legally he is allowed to treat this patient to the fullest extent. He will admit the patient to a hospital, treat the infection with antibiotics, and, when he considers it safe, he may empty the uterus with a dilatation and curettage. The gynecologist may have to report this case to the local police.

However, if an illegal abortion is performed by a physician, the attempt will be made by the abortionist to follow the procedures as one would in a therapeutic abortion. In early cases, a dilatation and curettage is done—even without anesthesia. In later cases, some abortionists who are physicians will use the intrauterine instillation of saline solution to bring on premature labor, but most will not interfere with a pregnancy that is more than three months gestation.

These operations are done almost anywhere. They may be performed in doctor's offices, hotel rooms, motel rooms, rooming houses, apartments, or in a patient's own home. Prices vary and are usually what the traffic will bear. Very few abortions cost less than $360 or more than $700. There have been extremes on either side of this price range. It seems that those who have the financial backing and wherewithal find it

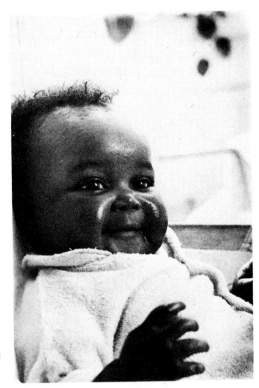

An increased number of black and bi-racial children have become available for adoption.

much easier to obtain the services required. I have heard of patients who have gone to Puerto Rico, Mexico, or Japan to undergo abortion. In Japan, where abortion is legalized, the operations are performed in clinics and all careful sterile operative techniques are followed.

## Legal Abortions

Philosophically, thoughts concerning abortion are changing. In this country we are becoming more aware of the problem as it exists, and we cannot erase from our minds the fact that one million women undergo illegal abortion every year. It is not only the woman who is involved; there are a husband, father, children, clergymen, doctor, and many others who are, in one way or another, a part of the problem.

In several states there have been repeals and revisions of abortion laws. Many states find their laws to be outdated (in several states, therapeutic abortions are still illegal), and such states as New York, Hawaii, and Colorado have passed legislation liberalizing their statutes.

We are slowly getting around to the idea that a woman has a right to prevent an unwanted pregnancy and, if that unwanted pregnancy should occur, to have it terminated. If this is the way we feel, then the people in this country should be more forceful in their appeals to the various legislatures. The medical profession and religious groups are not going to change the laws. Their efforts sometimes cloud the issue by making it possible for women to obtain abortions outside of the law. The abortion laws will be changed only when enough citizens work toward changing them.

Abortions are dangerous. It is far safer and wiser to use contraceptives than to have to face an unwanted pregnancy.

## Glossary

**Abortifacient:** a drug capable of producing abortion.
**Amenorrhea:** the absence of menses.
**Anesthesia:** medicaments used to render patients unconscious prior to an operation.
**Anteflexion:** the normal attitude of the uterus with the body of the uterus bent forward.
**Antibodies:** substances found in the body which can destroy foreign proteins.
**Antigen:** a protein capable of producing antibody reactions.

**Blastocyst:** early stage of the developing ovum.

**Bougie:** hard rubber surgical instrument used for probing.

**Caput:** head (in obstetrics, the baby's head at delivery).

**Catheter:** a rubber tube used to empty the bladder.

**Cervical os:** the opening into the cervix.

**Caesarean section:** a surgical procedure for delivery of a baby through an abdominal incision.

**Chorion:** the layer of the fetal membranes derived from the trophoblastic cells.

**Curette:** a surgical instrument used to scrape out tissue.

**Decidua:** the inner lining of the uterus during a pregnancy.

**Dilatation and curettage:** an operation for emptying the contents of the uterus.

**Embryo:** the developing ovum from about the third to the fifth week of gestation.

**Endometrial biopsy:** a surgical procedure, in which a sample of the inner lining of the uterus is taken.

**Endometrium:** the lining of the non-pregnant uterus.

**Episiotomy:** incision made to facilitate the delivery of a baby.

**Erosion of the cervix:** thinning of the covering of the cervix.

**Erythroblastosis fetalis:** a disease of the newborn, characterized by severe anemia, jaundice, and degeneration.

**Fetal membranes:** the sac-like membranes surrounding the developing fetus.

**Fetus:** the developing ovum, from about the fifth week of gestation to full term.

**Full term:** a pregnancy which has reached its completion.

**Hernia:** an abnormal protrusion of the intra-abdominal contents through an opening in the abdominal wall (through the inguinal canal, for example).

**Hypertrophy:** overgrowth.

**Immune globulin:** that fraction of the blood that contains antibodies and is capable of giving a temporary immunity to certain diseases (also called gamma globulin).

**In Utero:** existing in the uterus.

**In Vivo:** existing in the living state.

**Labia majora, labia minora:** portions of the external female genitalia.

**Lipoprotein:** a combination of protein and a lipoid or fatty substance.

**Multigravida:** a woman who has had previous pregnancies.

**Nullipara:** a woman who has not had any babies.

**Obstetrical forceps:** surgical instruments used to facilitate the delivery of a baby.

**Ovarian cyst:** a cystic tumor of the ovary.

**Oxytocin:** drug with the property of causing the uterus to contract.

**Perineum:** in the female, the region between the vaginal opening and the anus.

**Placenta:** the organ that connects the fetus to the uterus.

**Post-partum:** pertaining to the period after delivery of a child (also called puerperal).

**Prenatal:** before birth, i.e., during a pregnancy.

**Primigravida:** a woman who is pregnant for the first time.

**Retroflexion of the uterus:** a condition in which the body of the uterus bends backwards.

**Salpingitis:** an inflammation of the Fallopian tube or salpinx.

**Stenosis of the cervix:** tightening of the cervical canal.

**Therapeutic:** curative, as it pertains to a medical condition.

**Toxemia of pregnancy:** severe physiological changes in the pregnant woman characterized by high blood pressure, swelling of the tissues, and albumin in the urine (also called pre-eclampsia or eclampsia).

**Trophoblastic cells:** the outer layer of the developing ovum which has the capacity to invade the uterus.

**Vascularity:** blood supply.

**Xiphoid process:** the lower end of the sternum or breast bone.

**X-ray pelvimetry:** a technique for measuring the various diameters of the pelvis by use of x-ray.

## Questions for Study and Discussion

1. What is meant by the term "natural childbirth?"
2. What is the policy of most hospitals for allowing the father in the labor and delivery rooms?
3. Explain the process of the menstrual cycle.
4. Explain the various types of tests for pregnancy.
5. What are the two major functions of the reproductive system of the human male?
6. Discuss the normal sequence of events from the onset of labor to the birth of the baby.
7. Is parental understanding of growth and development characteristics of the child necessary in order to assure optimum health for the child?
8. Name some possible emergency situations at which time the knowledge of childbirth would be a necessity.
9. What is meant by the term "procreation"?
10. Explain the various kinds of abortion.
11. Why is it that some physicians risk their practices and a possible jail sentence to perform illegal abortions?

## References

DeLee, Joseph B. and Greenhill, J. P. *Principles and Practice of Obstetrics.* 13th ed. Philadelphia: W. B. Saunders, 1965.

Eastman, Nicholson J. *Williams Obstetrics.* 13th ed. New York: Appleton-Century-Crofts, 1966.

Papanicolaou, George N., Traut, Herbert F., and Marchetti, Andrew A. *The Epithelia of Woman's Reproductive Organs.* Cambridge, Mass.: Harvard University Press, 1948.

Williams, J. Whitridge. *Obstetrics.* 13th ed. New York: Appleton and Co., 1966.

Williams, Robert H. (Ed.). *Textbook of Endocrinology.* 4th ed. Philadelphia: W. B. Saunders, 1968.

# Index